Current Progress in Computed Tomography

Current Progress in Computed Tomography

Edited by Robert Meyer

hayle
medical

New York

Hayle Medical,
750 Third Avenue, 9th Floor,
New York, NY 10017, USA

Visit us on the World Wide Web at:
www.haylemedical.com

ISBN: 978-1-63241-579-0

Cataloging-in-Publication Data

Current progress in computed tomography / edited by Robert Meyer.
    p. cm.
Includes bibliographical references and index.
ISBN 978-1-63241-579-0
1. Tomography. 2. Radiography, Medical. I. Meyer, Robert.
RC78.7.T6 C87 2019
616.075 72--dc23

Table of Contents

Permissions

List of Contributors

Index

Preface

Computed tomography (CT) is a medical procedure that combines computer-processed combinations of X-ray measurements taken from different angles for producing cross-sectional images of specific areas of the scanned object. A three- dimensional volume of the interior of the object is generated using digital geometry processing. Computer tomography can be of different types, such as X-ray CT, single-photon emission computed tomography (SPECT) and positron emission tomography (PET). CT has applications in medical imaging, disease screening and preventive medicine. The detection of tumors, haemorrhages, infarctions, trauma, acute and chronic lung conditions, abdominal diseases, visualization of venous and arterial vessels, etc. are done using computed tomography scans. This book brings forth some of the most innovative concepts and elucidates the unexplored aspects of computed tomography. The ever growing need of advanced technology for medical diagnosis is the reason that has fueled the research in the field of CT in recent times. As this field is emerging at a rapid pace, the contents of this book will help the readers understand the modern concepts and applications of computed tomography.

The researches compiled throughout the book are authentic and of high quality, combining several disciplines and from very diverse regions from around the world. Drawing on the contributions of many researchers from diverse countries, the book's objective is to provide the readers with the latest achievements in the area of research. This book will surely be a source of knowledge to all interested and researching the field.

In the end, I would like to express my deep sense of gratitude to all the authors for meeting the set deadlines in completing and submitting their research chapters. I would also like to thank the publisher for the support offered to us throughout the course of the book. Finally, I extend my sincere thanks to my family for being a constant source of inspiration and encouragement.

Editor

Usefulness of Cone Beam Computed Tomography for the Diagnosis and Treatment of Oral and Maxillofacial Pathology

Márcio Diniz-Freitas, Javier Fernández-Feijoo,

Lucía García-Caballero, Maite Abeleira,

Mercedes Outumuro, Jacobo Limeres-Pose and

Pedro Diz-Dios

Abstract

Three-dimensional (3D) evaluation of oral and maxillofacial pathology, in comparison with two-dimensional (2D) radiological studies, offers many advantages that can assist in the diagnostic and in the preoperative evaluation of certain lesions and conditions of the jaws, reducing the risk of intraoperative and postoperative complications. The introduction of cone beam computed tomography (CBCT) represents an important technological advance in the context of oral and maxillofacial radiology as it permits the acquisition of high-quality 3D images and dynamic navigation over an area of interest in real time, with a short scan time and lower dose of radiation than conventional computed tomography (CT). The initial indications for CBCT have been extended by the progressive addition of new ones such as evaluation of the extent of osteonecrotic lesions of the jaw due to bisphosphonates, preoperative staging of oral cancer, and planning reconstructive surgery. As a consequence, this radiological technique represents an interesting complement to conventional radiology in those clinical situations in which 3D imaging can facilitate diagnosis and/or treatment.

Keywords: cone beam computed tomography, oral maxillofacial radiology, oral maxillofacial pathology

1. Introduction

Radiological evaluation of the size of a lesion, its density, thickness of the adjacent bone, and distance from anatomically nearby structures can assist in the diagnostic and in the preoperative evaluation of certain lesions and conditions of the jaws, reduce the risk of intraoperative and postoperative complications, and reduce surgical stress on the surgeon [1]. However, although two-dimensional (2D) radiological studies provide relevant information, in many situations they have limitations, such as indicating the location and size of a lesion in the buccolingual plane, showing characteristics of the surface (smooth or rough), and demonstrating changes that develop over time in order to evaluate progression of the lesion. As a consequence, three-dimensional (3D) studies are valuable in order to improve the diagnosis and treatment of these lesions.

Cone beam computed tomography (CBCT), also known as digital volumetric tomography (DVT) [2], volumetric computed tomography (VCT), or cone beam three-dimensional imaging (CB3D) [3], is a relatively new technology in the field of oral and maxillofacial radiology, but it is rapidly becoming established as the radiological technique of choice in numerous clinical situations [4]. CBCT enables a large quantity of data to be acquired with a short scan time and low dose of radiation compared with conventional computed tomography (CT). CBCT uses a conical X-ray beam (in contrast to the fan beam of conventional CT) and a special detector that, depending on the technology developed by the manufacturers, may be an image intensifier tube or an amorphous silicon flat-panel detector [4]. The X-ray source and reciprocal detector rotate synchronously around the head of the patient, in a single scan. Single projection images, known as "basis" images, are acquired at predetermined degree intervals. Software programs incorporating back-filtered projection are applied to the series of base images to generate a 3D volumetric data set, creating a spherical or a cylindrical volume called the "field of view" (FOV), which can be used to provide primary reconstruction images in three orthogonal planes (axial, sagittal, and coronal) [5].

The objective of this chapter is to provide a brief review of this new technology, its advantages and disadvantages, and its possible applications in the area of oral and maxillofacial pathology.

2. Clinical applications in dentistry

One of the main indications for CBCT is to determine bone availability for implant surgery [6]. However, the usefulness of CBCT imaging of the oral and maxillofacial region is continually increasing. Particularly useful indications include the diagnosis of bone disease (including maxillofacial fractures and deformities), preoperative evaluation of dental impaction, study of the temporomandibular joint, 3D cephalometric analysis in orthodontic practice, and diagnosis and surgical simulation in orthognathic surgery and in patients with cleft palate [7].

There now follows a summary of the most important studies on the use of CBCT in oral and maxillofacial pathology.

2.1. Disorders of tooth eruption

An important clinical application of CBCT is the diagnosis and planning of treatment for tooth eruption alterations. In this field, CBCT provides multiplanar visualization of the position of the tooth and its relationship with neighboring anatomical structures, as well as the presence of associated conditions, such as cystic degeneration of the dental follicle and root reabsorption of adjacent teeth, all of which are important factors in the therapeutic decision-taking process.

2.1.1. Dental inclusions

The extraction of impacted third molars is a common procedure in dental practice. In the majority of cases, it is a simple procedure with a minimal risk of damage to adjacent structures; however, in some cases, there is an intimate relationship between the roots of the mandibular third molars and the mandibular canal or the lingual cortical plate of the mandible, making it important to evaluate the topographical relationship between the third molar and these structures (**Figure 1**). Other characteristics that must be evaluated preoperatively are

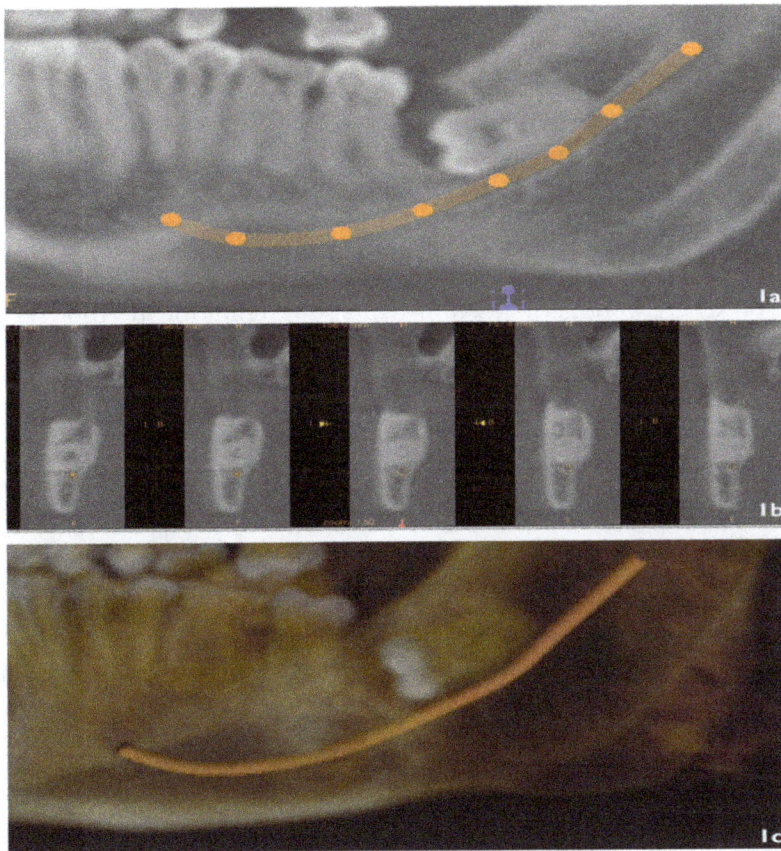

Figure 1. Inferior left third molar inclusion. (a) Detail of the panoramic reconstruction on CBCT in which the close relationship with the inferior alveolar nerve (IAN) canal (continuos line) is observed. (b) Cross-sectional images showing the three-dimensional location of the unerupted tooth and its relationship with the IAN (dark point). (c) Preoperative planning of surgical exodontia based on three-dimensional reconstruction (CS3D Imaging, CareStream, Rochester, NY).

angulation with respect to the sagittal plane, buccolingual inclination, size and shape of the crown, and the presence of local lesions. With respect to the roots of the tooth, the most important characteristic is their relationship with the mandibular canal, though it is also important to determine factors such as the number and shape of the roots and their stage of development in order to predict surgical difficulty [8, 9]. Oral and maxillofacial surgeons tend to use panoramic radiographs for evaluation of the morphology of impacted third molars and their relationship with the mandibular canal [10]. A number of radiological criteria suggestive of an intimate relationship between these two structures have been described in the literature. Sedaghatfar et al. [11] found that darkening of the root, interruption of the radiopaque lines that represent the roof and floor of the mandibular canal, divergence of the mandibular canal, and narrowing of the root on the panoramic radiograph were significantly associated with exposure of the inferior alveolar nerve after extraction of the mandibular third molars. Tantanapornkul et al. [12] found that these four criteria used independently were able to predict exposure of the nerve packet after third molars extraction, but in the multivariate analysis only interruption of the wall of the canal predicted nerve exposure. When the findings on the panoramic radiograph suggest an intimate relationship between the impacted tooth and the mandibular canal, some authors recommend complementary studies with CT or CBCT [13]. Using CBCT, Tantanapornkul et al. [12] found a sensitivity of 93% and a specificity of 77% for the prediction of inferior alveolar nerve exposure after third molar extraction, improving on the results obtained with panoramic radiographs. Exposure of the nerve correlated significantly with the presence of altered sensitivity in the postoperative follow-up. Recent studies based on images obtained by CBCT have shown that darkening of the root observed on the panoramic radiograph is more closely related with a reduction in the thickness or perforation of the lingual cortical plate than with the presence of an intimate relationship between the third molar and the mandibular canal. Thinning or perforation of the lingual cortical plate was confirmed on CBCT in 80% of cases in which darkening of the root was observed on panoramic radiograph [14]. When compared to a combination of 2D radiographs (panoramic radiography and cephalometric radiography), CBCT showed a higher detection quality of the relationship between the mandibular canal and the root tips of the third molars [15]. In addition, it has also been shown that CBCT is able to identify accessory roots and apical anomalies/curvatures not visible in the panoramic radiography [16].

Although two-dimensional imaging (panoramic and periapical radiography) is sufficient in most cases prior to the extraction of the lower third molars, CBCT may be indicated in cases where the two-dimensional image suggests one or more signs of close contact relationship between the third molar and the IDN, and if it is believed that the CBCT will change the treatment plan or the patient's prognosis [17].

With respect to the maxillary third molars, CBCT can be used to evaluate the relationship between the roots and the floor of the maxillary sinus [18] (**Figure 2**). Another advantage of CBCT in the preoperative evaluation of third molar surgery is the possibility of significantly decreasing the surgeon's level of stress in complex cases and reducing the duration of surgery.

The second most common dental impaction after the third molars is the maxillary canine, with a prevalence that varies between 1 and 2.5% [19]. Due to their functional and esthetic

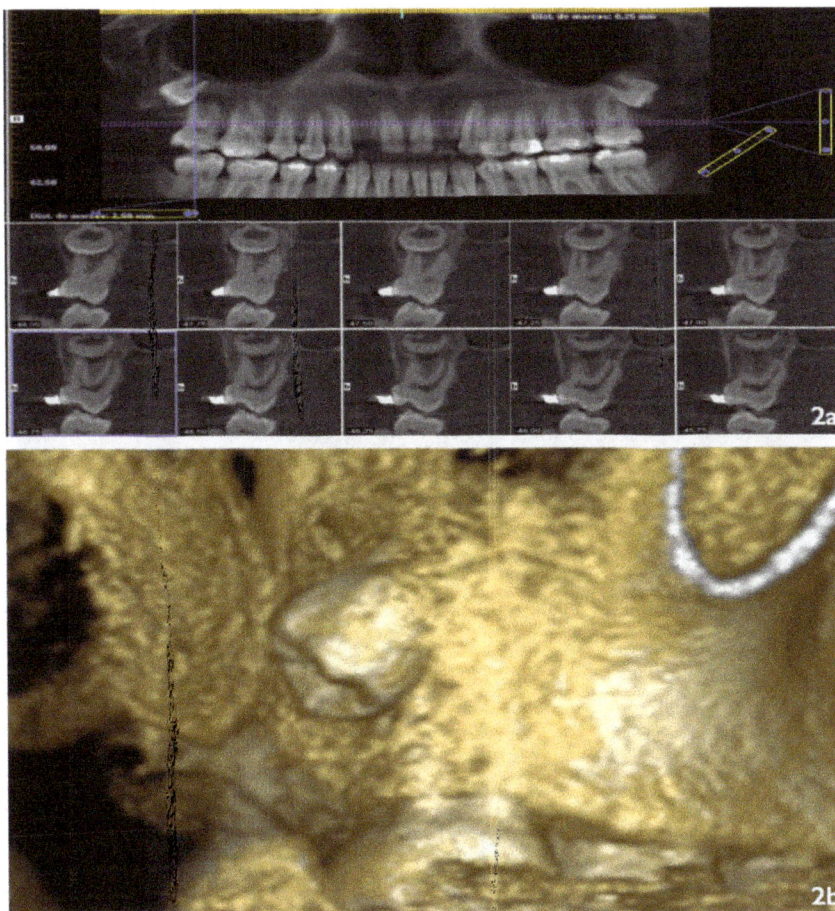

Figure 2. Third upper left molar inclusion. (a) View of the panoramic reconstruction and the cross-sectional images where an intimate relationship is observed with the roots of the second molar. (b) Preoperative planning of surgical exodontia based on three-dimensional reconstruction (I-CAT Vision, Imaging Sciences International, Hatfield, PA, USA).

relevance, the main objective in the treatment of impacted canines is their repositioning in the dental arch. Their 3D localization (**Figure 3**) is therefore important both for diagnosis and for the surgical-orthodontic management; this localization can be particularly difficult to explore with conventional radiological methods due to overlying anatomical structures [20]. CBCT can provide additional data not available with conventional 2D studies, such as the size of the follicle, the degree of inclination of the long axis of the tooth, facial-palatal position, the quantity of bone covering the tooth, the proximity and reabsorption of adjacent roots, and the stage of development of the tooth [21]. There are reports of the use of CBCT in the management of both maxillary- and mandibular-impacted canines [22]. Liu et al. [23] used CBCT to study the position and angulation of 210 impacted maxillar canines, the presence of reabsorption of the adjacent incisors, and the thickness of the dental follicle. These authors recommended complementary radiographic study using CBCT in those patients with impacted canines with marked displacement, possible reabsorption of adjacent incisors, or cystic degeneration of the dental follicle. Recently, How Kau et al. [24] proposed a new classification system—the KPG

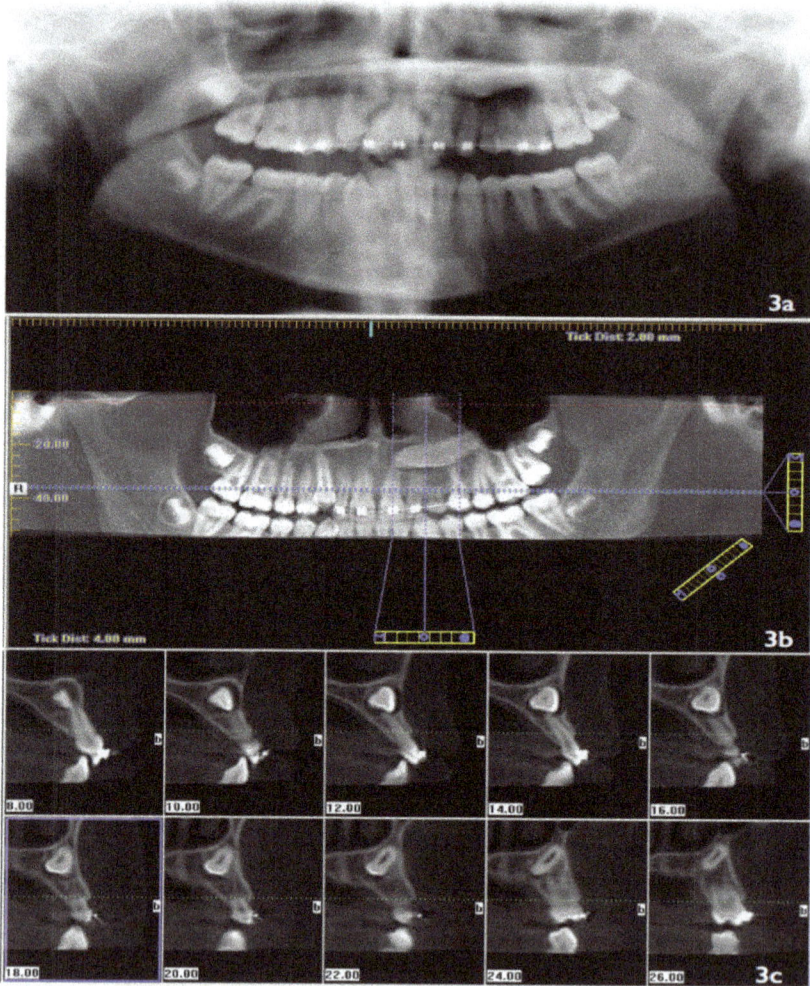

Figure 3. Left maxillary impacted canine. (a) Panoramic radiography; (b) cone beam computed tomography (CBCT) reconstruction obtained with I-CAT system (Imaging Sciences International, Hatfield, PA, USA); (c) cross-sectional images obtained with I-CAT system showing the three-dimensional location of the unerupted tooth and its relationship with adjacent anatomic structures.

index—based on the tridimensional localization of impacted canines provided by CBCT to predict the difficulty of treatment. However, this new classification system needs to be validated by prospective longitudinal studies. A recent systematic review concluded that CBCT is more accurate than conventional radiographs in localizing maxillary-impacted canine [25].

2.1.2. Supernumerary teeth

Supernumerary teeth are usually asymptomatic and are identified during routine radiological evaluation. Radiological study is useful to determine their position. Traditionally, such studies have used periapical, occlusal, and lateral skull radiographs. Periapical radiographs provide a detailed view of the anatomy of the tooth and, through the Clark's rule [26], can be used to establish the buccolingual and the palatal position of the tooth. However, these radiographs frequently do not enable a 3D evaluation to be made of the supernumerary tooth with respect to adjacent teeth and neighboring anatomical structures (**Figure 4**); this information can be important to determine the treatment plan. Liu et al. [27] used CBCT to study 487 patients with a total of 626 supernumerary teeth; in addition, panoramic and lateral skull radiographs had been performed previously in 50 of these patients with supernumerary teeth in the anterior region, allowing comparison of the visualization of the teeth and the adjacent bone structures with the three techniques. CBCT provided visualization qualified as "excellent" in practically all cases (there were only six cases in which visualization of the apices of the incisors was qualified as "reasonable"). CBCT was superior to the panoramic and lateral skull radiographs for all radiological criteria evaluated. Based on these results, the authors recommended that the evaluation of supernumerary teeth should routinely be performed by CBCT, particularly in those cases with multiple supernumerary teeth, malocclusions, or a high intramaxillary position. When extraction of supernumerary teeth is indicated, 3D localization by CBCT can help the surgeon in the choice of surgical access and identification of the tooth to be extracted, reducing trauma to the adjacent soft and hard tissues (**Figure 5**).

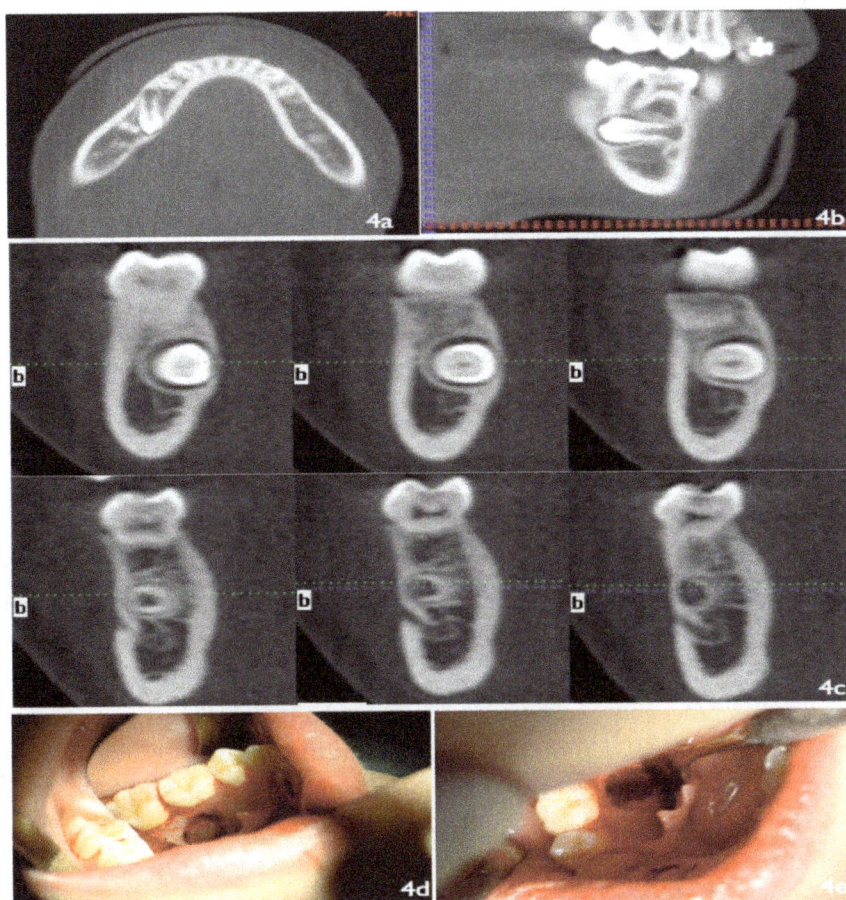

Figure 4. Supernumerary teeth in the posterior zone of the right inferior jaw. (a–c) Buccolingual localization and relationship with the mental foramen based on the multiplanar (MPR) reconstruction and cross-sectional images (I-Cat Vision). (d, e) Surgical removal of the supernumerary tooth.

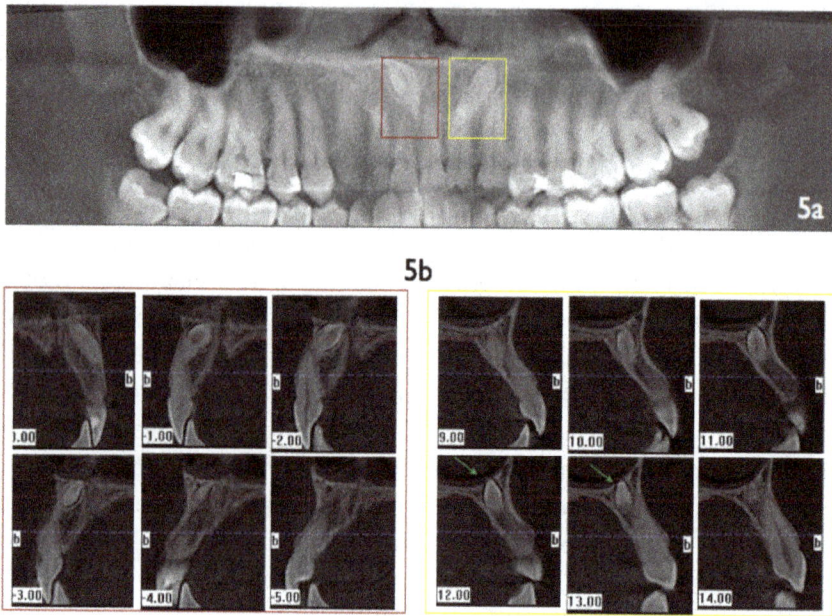

Figure 5. Supernumerary teeth in the anterior portion of the upper jaw. (a) Cone beam computed tomography (CBCT) reconstruction obtained with I-CAT system (Imaging Sciences International, Hatfield, PA, USA); (b) cross-sectional view of the supernumerary teeth and their relationship with adjacent anatomic structures. Notice a crown erupting in the nasal floor (arrows).

2.2. Periapical disease

Conventional radiographic techniques provide limited information about the origin, size, and situation of periapical lesions [28]. Superposition of adjacent anatomical and dental structures makes it necessary to perform a number of images from different angles [29]. It should be noted that the effective dose of radiation of two periapical radiographs in the area of the molars is of between 0.01 and 0.02 μSv [30], whereas the dose with limited CBCT is between 0.006 and 0.012 μSv [31].

Experimental studies have shown that CBCT is superior to digital or conventional intraoral radiography for the detection of chemically [32] or mechanically [33] induced periapical lesions. Lofthag-Hansen et al. [29] demonstrated the utility of limited CBCT for the detection of periapical pathosis not identified by conventional intraoral radiography. With CBCT, these authors found a larger number of teeth and roots involved and a larger number of lesions extending toward the maxillary sinus than on periapical radiographs. In 70% of the cases studied, the examiners considered that CBCT provided relevant additional diagnostic information in comparison with intraoral radiographs. The authors recommend the use of CBCT when there is a clinical suspicion of periapical disease and no pathology is detected on conventional radiographic techniques, as well as to plan periapical surgery for multi-rooted teeth. On the same subject, Estrela et al. [34] demonstrated that panoramic and periapical radiographs underestimated both the number and size of periapical lesions in comparison with CBCT. Estrela et al. [35] compared CBCT and intraoral radiographs for the diagnosis of periapical pathology in 596 patients with one or more endodontically treated teeth. Periapical pathology was detected in

60.9% of cases with CBCT and in 39.5% with intraoral radiographs. Based on these results, the authors proposed a new classification—the periapical index—for periapical pathosis based on the diameter of the lesion and on the expansion or destruction of cortical bone.

CBCT can also be used as a noninvasive diagnostic technique in periapical pathosis. Simon et al. [36] compared the diagnosis of large periapical lesions (granulomas vs. cysts) using CBCT and biopsy. These authors examined 17 lesions with a size equal to or greater than 1 cm × 1 cm, making a preoperative diagnosis based on the density of the lesions measured by CBCT. There was concordance between the preoperative diagnosis based on CBCT and the histological study in 13 of 17 cases. In four of the 17 lesions, the preoperative diagnosis by CBCT was of a cyst whereas the histological result was of chronic periapical granuloma. These results suggest that CBCT could be a rapid diagnostic method without invasive surgery and/or prolonged periods of observation to see if a nonsurgical therapy is effective.

Knowledge of the regional anatomy, such as, for example, root divergence and position in relation to the maxillary sinus or inferior alveolar nerve, and erosion of the vestibular and/or palatine/lingual cortical plate, can determine the surgical approach when planning periapical surgical treatment (**Figures 6 and 7**). After performing a descriptive study using CBCT to visualize the regional anatomy of the area of the upper first molars, Rigolone et al. [37] suggested the possibility of using a small vestibular access for apicoectomy of the palatal root of the maxillary first molars.

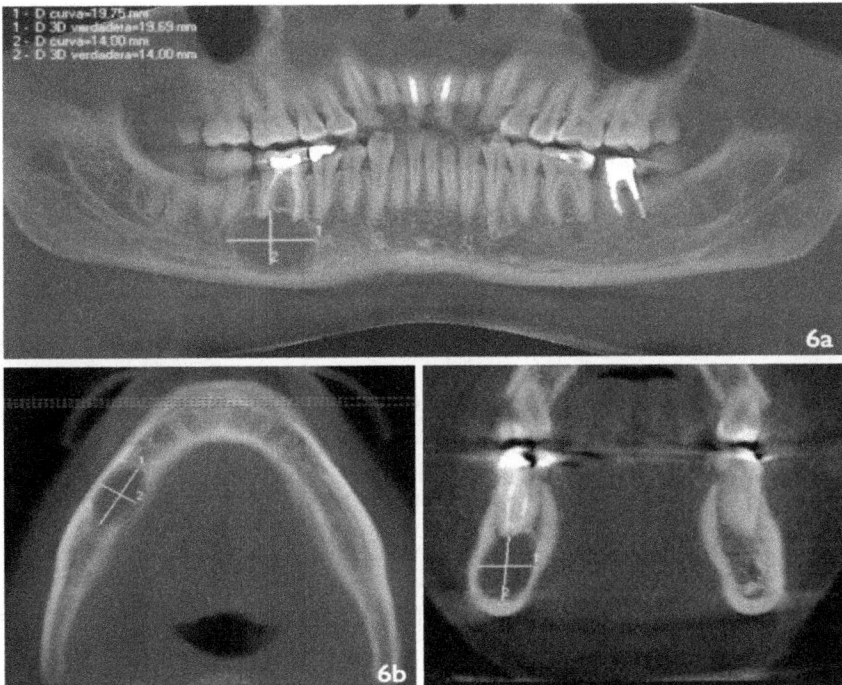

Figure 6. Well-defined radiolucent lesion at the apex of the lower right first molar. (a) Panoramic reconstruction of the CBCT. Two-dimensional measurement of lesion size (blue lines). (b, c) Measurement of the lesion in the axial and coronal sections.

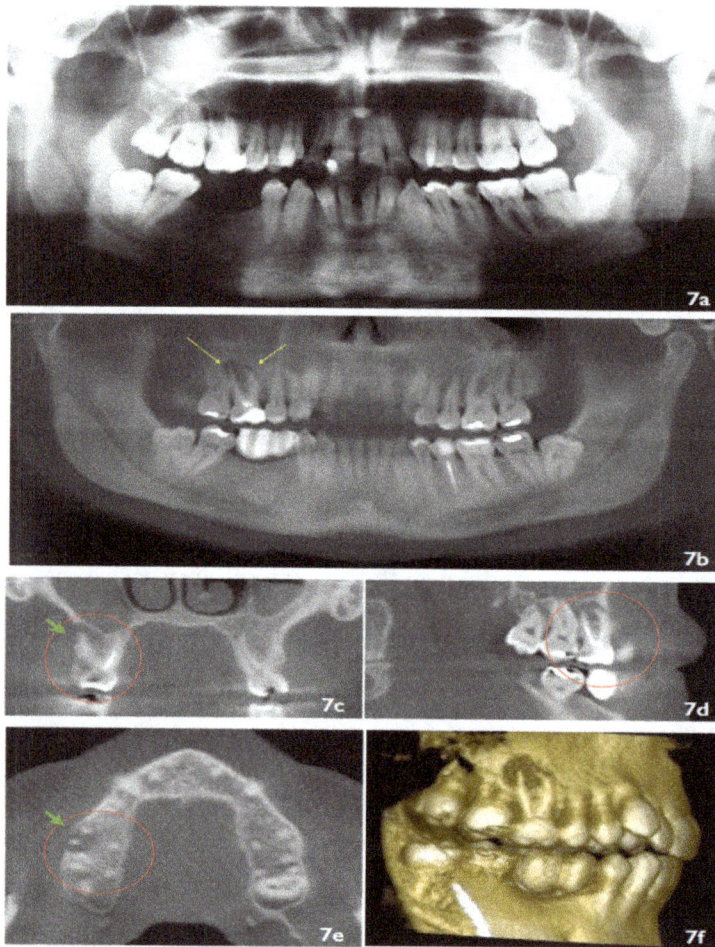

Figure 7. Preoperative evaluation of the lower right quadrant for dental implants treatment. (a) Panoramic radiography. (b) Panoramic reconstruction from cone beam computed tomography (CBCT) obtained with I-CAT system (Imaging Sciences International, Hatfield, PA, USA). Notice a periapical radiolucency in the first upper right molar poorly seen in the panoramic radiography and better identified in the CBCT (arrows). (c–e) Multiplanar reconstruction showing the limits of the periapical lesion (circle) and buccal alveolar plate destruction (arrow). (f) Three-dimensional-rendered model for case illustration.

In any case, there appears to be a degree of agreement by authors that CBCT should be reserved for those cases in which conventional radiological techniques are insufficient for providing diagnostic information about periapical pathosis.

2.3. Medication-related osteonecrosis of the jaws (MRONJs)

Medication-related osteonecrosis of the jaw (MRONJ) due to bisphosphonates was described by Marx in 2003 [38] and is characterized by exposure of the bone in the maxillofacial area (which can occur spontaneously or after a dental intervention) occurring in patients treated with antiresortives or antiangiogenics and that does not heal after 8 weeks. The diagnosis of MRONJ is based on clinical and/or radiological findings. The differential diagnosis includes lesions secondary to radiotherapy of the head and neck and malignant diseases of the jaw.

Radiological evaluation is used to confirm the diagnosis and determine the extent of the lesions. The radiological study must include orthopantomography (OPG) as first-line test, reserving magnetic resonance imaging (MRI), CT, and CBCT for those cases that require complementary tests to resolve the differential diagnosis [39]. A number of radiological signs suggestive of ONJ have been described, including an absence of bone healing and osteosclerosis at the cortical margins of dental sockets after tooth extraction, broadening of the periodontal ligament, osteolysis, altered medullary bone structure with increased density, and the formation of sequestra [40, 41] (**Figure 8**).

CBCT, as an alternative to CT, has become more widely accepted as a diagnostic technique for 3D imaging in jaw lesions [42, 43]. Although soft-tissue definition can be limited due to a poor contrast resolution, CBCT can provide detailed information about cortical thickness, medullary involvement, irregularities after tooth extraction, and density of the medullary bone; its use has been described in the diagnosis, follow-up, and treatment of patients with

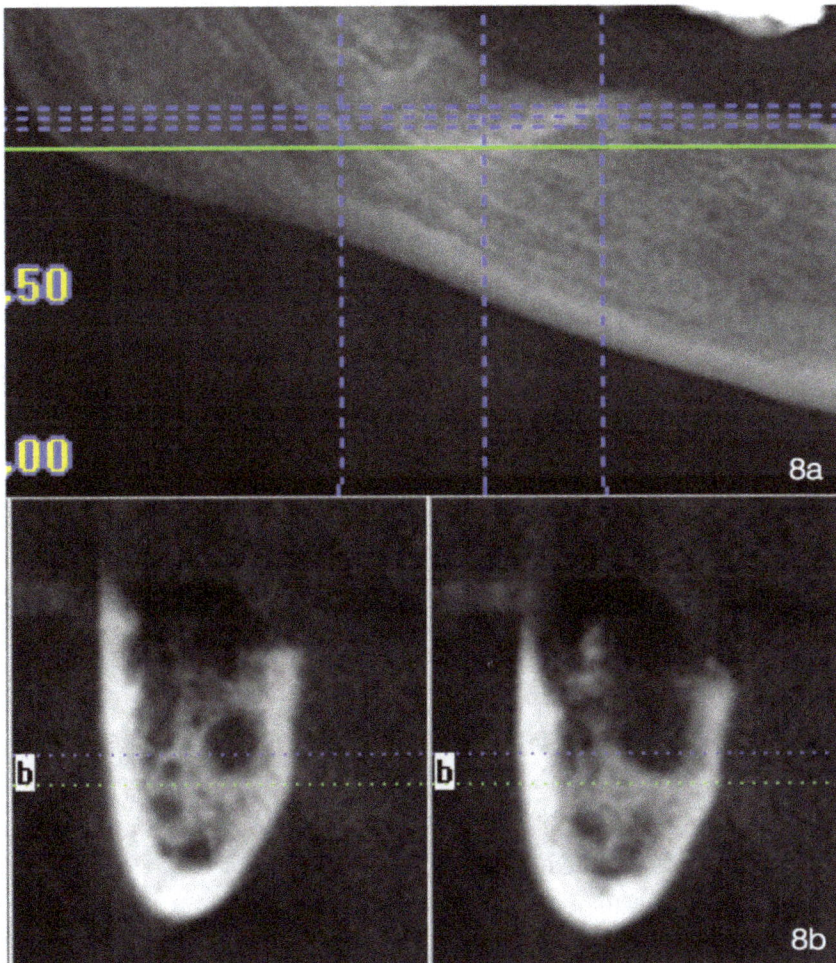

Figure 8. Medication-associated osteonecrosis of the jaws (MROJ). (a) Amplification of the zone of interest in the panoramic reconstruction. (b) Sectional views of the CBCT where the presence of osteolytic lesion is observed with small bone sequestra formation (I-CAT Vision, Imaging Sciences International, Hatfield, PA, USA).

MRONJ [44, 45]. Fullmer et al. [46] described the radiological findings of chronic suppurative osteomyelitis of the mandible on CBCT, including two cases with a history of bisphosphonate use. The authors suggested that the information provided by CBCT was not only of diagnostic utility but also that it was useful for preoperative evaluation of the true extent of the medullary bone involvement, and this information was easily transferred to 3D models that served as topographical references for the surgical treatment.

Flisher et al. [45] and Pautke et al. [41] used CBCT to locate areas of osteolysis and bone sequestra for their subsequent analysis with fluorescent lamps (Wood's lamp) to direct tetracycline absorption-guided surgical debridement. MRONJ is usually diagnosed in advanced stages, when it starts to become symptomatic [47], and CBCT can therefore facilitate early diagnosis and the identification of sequestra that could be undetectable clinically or on panoramic radiographs. According to these authors, CBCT is a useful screening technique for ONJ in patients on treatment with bisphosphonates and with additional risk factors.

Barragan-Adjemian et al. [48] analyzed 26 cancer patients treated with intravenous bisphosphonates, 18 of them presenting exposure of necrotic bone. CBCT revealed sclerotic and radiolucent bone lesions, and it was possible to measure them. The authors suggested that CBCT examination can be useful for evaluation of the extent of the lesions and for patient follow-up. Treister et al. [49] compared clinical and radiographic features of a series of seven subjects with MRONJ who were evaluated by both CBCT and panoramic radiography. Radiographic findings included sclerosis, cortical irregularity, lucency, mottling, fragmentation/sequestra formation, sinus communication, and persistent sockets. CBCT demonstrated a greater extent and quality of changes compared with panoramic radiography in nearly all cases. Other authors suggested that staging of osteonecrosis of the jaw requires computed tomography for accurate definition of the extent of bony disease [50]. Kämmerer et al. [51] have shown significant advantage of CBCT over panoramic radiography for surgeons with regard to therapeutic planning for MRONJ.

2.4. Oral cancer

The preoperative study of patients with oral cancer usually includes physical examination, blood tests, panendoscopy, and radiological examination. The radiological studies of choice are OPG, CT, and MRI. The technique of choice for visualization of tumor size in the soft tissues and for evaluation of cervical lymph node involvement is MRI, while CT is the technique of choice for evaluation of the presence and extent of bone invasion. The introduction of CBCT represents an alternative for the preoperative study of patients with oral cancer to evaluate the extent of jaw bone invasion.

Closmann and Schmidt [52] described the use of CBCT as a complementary examination for the preoperative evaluation of three patients with malignant lesions of the oral cavity (two squamous cell carcinomas and one osteosarcoma). Examination by CBCT was superior to that of OPG and MRI for evaluation of mandibular invasion and the extent of the lesion in the hard tissues, with the added advantage of lower cost and lower radiation dose than CT. The authors concluded that CBCT could be useful for the preoperative staging of oral cancer and for determining the extent of surgical resection necessary, as well as for planning reconstruction techniques.

In a study of 197 patients diagnosed with oral cancer, Linz et al. [53] have found that CBCT and bone scintigraphy (BS) showed the highest accuracy for the detection of bone invasion and showed better performance than panoramic radiography and CT/MRI. The authors concluded that for the evaluation of bone invasion, CBCT and BS might be the modalities of choice. However, CT and/or MRI remain essential for lymph node staging and for the detection of soft-tissue involvement.

3. Conclusions

The introduction of CBCT represents a great technological advance in the context of oral and maxillofacial radiology as it permits the acquisition of high-quality 3D images and dynamic navigation over an area of interest in real time, with a short scan time and lower dose of radiation than conventional CT. The initial indications of CBCT have been extended by the progressive addition of new ones such as evaluation of the extent of osteonecrotic lesions of the jaw due to bisphosphonates, preoperative staging of oral cancer, and planning reconstructive surgery. As a consequence, this radiological technique represents an interesting complement to conventional radiology in those clinical situations in which 3D imaging can facilitate diagnosis and/or treatment.

Author details

Márcio Diniz-Freitas*, Javier Fernández-Feijoo, Lucía García-Caballero, Maite Abeleira, Mercedes Outumuro, Jacobo Limeres-Pose and Pedro Diz-Dios

*Address all correspondence to: marcio.diniz@usc.es

Special Needs Unit and OMEQUI Research Group, School of Medicine and Dentistry, Santiago de Compostela University, Santiago de Compostela, Galicia, Spain

References

[1] Nakagawa Y, Kobayashi K, Ishii H, Mishima A, Ishii H, Asada K, Ishibashi K. Preoperative application of limited cone beam computerized tomography as an assessment tool before minor oral surgery. International Journal of Oral and Maxillofacial Surgery. 2002;**31**:322-327

[2] Patel S. New dimensions in endodontic imaging: Part 2. Cone beam computed tomography. International Journal of Endodontics. 2009;**42**:463-475

[3] Molteni R. The so-called cone beam computed tomography technology (orCB3D, rather!). Dentomaxillofacial Radiology. 2008;**37**:477-478

[4] Whaites E. Essentials of Dental Radiography and Radiology. 3rd ed. Churchill Livingstone, Edinburgh; 2002

[5] Scarfe WC, Farman AG, Sukovic P. Clinical applications of CBCT in dental practice. JCDA. 2006;**72**(1):75

[6] . Guerrero ME, Jacobs R, Loubele M, Schtyser F, Suetens P, van Steenberghe D. State-of-art on cone beam CT imaging for preoperative planning of implant placement. Clinical Oral Investigations. 2006;**10**:1-7

[7] Quereshy FA, Savell TA, Palomo JM. Applications of cone beam computed tomography in the practice of oral and maxillofacial surgery. Journal of Oral and Maxillofacial Surgery. 2008;**66**:791-796

[8] Flyagare L, Öhman A. Preoperative imaging procedures for lower wisdom teeth removal. Clinical Oral Investigations. 2008;**12**:291-392

[9] Danforth RA, Peck J, Hall P. Cone beam volume tomography: An imaging option for diagnosis of complex mandibular third molar anatomical relationships. CDA Journal. 2003;**31**:847-852

[10] Koong B, Pharoah MJ, Bulsara M, Tenannant M. Methods of determining the relationship of the mandibular canal and third molars. A survey of Australian oral and maxillofacial surgeons. Australian Dental Journal 2006;**51**:164-168

[11] Sedaghatfar M, August MA, Dodson TB. Panoramic radiographic findings as predictors of the inferior alveolar nerve exposure following third molar extraction. Journal of Oral and Maxillofacial Surgery. 2005;**63**:3-7

[12] Tantanapornkul W, Okouchi K, Fujiwara Y, Yamashiro M, Maruoka Y, Ohbayashi N, Kurabayashi T. A comparative study of cone-beam computed tomography and conventional panoramic radiography in assessing the topographic relationship between the mandibular canal and impacted third molars. Oral Surgery, Oral Medicine, Oral Pathology, Oral Radiology and Endodontology. 2007;**103**:253-259

[13] Friedland B, Donoff B, Dodson TB. The use of 3-dimensional reconstructions to evaluate the anatomic relationship of the mandibular canal and impacted mandibular third molars. Journal of Oral and Maxillofacial Surgery. 2008;**66**:1678-1685

[14] Tantanapornkul W, Okouchi K, Bhakdinaronk A, Ohbayashi N, Kurabayashi. Correlation of darkening of impacted mandibular third molar root on digital panoramic images with cone beam computed tomography findings. Dentomaxillofacial Radiology. 2009;**38**:11-16

[15] Neugebauer J, Shirani R, Mischkowski RA, Ritter L, Scheer M, Keeve E, Zöller JE. Comparison of cone-beam volumetric imaging and combined plain radiographs for localization of the mandibular canal before removal of impacted lower third molars. Oral Surgery, Oral Medicine, Oral Pathology, Oral Radiology and Endodontology. 2008;**105**:633-642

[16] Pippi R, Santoro M, D'Ambrosio F. Accuracy of cone-beam computed tomography in defining spatial relationships between third molar roots and inferior alveolar nerve. European Journal of Dentistry. 2016 Oct–Dec;10(4):454-458

[17] Matzen LH, Wenzel A. Efficacy of CBCT for assessment of impacted mandibular third molars: A review-based on a hierarchical model of evidence. Dentomaxillofacial Radiology. 2015;44(1):20140189

[18] Lopes LJ, Gamba TO, Bertinato JV, Freitas DQ. Comparison of panoramic radiography and CBCT to identify maxillary posterior roots invading the maxillary sinus. Dentomaxillofacial Radiology. 2016;45(6):20160043

[19] Cooke J, Wang HL. Canine impactions: Incidence and management. International Journal of Periodontics and Restorative Dentistry. 2006;26:483-491

[20] Maverna R, Gracco A. Different diagnostic tools for the localization of impacted maxillary canines: Clinical considerations. Progress in Orthodontics. 2007;8:28-44

[21] Walker L, Enciso R, Mah J. Three-dimensional localization of maxillary canines with cone-beam computed tomography American Journal of Orthodontics and Dentofacial Orthopedics. 2005;128:418-423

[22] Mah J, Enciso R, Jorgensen M. Management of impacted cuspids using 3-D volumetric imaging. Journal of the California Dental Association. 2003;31:835-841

[23] Liu DG, Zhang WL, Zhang ZY, Wu YT, Ma XC. Localization of impacted maxillary canines and observation of adjacent incisor resorption with cone-beam computed tomography. Oral Surgery, Oral Medicine, Oral Pathology, Oral Radiology and Endodontology. 2008;105:91-98

[24] How Kau C, Pan P, Gallerano RL, English JD. A novel 3D classification system for canine impactions—the KPG index. International Journal of Medical Robotics. 2009;5:291-6 (In press)

[25] Eslami E, Barkhordar H, Abramovitch K, Kim J, Masoud MI. Cone-beam computed tomography vs conventional radiography in visualization of maxillary impacted-canine localization: A systematic review of comparative studies. American Journal of Orthodontics and Dentofacial Orthopedics. 2017 Feb;151(2):248-258

[26] Clark CA. A method of ascertaining the relative position of unerupted teeth by means of film radiographs. Proceedings of the Royal Society of Medical Odontology Section. 1910;3:87-90

[27] Liu DG, Zhang WL, Zhang ZY, Wu YT, Ma XC. Three-dimensional evaluations of supernumerary teeth using cone-beam computed tomography for 487 cases. Oral Surgery, Oral Pathology, Oral Medicine, Oral Radiology and Endodontology. 2007;103:403-411

[28] Shoha RR, Downson J, Richards AG. Radiographic interpretation of experimentally produced bony lesions. Oral Surgery, Oral Pathology, Oral Medicine, Oral Radiology and Endodontology. 1974;38:294-303

[29] Lofthag-Hansen S, Huumonen S, Gröndahl HG. Limited cone beam CT and intraoral radiography for the diagnosis of periapical pathology. Oral Surgery, Oral Pathology, Oral Medicine, Oral Radiology and Endodontology. 2007;**103**:114-119

[30] Ekestube A, Thilander-Klang A, Lith A, Gróndahl HG. Effective and organ doses from scanography and zonography: A comparison with periapical radiography. Dentomaxillofacial Radiology. 2004;**33**:87-92

[31] Iwai K, Arai Y, Hashimoto K, Nishizawa K. Estimation of effective dose from limited cone beam X-ray CT examination. Japanese Dental Radiology. 2000;**40**:251-259

[32] Özen T, Kamburoglu K, Cebeci ALI, Yüskel SP, Paksoy CS. Interpretation of chemically created periapical lesions using 2 different dental cone-beam computerized tomography units, an intraoral digital sensor, and conventional film. Oral Surgery, Oral Medicine, Oral Pathology, Oral Radiology and Endodontology. 2009;**107**:426-432

[33] Stravropoulos A, Wenzel A. Accuracy of cone beam dental CT, intraoral digital and conventional film radiography for the detection of periapical lesions. An ex vivo study in pig jaws. Clinical Oral Investigations. 2007;**11**:101-116

[34] Estrela C, Bueno MR, Leles CR, Azevedo B, Azevedo JR. Accuracy of cone beam computed tomography and panoramic and periapical radiography for detection of apical periodontitis. Journal of Endodontology. 2008;**34**:273-279

[35] Estrela C, Bueno MR, Azevedo BC, Azevedo JR, Pécora JD. A new periapical index based on cone beam computed tomography. Journal of Endodontology. 2008;**34**:1325-1331

[36] Simon JHS, Enciso R, Malfaz JM, Rogers R, Bailey-Perry M, Patel A. Differential diagnosis of large periapical lesions using cone-beam computed tomography measurements and biopsy. Journal of Endodontology. 2006;**32**:833-837

[37] Rigolone M, Pasqualini D, Bianchi L, Berutti E, Bianchi SD. Vestibular surgical access to the palatine root of the superior first molar:"Low-dose cone-beam" CT analysis of the pathway and its anatomic variations. Journal of Endodontology. 2003;**29**:773-775

[38] Marx RE. Pamidronate (Aredia) and zoledronate (Zometa) induced avascular necrosis of the jaws: A growing epidemic. Journal of Oral and Maxillofacial Surgery. 2003;**61**: 1115-1117

[39] Rizzoli R, Burlet N, Cahall D, Delmas PD, Eriksen EF, Felsenberg D, Grbic J, Jontell M, Landesberg R, Laslop A, Wollenhaupt M, Papapoulos S, Sezer O, Sprafka M, Reginster JY. Osteonecrosis of the jaw and bisphosphonate treatment for osteoporosis. Bone. 2008;**42**:841-847

[40] Groetz K, Al-Nawas B. Persisting alveolar sockets—A radiologic symptom of BP-ONJ. Journal of Oral and Maxillofacial Surgery. 2006;**64**:1571-1572

[41] Pautke C, Bauer F, Tischer T, Kreutzer K, Weitz J, Kesting M, Hölze F, Kolk A, Stüezenbaum SR, Wolf KD. Fluorescence-guided bone resection in bisphosphonate associated osteonecrosis of the jaws. Journal of Oral and Maxillofacial Surgery. 2009;**67**:471-476

[42] Sukovic P. Cone beam computed tomography in craneofacial imaging. Orthodontics & Craniofacial Research. 2003;6:31-36s; discussion 179-82s

[43] Hashimoto K, Arai Y, Iwai K, Araki M, Kawashima S, Terakado M. A comparison of a new limited cone beam computed tomography machine for dental use with a multide-tector row helicoidal CT machine. Oral Surgery, Oral Medicine, Oral Pathology, Oral Radiology and Endodontology. 2003;95:371-377

[44] Kumar V, Pass B, Guttenberg SA, Ludlow J, Emery RW, Tyndall DA, Padilla RJ. Bisphosphonate-related osteonecrosis of the jaws: A report of three cases demonstrating variability in outcomes and morbidity. JADA. 2007;138:602-609

[45] Flisher K, Phelan J, Norman RG, Glickman RS. Tetracycline-guided debridement and cone beam computed tomography for the treatment of bisphosphonate-related osteonecrosis of the jaw: A technical note. Journal of Oral and Maxillofacial Surgery. 2008;66:2646-2653

[46] Fullmer JM, Scarfe WC, Kushner GM, Alpert B, Farman AG. Cone beam computed tomographic findings in refractory chronic suppurative osteomyelitis of the mandible. British Journal of Oral and Maxillofacial Surgery. 2007;45:364-371

[47] Chiandussi S, Biassoto M, Dore F, Rinaldi A, Rizzardi C, Cavalli F, Cova MA, Di Lenarda R. Clinical and diagnostic imaging of bisphosphonate-associated osteonecrosis of the jaws. Dentomaxillofacial Radiology. 2006;35:236-243

[48] Barragan-Adjemian C, Lausten L, Ang DB, Johnson M, Katz J, Bonewald LF. Bispho-sphonates-related osteonecrosis of the jaw: Model and diagnosis with cone beam computerized tomography. Cells Tissue Organ. 2009;189:284-288

[49] Treister NS, Friedland B, Woo SB. Use of cone-beam computerized tomography for evaluation of bisphosphonate-associated osteonecrosis of the jaws. Oral Surgery, Oral Medicine, Oral Pathology, Oral Radiology and Endodontology. 2010;109:753-784

[50] Bedogni A, Fedele S, Bedogni G, Scoletta M, Favia G, Colella G, et al. Staging of osteone-crosis of the jaw requires computed tomography for accurate definition of the extent of bony disease. British Journal of Oral and Maxillofacial Surgery. 2014 Sep;52(7):603-608

[51] Kämmerer PW, Thiem D, Eisenbeiß C, Dau M, Schulze RK, Al-Nawas B, Draenert FG. Surgical evaluation of panoramic radiography and cone beam computed tomography for therapy planning of bisphosphonate-related osteonecrosis of the jaws. Oral Surgery, Oral Medicine, Oral Pathology, Oral Radiology. 2016 Apr;121(4):419-424

[52] Closmann JJ, Schmidt BL. The use of cone beam computed tomography as an aid in eval-uating and treatment planning for mandibular cancer. Journal of Oral and Maxillofacial Surgery. 2007;65:766-771

[53] Linz C, Müller-Richter UD, Buck AK, Mottok A, Ritter C, Schneider P, et al. Performance of cone beam computed tomography in comparison to conventional imaging techniques for the detection of bone invasion in oral cancer. International Journal of Oral and Maxillofacial Surgery. 2015 Jan;44(1):8-15

OncoSpineSeg: A Software Tool for a Manual Segmentation of Computed Tomography of the Spine on Cancer Patients

Silvia Ruiz-España and David Moratal

Abstract

The organ most commonly affected by metastatic cancer is the skeleton, and spine is the site where it causes the highest morbidity. Computer-aided diagnosis (CAD) for detecting and assessing metastatic disease in bone or other spine disorders can assist physicians to perform their decision-making tasks. A precise segmentation of the spine is important as a first stage in any automatic diagnosis task. However, it is a challenging problem to segment correctly an affected spine, and it is a crucial step to assess quantitatively the results of segmentation by comparing them with the results of a manual segmentation, reviewed by one experienced radiologist. This chapter presents the design of a MATLAB-based software for the manual segmentation of the spine. The software tool has a simple and easy to use interface, and it works with either computed tomography or magnetic resonance imaging (MRI). A typical workflow includes loading the image volume, creating multi-planar reconstructions, manually contouring the vertebrae, spinal lesions, intervertebral discs and spinal canal with availability of different segmentation tools, classification of the bone into healthy bone, osteolytic metastases, osteoblastic metastases or mixed lesions, being also possible to classify an object as a false-positive and a 3D reconstruction of the segmented objects.

Keywords: computed tomography, magnetic resonance imaging, manual segmentation, metastatic disease, spinal canal, intervertebral discs, vertebrae

1. Introduction

Spine is a structure commonly involved in several prevalent diseases causing, in most of the cases, back pain [1]. Back pain is an important public health problem in industrialized countries [1], and it is a common cause of disability, activity limitation, work absenteeism and economic burden [2].

Moreover, spinal metastases affect many patients with advanced cancer since the bone is the most common spot of metastatic recurrence and the spine the most frequent place of bone metastases [3]. Bone metastasis is typically referred as osteolytic or osteoblastic. Osteolytic or lytic lesions are associated with bone resorption; there is a scarce new bone formation and focal bone destruction. Osteoblastic or blastic lesions are associated with an increased osteoblastic activity; these lesions seem to have little or no resorptive component. The structure of the new bone grows abnormally and causes the bone to be weak [4]. Metastatic spine is prone to several complications such as fractures and spinal cord compression due to weakness [4, 5].

Nowadays, spinal imaging studies are increasing worldwide [6], and computer-aided diagnosis (CAD) is beginning to be a part of the routine clinical work, being applied in the detection and differential diagnosis of abnormalities. Hence, its demand over the past decade has increased as a way to assist radiologists in the imaging diagnosis of back pain [7, 8]. Automatic reliable methods to quantify and classify spinal disorders, and an early detection of metastatic disease to prevent complications, are an unmet need. However, an accurate segmentation of the spine is an essential step prior to any diagnosis task. For this reason, considerable research effort has been directed towards the development of automatic or semi-automatic algorithms for the segmentation of the spine in computed tomography (CT) or magnetic resonance imaging (MRI) [9]. There are methods that do not include prior information in the process of segmentation as this kind of data is not always available. These algorithms mainly rely on the information extracted from the acquired images, for example, the application of intensity thresholds, watershed, level-set and direct graph methods [10–13]. However, other methods incorporate higher-level knowledge of the object of interest to facilitate or improve the segmentation results. Most of them are based on deformable models [14–17]. For example, using an active shape model, a statistical representation of the object is performed. The active shape model is used to identify objects, within other images, considered as the same class by using landmark points [18, 19]. Some algorithms also integrate image patches, such as intensity or texture, into the statistical model. These methods are known as active appearance models [20]. Using an atlas-based segmentation is also a way to introduce anatomical information related to the position of an organ [21–23]. The raw data values that are stored in an image are not always sufficiently informative, especially in the case of organs whose limit surface is not clearly defined in terms of signal value. In these cases, the only way to classify appropriately a voxel is taking into account its spatial location, either in absolute co-ordinates or, more commonly, given its spatial relationship with other already segmented structures. This is exactly the kind of information that can be provided by an atlas.

Unfortunately, the segmentation process involves four image-related problems. They are partial volume effect, intensity inhomogeneity, intensity similarity and noise. These problems and the differences in body structures among individuals make the segmentation process a very challenging task. Therefore, in order to obtain an accurate and robust segmentation, it is a crucial step to assess quantitatively the results of segmentation by comparing them with the results of a manual segmentation, made by experts. Some free softwares developed for image analysis or as automatic (semi-automatic) medical image segmentation tools can be also used for manual segmentation. For instance, Heilberg et al. developed a cardiovascular image analysis software package called segment. The main features of this software include loading Digital Imaging and Communications in Medicine (DICOM) images from all major MRI vendors, display of multiple image stacks at the same time, automated segmentation of the left ventricle, flow quantification, region of interest analysis, myocardial viability analysis and image fusion tools. The software also incorporates all the necessary tools to perform a manual segmentation [24]. Casero et al. developed a new spline tool for the open source software platform Seg3D [25] in order to perform the manual segmentation of the annulus of the cardiac valves. In this work, they review two manual segmentation approaches, slice-by-slice and manual segmentation interpolating a sparse set of landmarks [26]. However, these softwares are mainly focused on cardiovascular image analysis.

In this chapter, we present a software tool for performing the manual segmentation of vertebrae, intervertebral discs, spinal metastases and spinal canal. To the best of our knowledge, there is no free software for the manual segmentation of the spine. For this reason, it has been designed to get references with which users can compare automatic segmentations. The software tool can be divided into six main modules, and a general approach is shown in **Figure 1**.

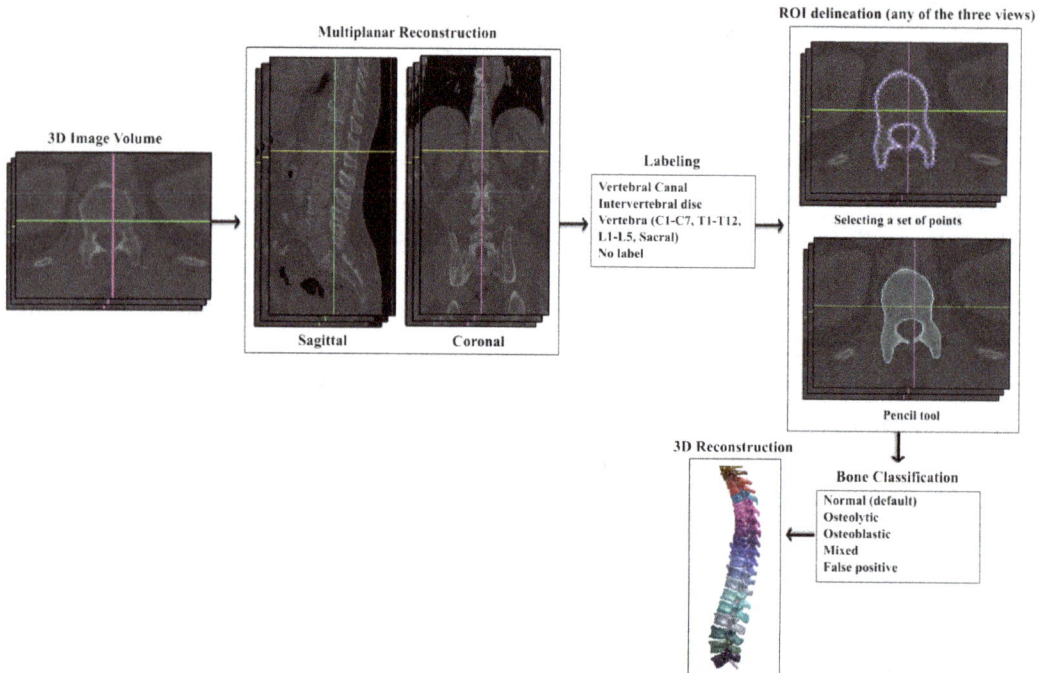

Figure 1. General approach of the manual segmentation software developed. After loading a 3D image volume, a multi-planar reconstruction from the original axial planes is performed. Next, it is necessary to label the structure to be segmented. Segmentation can be performed in any of the three views and in two different ways. Following segmentation, it is possible to classify the segmented bone. Finally, a 3D reconstruction can be obtained.

2. Software description

2.1. Software platform and data

The software tool presented in this work is called OncoSpineSeg, and its main interface is shown in **Figure 2**. The graphical user interface and all the implemented functions have been developed under MATLAB 7.10 (R2010a) (The Mathworks, Inc., Natick, MA, USA). Using MATLAB, the code can be written in a straightforward manner, which allows easily modifying, extending or integrating new functions. It can be executed under Windows, Linux or Mac OS.

The software has been tested with CT imaging and also with MRI. Both modalities are widely used for the diagnosis of spinal disorders. MRI is the preferred modality for the diagnosis of intervertebral disc pathology and spinal stenosis because it provides better contrast resolution to differentiate soft tissues [27, 28]. However, bony structures are more clearly identified in CT scans being possible to distinguish between cortical and trabecular bones and allowing accurate diagnosis of vertebral lesions [29].

The software supports the classical formats encountered in medical applications, e.g. DICOM, Neuroimaging Informatics Technology Initiative (Nifti), Raw, Meta-Image or the Visualization Toolkit (VTK). When 3D data are loaded, relevant information such as image data, resolution, acquisition details or patient identification is stored as a structure to be included in the final segmentation output file. The final output file will also contain the manual segmentation.

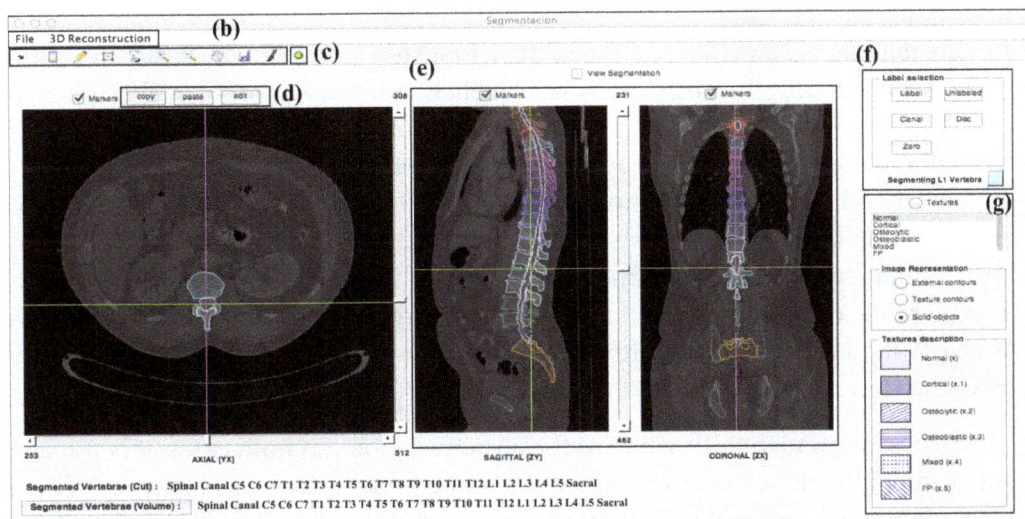

Figure 2. Main interface of OncoSpineSeg. (a) To load the 3D data volume, a saved segmentation, or to perform a 3D reconstruction. (b) To prepare images for segmentation and to perform manual segmentation. (c) To get information about the objects, which have been already segmented. (d) To copy and paste different objects and to edit the contour or label of a segmented object. (e) Multi-planar reconstruction. The straight vertical and horizontal lines are the position markers. (f) To label the structure to be segmented. (g) To classify the segmented bone ('textures' menu). There are three different options for the representation of the segmented objects, and there is information about the texture patterns associated with the different bone types available in the 'textures' menu.

After loading a 3D image volume, a multi-planar reconstruction (MPR) is performed. Sagittal and coronal cross sections are reconstructed from original axial planes. In this way, it allows an easy and a fast mutual cross-correlation of any object with the other views. The software has available position markers that allow the user to move through the volume data only by clicking with the mouse button at the desired position over any of the three planes. It is also possible scrolling between image slices using a set of sliders.

The software tool allows loading a second dataset. That is, it is also possible to load a saved segmentation in order to easily fix mistakes, using the editing tool, or finish an incomplete segmentation. This will be explained in Section 2.3.

2.2. Tools for image segmentation preparation

In spite of high contrast of MRI and CT images, there are often unclear object boundaries or similar structures in close vicinity, which impede obtaining an exact segmentation.

Classic image processing tools have been developed to facilitate manual segmentation. By using these tools, it is possible to adjust image details such as contrast and brightness or to zoom into specific regions of the image, according to mouse movements. Zoom is applied to all sections, axial, sagittal and coronal, at the same time.

Position markers are also useful for image preparation because they allow users to move between image slices and select the most appropriate region to segment each structure.

2.3. Slice-by-slice manual segmentation

Prior to start manual segmentation, a mandatory first step is to label the structure, which is going to be segmented. If the structure is not labelled, the process of manual segmentation will not be available and the user will receive information about how to proceed. In the presented tool, there is a module for this purpose, which opens up an anatomical image displaying the anterior and lateral views of an artificial spine. Only by clicking on the vertebra, we want segmentation of the specific label to be automatically set. It is also possible to select a label for the intervertebral discs and the spinal canal. A 'NO LABEL' label can also be used, allows segmenting a structure without any specific information. A default colour is assigned to each one of the available labels, although these colours can be changed. Any performed change will be stored and saved with the segmentation results.

There are two ways to manually segment the structures, and, in both cases, it is possible to segment in any of the three views (axial, sagittal and coronal), shown in **Figure 1**. In the first way, the region of interest is specified by placing a set of points using the mouse. Once the regions have been specified, they can interactively be dragged, or resized by deleting or adding new points. Then, the set of points is interpolated with a spline curve. In the second way, the region of interest is manually drawn, as using a pencil. To facilitate the segmentation task, the software permits the user to copy one or several contours and paste them upwards and downwards through the slices. The user has the possibility of using the editing tool, anytime, to edit any contour, as well as its label, to accommodate them to a more precise segmentation or to change its identification. If it is necessary to perform the segmentation again, it is possible to undo the last segmentation or delete all or just some specific contours.

The segmented objects are shown in all three views: axial, sagittal and coronal. In the axial view, it is only possible to see the segmentations performed in the current slice. However, in the sagittal and coronal views, the segmentations performed in all other slices are shown at the level indicated by the markers. An example of slice-by-slice segmentation of the vertebrae and the spinal canal in CT images is shown in **Figure 3**.

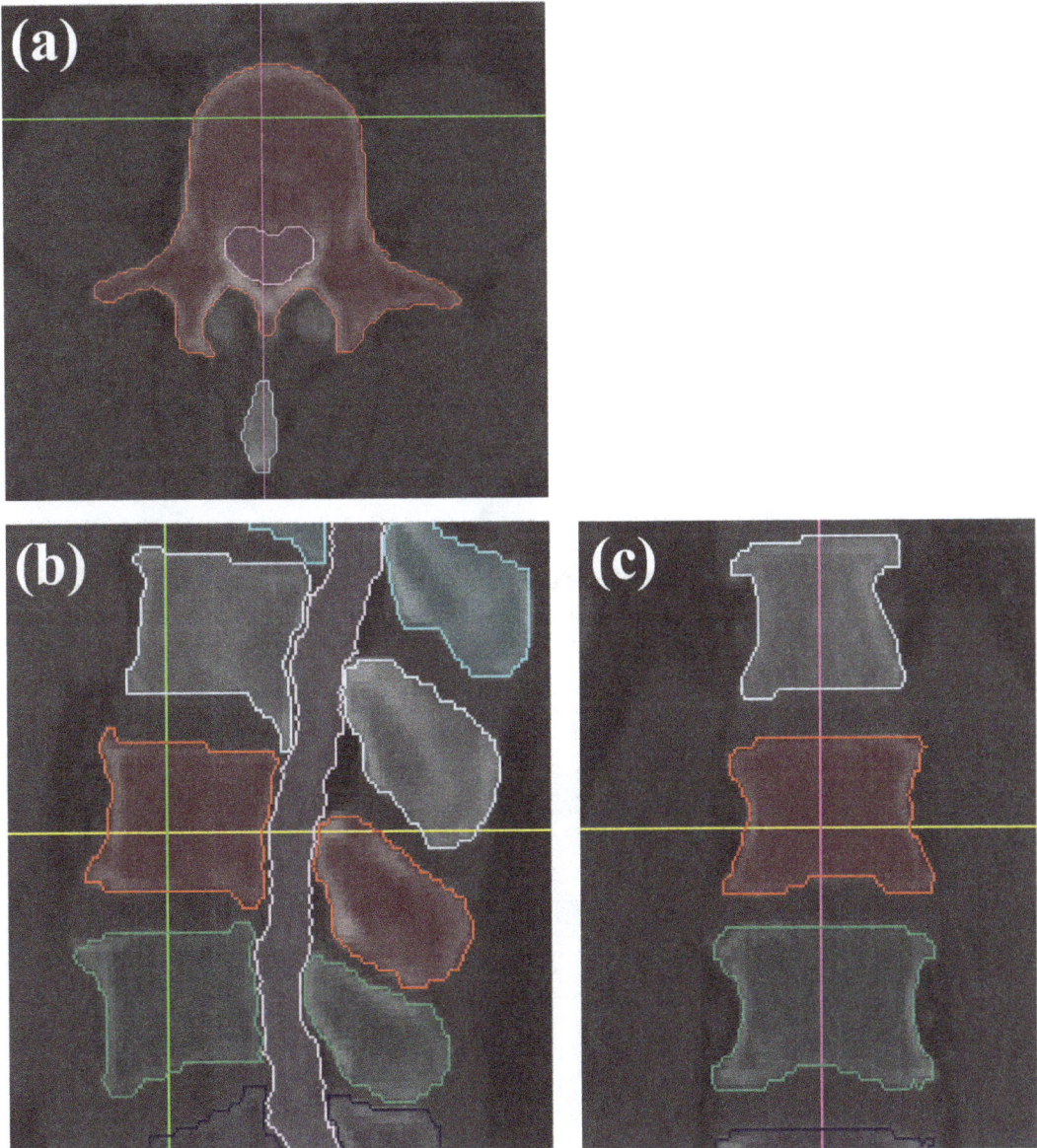

Figure 3. (a) Manual segmentation of a slice corresponding to the vertebra L3 and to the spinal canal. (b) and (c) show the corresponding slices to the vertebra for the sagittal and coronal views, respectively, as selected by the markers.

Another example of manual segmentation is shown in **Figure 4**. In this case, all intervertebral discs of the lumbar region have been segmented in MRI.

The software offers, constantly, information about the objects segmented in the current slice and the objects already segmented within the whole volume. Mask values and labels are already accessible after segmentation. All masks corresponding to the segmented objects are stored in a volume data. As stated previously, the structure of the final file has different fields for storing important information. Details such as image data, spatial resolution, acquisition details, patient identification and user's name, besides all previously reported segmentation data (masks, labels and colours assigned to each label), will be stored as a .mat.

2.4. Bone classification

Once the segmentation of the structures has been performed, it is possible to classify the segmented bone. In the right side of the software interface, a menu called 'textures' is available. This menu permits to categorize the bone into healthy bone (default mode), osteolytic metastases, osteoblastic metastases or a mixture of osteolytic and osteoblastic lesions. It is also possible to classify an object as a false-positive (i.e. osteophytes).

According to the selected bone lesion, different texture patterns are applied, as shown in **Figure 5**. In addition, in the right side of the software interface, a panel called 'texture description' can be found where there is information about the textures associated with the different available bone types. In this way, the user can easily differentiate among the different spinal lesions.

There are different ways to visualize the structures, which have been segmented and classified. A menu called 'image representation' is available for this purpose. Inside the menu

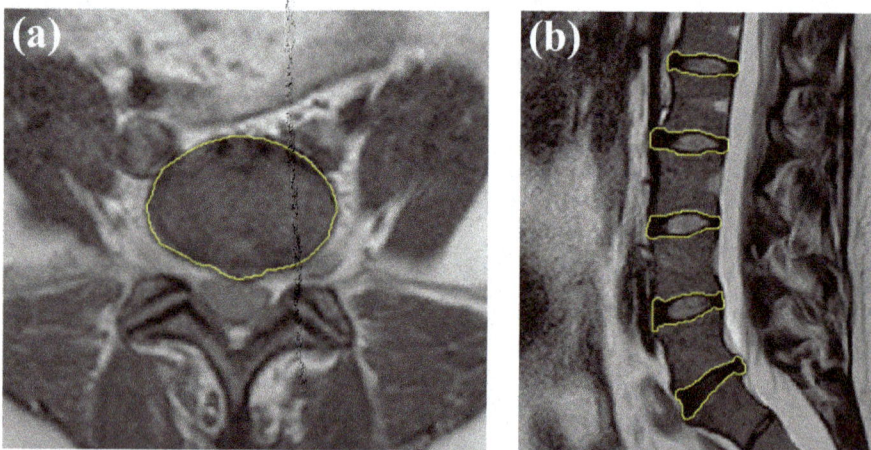

Figure 4. (a) Manual segmentation of a slice corresponding to the intervertebral disc L5-S1 in the axial view of an MR image. (b) Shows the segmentation of all lumbar intervertebral discs in the sagittal view. External contours are shown with a solid line.

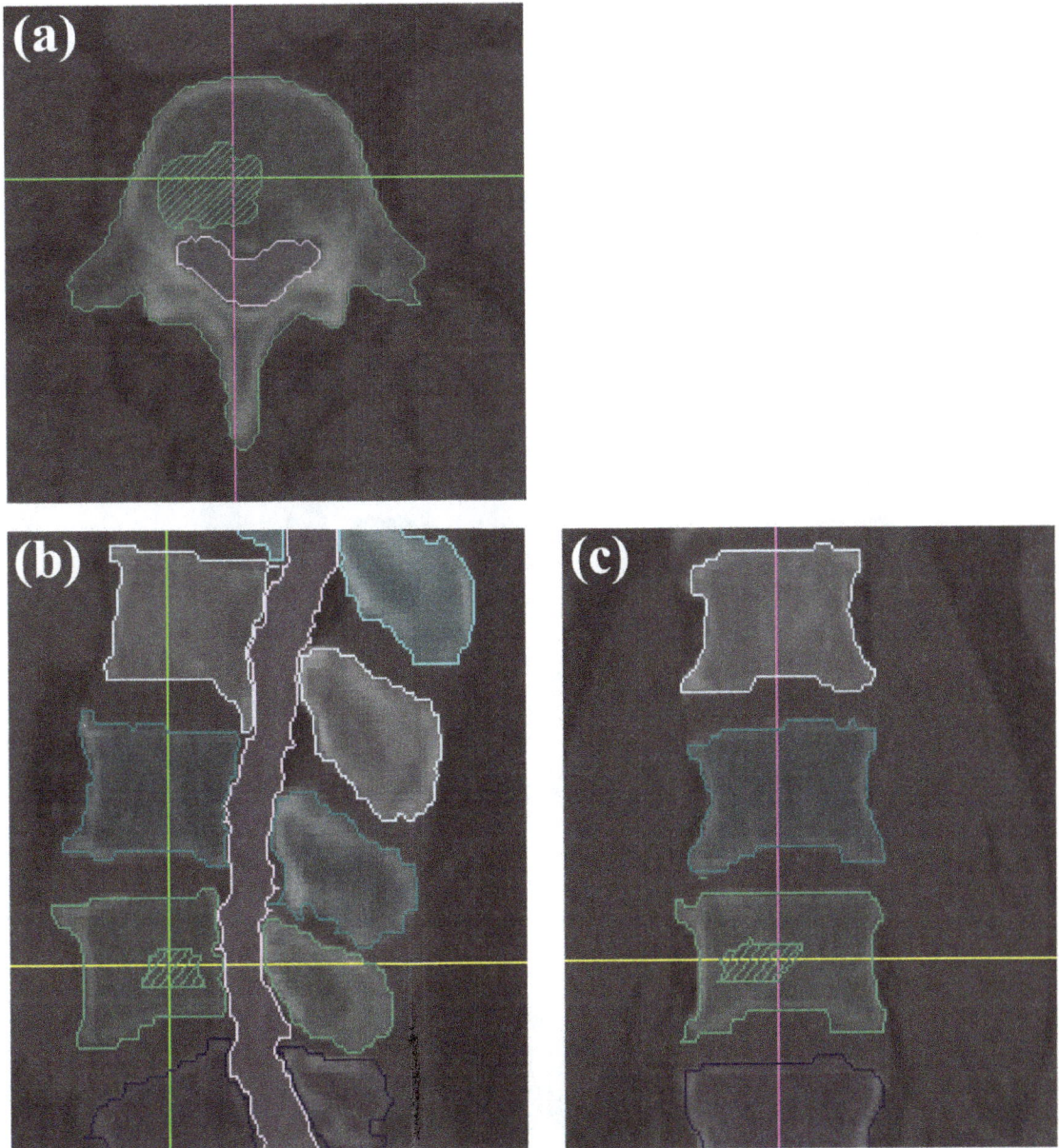

Figure 5. (a) Manual segmentation of a slice corresponding to the vertebra L4 and to the spinal canal. The striped region corresponds to an osteolytic metastasis. The segmentation of all the slices corresponding to the vertebra L4 is shown in the point indicated by the markers, in sagittal section (b) and coronal section (c).

there are three visualization options: selecting 'external contours' allows to show only the segmentation of the spine without any lesion, 'texture contours' permits us to visualize the segmentation contour of the spine and all the spinal lesions and, finally, 'solid objects' allows to depict segmentation of the spine and the spinal lesions with their corresponding texture patterns.

At this point, a complete spine segmentation has been performed, and it can be used as a reference to assess the accuracy of automatic segmentation methods, or to evaluate metastatic involvement.

2.5. 3D reconstruction

3D reconstruction provides accurate information of the 3D structure of the whole spine, which can be very important as some clinical applications often use some parameters obtained from these 3D reconstructions.

The software uses a volume rendering algorithm to reconstruct an isosurface from the volumetric dataset containing the segmentation results. It also smooths the resulting isosurfaces, applies a colour, which corresponds to colours assigned during labelling, and displays the 3D object. The resulting image can be easily rotated, zoomed or saved. An example of a 3D reconstruction is shown in **Figure 6**.

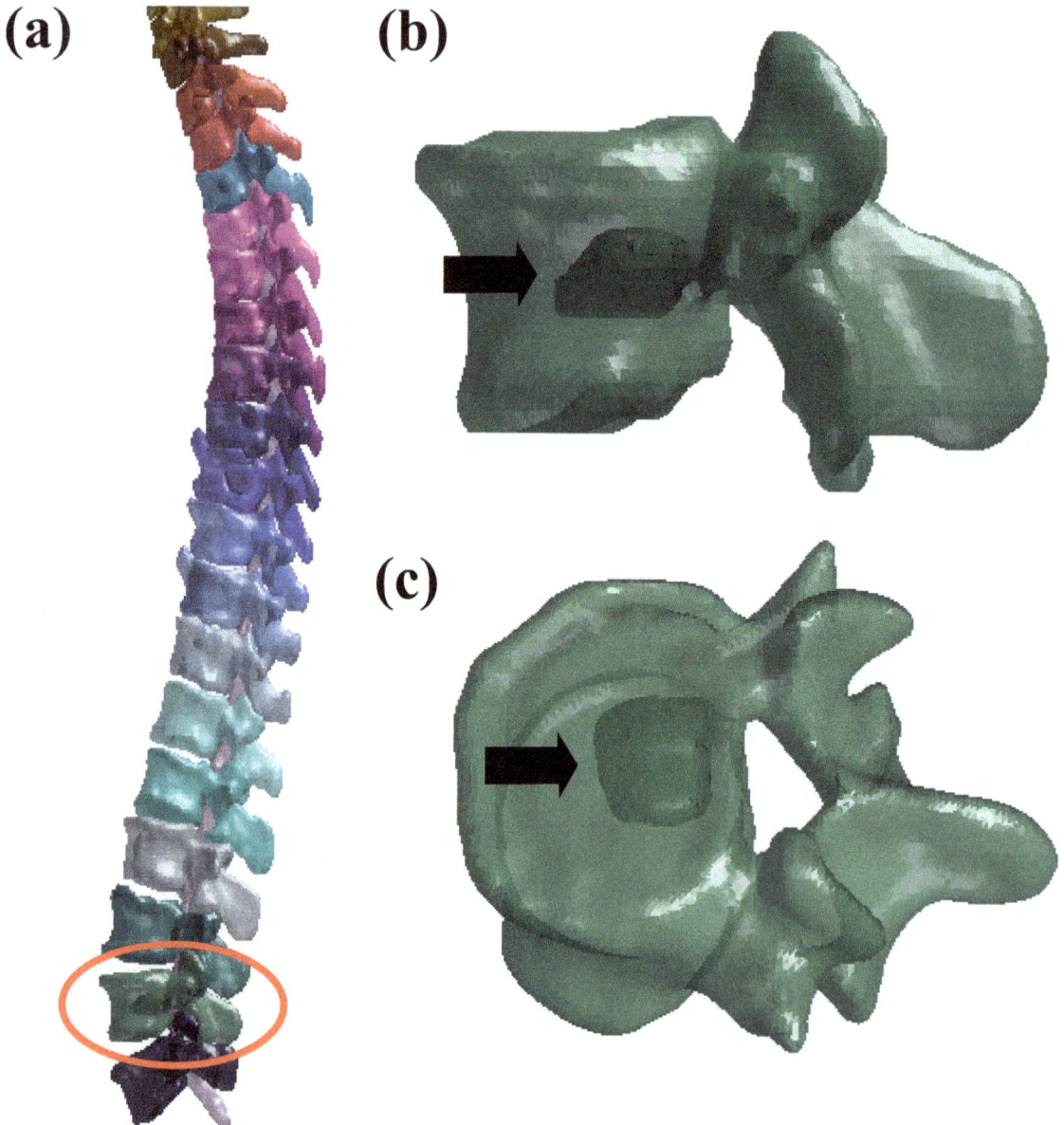

Figure 6. (a) 3D reconstruction of a whole spine with a spinal metastasis. The vertebra with the circle is zoomed in (b) and (c) where a metastasis can be distinguished (arrow).

3. Conclusions and future work

A software tool called OncoSpineSeg has been presented. This tool permits to manually segment an MRI or CT dataset, showing vertebral bodies, spinal metastases, intervertebral discs and spinal canal.

OncoSpineSeg has been fully developed using MATLAB in a straightforward manner, which allows the user not only modify or integrate new functions but also easily adapt the software to detect other spinal lesions or segment other structures. All the needed tools to facilitate the workflow have been implemented, such as the contour editing mode to fix mistakes or redraw inaccurate contours without the necessity of drawing again the complete contour. In addition, it offers a simple, intuitive and easy to use interface.

Slice-by-slice segmentation is a time-consuming process. However, it is widely known the importance of having image sets, manually segmented by experts, for reference. For this reason, and in order to facilitate the advance of research on this topic, we expect to share OncoSpineSeg through internet under a free to download open source license. We also expect to provide a database of several spine CT volumes and the manual segmentation of the vertebral bodies and spinal canal. In addition, OncoSpineSeg will be also available in source code to allow modifications and extensions.

Acknowledgements

The authors thank the financial support of the Spanish Ministerio de Economía y Competitividad (MINECO) and the FEDER funds under Grants TEC2012-33778 and BFU2015-64380-C2-2-R. The authors thank Dr. Estanislao Arana for his collaboration.

Author details

Silvia Ruiz-España and David Moratal*

*Address all correspondence to: dmoratal@eln.upv.es

Center for Biomaterials and Tissue Engineering, Universitat Politècnica de València, Valencia, Spain

References

[1] Loney PL, Stratford PW. The prevalence of low back pain in adults: A methodological review of the literature. Physical Therapy. 1999;**79**:384-396

[2] Hoy D, Brooks P, Blyth F, Buchbinder R. The epidemiology of low back pain. Best Practice and Research Clinical Rheumatology. 2010;**24**(6):769-781. DOI: 10.1016/j.berh.2010.10.002

[3]   Oliveira MF, Rotta JM, Botelho RV. Survival analysis in patients with metastatic spinal disease: The influence of surgery, histology, clinical and neurologic status. Arquivos de Neuro-Psiquiatria. 2015;**73**(4):330-335. DOI: 10.1590/0004-282X20150003

[4]   Mundy GR. Metastasis to bone: Causes, consequences and therapeutic opportunities. Nature Reviews Cancer. 2002;**2**(8):584-593. DOI: 10.1038/nrc867

[5]   Hortobagyi GN, Theriault RL, Lipton A, Porter L, Blayney D, Sinoff C, et al. Long-term prevention of skeletal complications of metastatic breast cancer with pamidronate. Journal of Clinical Oncology. 1998;**16**(6):2038-2044. DOI: 10.1200/JCO.1998.16.6.2038

[6]   Chou R, Qaseem A, Owens DK, Shekelle P. Diagnostic imaging for low back pain: Advice for high-value health care from the American College of Physicians. Annals of Internal Medicine. 2011;**154**(3):181-189. DOI: 10.7326/0003-4819-154-3-201102010-00008

[7]   Doi K. Computer-aided diagnosis in medical imaging: Historical review, current status and future potential. Computerized Medical Imaging and Graphics. 2007;**31**(4-5):198-211. DOI: 10.1016/j.compmedimag.2007.02.002

[8]   Ruiz-España S, Arana E, Moratal D. Semiautomatic computer-aided classification of degenerative lumbar spine disease in magnetic resonance imaging. Computers in Biology and Medicine. 2015;**62**:196-205. DOI: 10.1016/j.compbiomed.2015.04.028

[9]   Alomari RS, Ghosh S, Koh J, Chaudhary V. Vertebral column localization, labeling, and segmentation. Spinal Imaging and Image Analysis. 2015;**18**:193-229. DOI: 10.1007/978-3-319-12508-4

[10] Yao J, O'Connor SD, Summers RM. Automated spinal column extraction and partitioning. In: Proceedings of the IEEE International Symposium on Biomedical Imaging: From Nano to Macro (ISBI 2006); 2006. pp. 390-393. DOI: 10.1109/ISBI.2006.1624935

[11] Kang Y, Engelke K, Kalender WA. A new accurate and precise 3-D segmentation method for skeletal structures in volumetric CT data. IEEE Transactions on Medical Imaging. 2003;**22**(5):586-598. DOI: 10.1109/TMI.2003.812265

[12] Lim PH, Bagci U, Bai L. Introducing Willmore flow into level set segmentation of spinal vertebrae. IEEE Transactions on Bio-Medical Engineering. 2013;**60**(1):115-122. DOI: 10.1109/TBME.2012.2225833

[13] Ruiz-España S, Díaz-Parra A, Arana E, Moratal D. A fully automated level-set based segmentation method of thoracic and lumbar vertebral bodies in computed tomography images. In: Proceedings of the IEEE Engineering in Medicine and Biology Society; EMBC 2015; 2015. pp. 3049-3052

[14] Ma J, Lu L, Zhan Y, Zhou X, Salganicoff M, Krishnan A. Hierarchical segmentation and identification of thoracic vertebra using learning-based edge detection and coarse-to-fine deformable model. In: Proceedings of the Medical Image Computing and Computer-Assisted Intervention (MICCAI 2010); 2010. pp. 19-27. DOI: 10.1007/978-3-642-15705-9_3

[15] Kim Y, Kim D. A fully automatic vertebra segmentation method using 3D deformable fences. Computerized Medical Imaging and Graphics. 2009;**33**(5):343-352. DOI: 10.1016/j.compmedimag.2009.02.006

[16] Klinder T, Ostermann J, Ehm M, Franz A, Kneser R, Lorenz C. Automated model-based vertebra detection, identification, and segmentation in CT images. Medical Image Analysis. 2009;13(3):471-482. DOI: 10.1016/j.media.2009.02.004

[17] Korez R, Ibragimov B, Likar B, Pernus F, Vrtovec T. A Framework for automated spine and vertebrae interpolation-based detection and model-based segmentation. IEEE Transactions on Medical Imaging. 2015;34(8):1649-1662. DOI: 10.1109/TMI.2015. 2389334

[18] Rasoulian A, Rohling R, Abolmaesumi P. Lumbar spine segmentation using a statistical multi-vertebrae anatomical shape+pose model. IEEE Transactions on Medical Imaging. 2013;32:1890-1900. DOI: 10.1109/TMI.2013.2268424

[19] Castro-mateos I, Pozo JM, Pereañez M, Lekadir K, Lazary A, Frangi AF. Statistical inter-space models (SIMs): Application to robust 3D spine segmentation. IEEE Transactions on Medical Imaging. 2015;34(8):1663-1675. DOI: 10.1109/TMI.2015.244391

[20] Roberts MG, Cootes TF, Pacheco E, Oh T, Adams JE. Segmentation of lumbar vertebrae using part-based graphs and active appearance models. In: Proceedings of the Medical Image Computing and Computer-Assisted Intervention (MICCAI 209). 2009;12(Pt 2):1017-1024. DOI: 10.1007/978-3-642-04271-3_123

[21] Forsberg D. Atlas-based registration for accurate segmentation of thoracic and lumbar vertebrae in CT data. Recent Advances in Computational Methods and Clinical Applications for Spine Imaging. 2015;20:49-59. DOI: 10.1007/978-3-319-14148-0_5

[22] Hardisty M, Gordon L, Agarwal P, Skrinskas T, Whyne C. Quantitative characterization of metastatic disease in the spine. Part I. Semiautomated segmentation using atlas-based deformable registration and the level set method. Medical Physics. 2007;34(8):3127. DOI: 10.1118/1.2746498

[23] Ruiz-España S, Domingo J, Díaz-Parra A, Dura E, D'Ocón-Alcañiz V, Arana E, et al. Automatic segmentation of the spine by means of a probabilistic atlas with a special focus on ribs supression. Preliminary results. In: Proceedings of the IEEE Engineering in Medicine and Biology Society (EMBC 2015); 2015; IEEE. pp. 2014-2017

[24] Heiberg E, Sjögren J, Ugander M, Carlsson M, Engblom H, Arheden H. Design and validation of segment—Freely available software for cardiovascular image analysis. BMC Medical Imaging. 2010;10:1. DOI: 10.1186/1471-2342-10-1

[25] Scientific Computing and Imaging Institute (SCI). Seg3D: Volumetric Image Segmentation and Visualization [Internet]. Available from: http://www.sci.utah.edu/cibc-software/seg3d.html [Accessed: 12 November, 2016]

[26] Casero R, Burton RA, Quinn T, Bollensdorff C, Hales P, Schneider JE, et al. Cardiac valve annulus manual segmentation using computer assisted visual feedback in three-dimensional image data. In: Proceedings of the IEEE Engineering in Medicine and Biology Society (EMBC 2010); 2010; IEEE. pp. 738-741. DOI: 10.1109/IEMBS.2010.5626303

[27] Brayda-Bruno M, Tibiletti M, Ito K, Fairbank J, Galbusera F, Zerbi A, et al. Advances in the diagnosis of degenerated lumbar discs and their possible clinical application. European Spine Journal. 2014;**23**(3):S315–S323. DOI: 10.1007/s00586-013-2960-9

[28] Larroza A, Bodí V, Moratal D. Texture analysis in magnetic resonance imaging: Review and considerations for future applications. In: Constantinides C, editor. Assessment of Cellular and Organ Function and Dysfunction Using Direct and Derived MRI Methodologies. Rijeka, Croatia: InTech; 2016. DOI: 10.5772/64641

[29] Quattrocchi CC, Santini D, Delláia P, Piciucchi S, Leoncini E, Vincenzi B, et al. A prospective analysis of CT density measurements of bone metastases after treatment with zoledronic acid. Skeletal Radiology. 2007;**36**(12):1121-1127. DOI: 10.1007/s00256-007-0388-1

Cone Beam Computed Tomography in Orthodontics

Emine Kaygısız and Tuba Tortop

Abstract

Cone beam computed tomography (CBCT) is an important source of three-dimensional volumetric data in clinical orthodontics. Due to the progress in the technology of CBCT, for orthodontic clinical diagnosis, treatment and follow-up, CBCT supply much more reliable information compared to conventional radiography. The most justified indications for the use of CBCT in orthodontics are the existence of impacted and transposed teeth. For the management of the impacted teeth, CBCT enhances the ability to localize these teeth accurately and to assess root resorption of adjacent teeth. Patients with craniofacial anomalies like cleft palate cases, the abnormalities of the temporomandibular joint contributing malocclusion, evaluation of airway morphology in obstructive sleep apnea cases, patients needing maxillary expansion or planning orthognathic surgery in severe skeletal discrepancies are also listed among the indications of using CBCT in orthodontics. CBCT is useful in identifying optimal site location for temporary skeletal anchorage device. The use of CBCT for the assessment of treatment outcomes and evaluation of cervical vertebral maturation are still controversial issues. It should be kept in mind that before using CBCT, justification and evaluation of risks and benefits are needed. In order to minimize the radiation dose, the exam should include only the areas of interest.

Keywords: cone beam computed tomography, orthodontics, impacted canine, orthodontic treatment planning, root resorption

1. Introduction

The key of a successful orthodontic treatment is an accurate diagnosis, growth evaluation and treatment planning. Diagnostic records for an orthodontic treatment planning generally begin with history and intraoral and extraoral examination of the patient. Dental casts, intraoral and extraoral photographs are also routine diagnostic materials. Imaging is a necessary diagnostic tool in the practice of orthodontics. For radiographic evaluation, panoramic radiograph, periapical views, upper occlusal radiograph and lateral cephalometric radiograph are obtained if indicated. Imaging should answer the questions that cannot be solved clinically. By using radiographic examination, it is possible to confirm or rule out clinical findings [1].

In recent years, orthodontists have begun to use three-dimensional (3D) cone beam computed tomography (CBCT) images to overcome the inadequateness of two-dimensional (2D) radiographic records. When computed tomography was first introduced into the dental field, because of the high radiation dose, it is not preferred for orthodontic diagnosis. The technology has been evolving ever since, resulting in a reduction in radiation dose and relatively low cost of CBCT systems, so they become popular to visualize the craniofacial complex in three dimensions.

In some studies, it has been suggested that different options for orthodontic treatment plans in some specific cases may change due to use of CBCT [2–4]. Orthodontists should know how to use the radiographic records and what they offer, before deciding which tool they will use [1].

2. Advantages and disadvantages of using CBCT in orthodontics

Although there has been considerable interest in using CBCT as a part of routine orthodontic management, diverse results about the advantages, disadvantages and indications were noted in the literature.

The review of recent literature reveals some advantages [1, 5–15] and disadvantages [16–20] as following:

2.1. Advantages

- Accuracy of image geometry is increased, and real size 3D image is obtained by CBCT. Unlike lateral cephalometric radiographs, CBCT image is more similar to the patient, more accurate and distortion-free.

- It eliminates the magnification, overlapping and distortion of structures.

- It is possible to assess the image from the three planes.

- CBCT images allow to make localized and specific transversal cuts to assess areas of clinical interest.

- For a proper diagnosis and treatment planning, sometimes temporomandibular, postero-anterior cephalograms, periapical, occlusal and bite-wing radiographs are also required besides the routine panoramic and lateral cephalometric examination. But, by using CBCT technology, it is possible to produce several types of radiographic images and to construct study casts from a single scan.

- The reorientation of the images, on the contrary to the lateral cephalometric radiograph, is possible.

- The ease of landmark identification and high precision of superimposed images have been reported.

- By the use of CBCT, less variability and more reproducibility of transverse measurements were demonstrated compared to conventional 2D. CBCT images were reported to be more reliable than posteroanterior cephalograms and offer an unobstructed view for diagnosis of maxillary transverse discrepancies.

- The unerupted tooth sizes, bone dimensions and even soft tissue anthropometric measurements can be assessed precisely by CBCT.

- The fine adjustment of the head position is not essential for CBCT.

- The use of CBCT in orthodontics greatly enhances evaluation of impacted canines and offers comprehensive information.

- The detection of root resorption is reported to be highly accurate with CBCT scanners.

- An occlusal view of the maxilla from CBCT can be used for the customized transpalatal arch design. This might prevent interfering of the wire to the path of eruption of impacted tooth.

2.2. Disadvantages

- The amount of generated radiation is the biggest controversy about the use of CBCT in dental imaging. Although the radiation dose of the CBCT is lower than the medical spiral CT, it is still higher than that of a 2D cephalogram.

- Difficulty in differentiating various soft tissues in the image due to the poor low-contrast resolution compared to medical CT is one of the disadvantages.

- An adequate method to digitize and analyze 3D radiographic images is not still improved.

- The lack of 3D standard population norms has also restricted CBCT from routine orthodontic use.

- Landmark identification on coronal, sagittal and axial views of CBCT is more time consuming to carefully select the best slice.

- The diagnostic accuracy for caries detection with CBCT is less than with conventional periapical radiographs.

3. The usage of CBCT in orthodontics

Many orthodontists interested in using CBCT during their routine diagnosis and treatment planning because of the additional diagnostic information. This brings the risk of unnecessary ionizing radiation. So, it is mandatory to determine exact indications for the use of CBCT in orthodontics.

3.1. Impacted and transposed teeth

Tooth impaction is a commonly observed dental anomaly which needs orthodontic treatment. The most frequent impacted teeth were mandibular wisdom teeth, which were followed by maxillary and mandibular canines [21]. Radiographic examinations play a more critical role than clinical examination especially in the initial diagnosis and treatment planning of impacted teeth. For several years, radiographic evaluation of these teeth was done by using panoramic, periapical, occlusal or lateral cephalograms. These conventional two dimensional radiographs are inadequate in accurately visualizing the location, angulation, spatial position and relationships of the impacted tooth in three dimensions. So, the most justified indications for the use of CBCT in orthodontics are the existence of impacted and transposed teeth (**Figure 1a–c**).

For the management of the impacted teeth, CBCT enhances the ability to localize these teeth accurately, evaluate their proximity to other teeth and structures, determine the alveolar width and follicle size, the presence of pathology and assess root resorption of adjacent teeth, assist in planning surgical access and bond placement, besides determining optimal direction for the extrusion of these teeth into the oral cavity [22–25]. In particular, for impacted teeth, if exposure or forced eruption is planned, it would be possible to determine not only the position of tooth and dilacerated root but also the alveolar boundary conditions. Additionally, it would be much easier to prepare the space needed for the impacted tooth as it is possible to obtain a more accurate size from CBCT images.

Haney et al. [26] reported an approximate 20% lack of agreement among clinicians on the location (palatal versus labial) of the tooth tip between the routine 2D radiographs and 3D CBCT images. Also large differences in treatment approaches were demonstrated when the two imaging methods were compared [27]. On the other hand, in another study, it was reported that the determination of canine position was not significantly different when using panoramic and CBCT systems [3].

Using CBCT improves the clinician confidence in diagnosis and treatment plan as it is helpful in defining the surgical access site, bond position and in designing mechanics [25, 26]. The orthodontists have a different perception of localization and can determine the shortest way for the impacted tooth in three planes of space while avoiding damage to neighboring teeth.

In some studies, it was suggested that orthodontic treatment planning for impacted tooth showed no differences when using 2D- or 3D-based information. On the contrary, findings of some other studies showed that orthodontists changed their treatment planning derived from conventional radiographs for 25% of the impacted teeth when they viewed CBCT images [26, 28]. Alqerban et al. [4, 29] concluded that CBCT allows clinicians to obtain 3D images with visualization of craniofacial structures and significantly increases the orthodontists' confidence level, with more information on canine localization and detection of possible root resorption on adjacent incisors [30].

When the impacted tooth did not move, CBCT is indicated. Becker et al. [31] reported that invasive cervical root resorption is a rare insidious and aggressive form of external

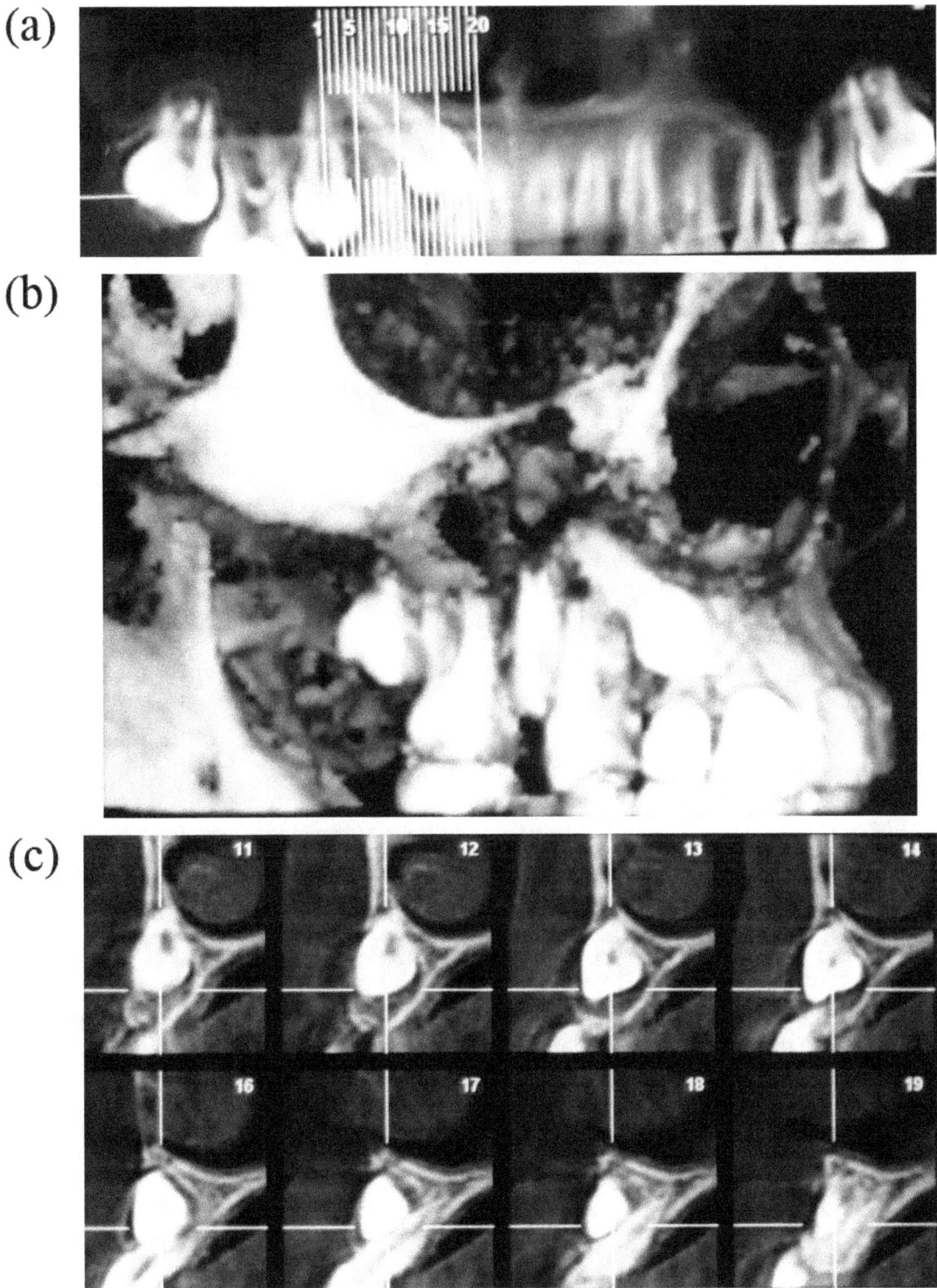

Figure 1. (a) Panoramic view of a maxillary impacted canine. Note that in this case, FOV was restricted only to maxilla. (b) Determination of vestibular location of a maxillary impacted canine. (c) Evaluation of proximity between impacted canine and root of lateral incisor by CBCT.

root resorption and an overlooked cause of failure of orthodontic resolution of impacted canines.

CBCT minimizes superimposition artifacts and provides superior visualization of roots [24, 32]. In extraction cases with an impacted tooth, it is a much more important to decide which tooth to extract, a tooth with a resorbed root or a healthy premolar? Using CBCT images will contribute to a logical clinical outcome, as it provides superior information on root resorption.

Overall, it could be considered to increase efficiency and enhance success rates for the treatment of impacted teeth when the treatment and biomechanics are customized by using CBCT [33].

Field of view (FOV) must be determined according to the needs of the case. If the only problem is an impacted tooth, it would be logical to localize the FOV as the impacted tooth, adjacent teeth and surrounding alveolar structure. In fact, in a recent study, Wriedt et al. [30] recommended small volume FOV CBCT for impacted maxillary canines if the canine inclination on a conventional 2D panoramic radiograph exceeds 30° relative to a perpendicular midline, when adjacent root resorption is suspected, and/or when canine root dilaceration is suspected on conventional panoramic radiographs. But if an orthognathic surgical treatment plan is predicted, cephalometric and panoramic radiograph need must be considered while determining FOV. It is advisable to refer the patient to an oral and maxillofacial radiologist with a note including clinically significant findings and request a report on the region of interest [27].

Maxillary lateral incisor root resorption is most commonly associated with canine impaction. It often remains asymptomatic, limiting early diagnosis. However, early diagnosis is important, because the presence or absence of root resorption will determine the treatment strategy. Furthermore, advanced root resorption can make treatment impossible [34]. Improvement in diagnostic measures for early detection and prevention is therefore essential for ensuring correct treatment, and it might also reduce treatment time, complexity, complications and costs. It has been suggested that by using 3D images, overlapping of structures can be avoided.

Dental transposition represents a multifactorial condition. In the etiology of transposition, both genetic and environmental factors play an important role [35]. For the diagnosis and treatment planning of transposed teeth, several significant variables can be derived from CBCT imaging, especially, critical when deciding whether patient requires extraction or not. So, it would be much easier to evaluate adequately the quality and shape of teeth, location of roots and limitations of the alveolar boundary conditions around the transposed teeth by using CBCT. Kapila et al. [28] recommended to be selective about which cases may benefit from CBCT scans for assessing boundary conditions. Cases with compromised periodontal or gingival conditions, patients with narrow alveolar bone in which it would be critical to manage buccolingual displacements or angulations of teeth, and cases who need shifting position of the teeth are listed as cases that will benefit from CBCT scans.

3.2. Supernumerary teeth

A supernumerary tooth may closely resemble the teeth of the group to which it belongs [36]. In supernumerary cases, radiographic examination aims to determine the localization and the morphology of the supernumerary teeth. As it is critical to decide which teeth to be extracted and which teeth to be retained, CBCT helps to precisely evaluate the position and morphology of these teeth. It is also possible to detect any contact between the supernumerary teeth and adjacent teeth and to evaluate their relation with other anatomical structures. The information obtained from CBCT images also facilitates the determination of the optimal surgical access to these teeth in order to minimize harm to adjacent teeth and to surrounding tissue [37] (**Figure 2**).

3.3. Root resorption

Root resorption is a condition occurs in response to a variety of stimuli resulting in a loss of dentin, cementum or bone [36]. Panoramic radiographs have a week diagnostic efficacy in determining external root resorption. So, root resorption has traditionally been evaluated by periapical radiographs. Nevertheless, in recent years, it is suggested that CBCT can detect precise images of small root defects with a greater sensitivity and specificity compared to 2D radiographs [3, 24]. In a meta-analysis, Yi et al. [38] reported that CBCT is superior to periapical radiographs in the accuracy of diagnosing external root resorption. They emphasized that periapical radiographs provide limited information of external root resorption in the buccal and lingual root surface.

External root resorption of maxillary lateral incisor is a common finding that associates with canine impaction. Early diagnosis is difficult as it is asymptomatic and advanced root resorption makes the treatment planning more complex. In a study evaluating efficacy of CBCT for the diagnosis of root resorption associated with impacted canines, improved detection rates of root resorption (63%) were reported [39]. By using CBCT, it is possible to visualize of root resorptions on buccal and lingual surfaces. This might be critical for the extraction decision during treatment planning. In another study, it was suggested that the combination of thin slices and high resolution caused overestimation of the cavities for moderate root resorption cases [3].

The main problem is to decide how and when a clinician justify taking CBCT scan when a patient has undergone root resorption. Yi et al. [38] suggested that patients with clinically suspected root resorption be first evaluated by periapical radiographs. If positive results are obtained, for further examination, CBCT should be considered.

Alqerban et al. [10] reported that all CBCT systems used in their study showed high accuracy in the detection of root resorption, and there was no significant difference among CBCT systems in the detection of the severity of root resorption. Limitations of using CBCT for external root

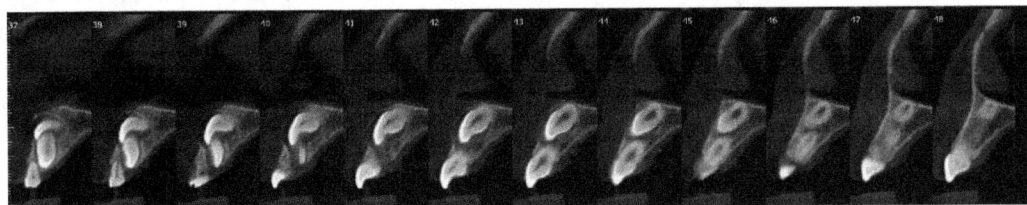

Figure 2. Evaluation of position of a supernumerary tooth and impacted incisor and their relation with neighboring structures.

resorption are the detection of small resorptions in the apical third and the high dose of radiation required [3].

3.4. Evaluation of root angulation and length

CBCT imaging becomes a preferred method for diagnosis by orthodontists because of its
three dimensional rendering capability. Root position and morphology are critical issues for
an orthodontist as it may affect the final occlusion. Root anatomy, such as short or dilacerated, is a determinant factor for the amount and direction of a tooth movement. Furthermore,
because of the concerns about external root resorption, orthodontists need to get precise measurements of root angulation and length before treatment. Using CBCT images also provide
detailed information about dysmorphic roots. Root positioning and morphology might be
indicators of a disease. Of course, all root anomalies are not identical, but when supported
with genetic testing, CBCT imaging will be helpful in interpreting anomalous root morphology in syndromic cases [40].

3.5. Tooth-bone relationship

In bimaxillary protrusion cases, Class 3 patients with an initial symphysis bone width,
cases with preexisting periodontal disease, after maxillary expansion treatment, CBCT provides valuable information about tooth-bone relationships, and it might reduce the risk
factor for dehiscence. While assessing deficiencies of buccolingual thickness in the alveolar
ridge of patients subjected to critical tooth movement, high resolution and a limited FOV
is recommended [41].

3.6. Cleft lip and palate (CLP) cases

Patients with CLP are treated by interdisciplinary teams from infancy until adulthood.
Several types of surgical procedures are used to reconstruct the anatomy of the alveolar
ridge, dentofacial region, lips and nose. The SEDENTEXCT Consortium stated, in regard
to the radiation dose, that "the application of CBCT in cleft lip and palate patients was
found to be the simplest to support" in dentistry [42]. However, in a recent systematic
review, it was suggested that further investigation is necessary to determine the influence
of this new 3D facial imaging modality on treatment planning, treatment outcome and
treatment evaluation.

The preoperative CBCT may provide reliable estimates on how much expansion and graft
material will be needed, aid in appropriate selection of an autogenous graft donor site
before surgery and enable the visualization of the three-dimensional morphology of the
bone bridge, the relationship between the bone bridge and roots of the neighboring teeth.
For alveolar bone graft success, determination of the buccal-palatal width of the bone
in CLP cases, the use of CBCT is recommended [43] (**Figure 3**). Pharyngeal space, the
results of bone grafting, and the effect of nasoalveolar molding can be evaluated with a
post-treatment CBCT.

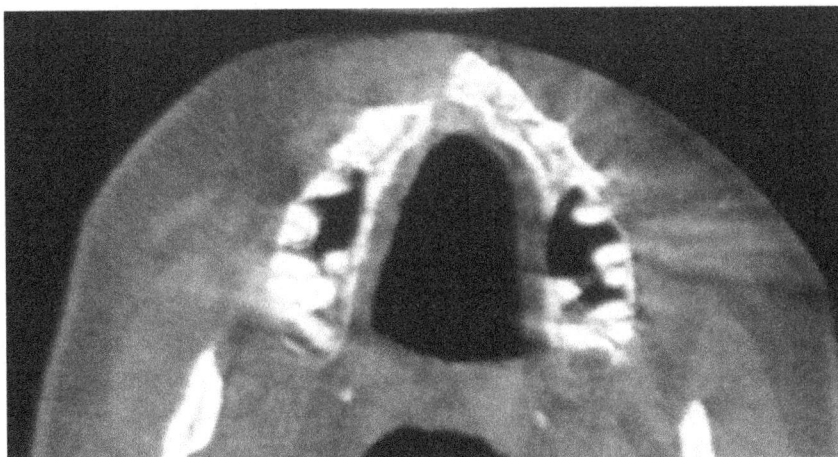

Figure 3. Preoperative CBCT view of a CLP case showing the graft site.

3.7. Temporomandibular joint (TMJ) morphology and pathology contributing to malocclusion

The changes in the size, form and special and functional relationships of the TMJ components might cause pathological TMJ conditions. TMJ disorders which occurred during active growth period might alter jaw, tooth positions and occlusion. Even though signs and symptoms of disturbances in the masticatory system are common, understanding the cause can be very complex. A proper diagnosis is possible, if only a through history and examination were achieved. Various types of imaging techniques can be used to gain additional information regarding the health and function of TMJs. CBCT is indicated for orthodontic cases that require analysis of TMJ bone components accompanied by signs and symptoms [44, 45]. One of the greatest advantages of CT scan is evaluating the condyle-disk relationship [46]. In comparison with panoramic radiograph and linear tomography, CBCT proves more accurate in diagnosing erosion of the condyle [47]. Soft tissue imaging is possible, but bony tissues are best imaged with CT scans [48]. As magnetic resonance imaging enables visualizing the non-mineralized soft tissues, it is preferable for the diagnosis of internal derangements of TMJ. However, it is not possible to observe dynamic joint movements.

Besides the evaluation of TMJ disorders, CBCT has been used to evaluate the condylar changes after orthodontic treatment. It allows volumetric evaluation of TMJ and provides better landmark identification on curved surfaces like condyle. Literature review showed that CBCT evaluation was preferred to determine respond of TMJ to mandibular advancement [49] or extraction treatment [50] and effects of the distraction splint therapy in mandibular asymmetry cases.

3.8. Airway morphology and obstructive sleep apnea (OSA)

Sleep-disordered breathing is a spectrum of conditions with abnormal respiratory pattern, and OSA is the severe end of that spectrum. Orthodontics takes place in the management of OSA by using mandibular advancement appliances and by planning orthognathic surgery in these cases. It is also crucial to evaluate the dimensional changes in the nasopharyngeal area and airway obstruction in CLP [51]. Until recent years, lateral cephalometric radiography was used for the evaluation of the upper airway. But, changes which occur in the transverse dimension cannot be visualized. Three-dimensional analysis and evaluation of airway have got a significant attention in the literature. CBCT allows orthodontists to measure cross-sectional area, minimum cross section and total volume of the patient's airway accurately. Also, it has been used to investigate the effects of orthodontic treatments and orthognathic surgery on airway dimensions.

Studies of the upper airway based on CBCT scans are considered to be reliable in providing important information about the morphology of the pharyngeal airway; however, they have limitation in distinguishing different types of soft tissues [52]. Variations in airway dimensions and morphology due to patient's swallowing movement and head posture are also among the limitations of this technique [53].

3.9. Maxillary transverse dimension and maxillary expansion

In the treatment of transverse maxillary deficiencies, it is important to assess transverse dimension as early as possible and accurately diagnose the need for transverse maxillary expansion using proper diagnostic tools. Before CBCT, post-treatment skeletal changes on patients treated with RME were measured on dental casts, lateral and posterior-anterior cephalometric and occlusal radiographs. Researches to date on rapid maxillary expansion have focused on determining treatment outcomes like dental tipping, alveolar bone bending, skeletal expansion and soft tissue changes, rather than the benefits of CBCT in diagnosis and treatment planning. Nowadays, it is claimed that CBCT images appear to be more reliable than posteroanterior cephalograms, offer an unobstructed view for the assessment of transversal intermaxillary discrepancies and provide much greater resolution and minimal image distortion [15]. However, the radiation dosage and its effect on growing patients must be taken into account.

The mid-palatal suture becomes more fused after the completion of the adolescent growth spurt [54], as prediction of mid-palatal suture maturation is possible by using CBCT [55]. It is a reliable diagnostic tool, while planning surgically assisted rapid maxillary expansion (SARME) in skeletally mature patients or using bone-borne devices, which have recently gained popularity. It is possible to determine treatment outcomes of SARME and also permits the detection of the complications, such as tooth tilting of the anchoring teeth and bone fenestration due to periodontal stress [56].

3.10. Temporary anchorage device (TAD) placement

In recent years, TADs are considered as a prerequisite for the resistance of unwanted tooth movements during the treatment of various orthodontic problems without patient compliance. The most common indications for treatment with TADs are molar protraction followed by indirect skeletal anchorage for space closure, intrusion of supraerupted teeth, intrusion of anterior to manage anterior open bite, anterior en-masse retraction, molar uprighting, intrusion of maxillary cant, molar distalization, traction on impacted canine, and attachment for protraction facemask. CBCT images can be helpful to anchor the miniscrew and mini-plate securely in the surrounding bone and to visualize neighboring structures for avoiding damage or complications during TAD placement and be useful in identifying optimal site location (**Figure 4**).

CBCT technology enables us to evaluate the interradicular distance and thickness, transverse bone thickness, bone density and thickness, cortical bone dimensions and quality. Even though anterior palate offers the greatest bone thickness, Holm et al. [57] recommended a CBCT evaluation for maximum screw length, as there is considerable variation of bone thickness between individuals. Before placing a miniscrew by using CBCT, it is also possible to define even cranial and caudal boundaries, besides alveolar boundary conditions, and eliminate the risk of bone and root perforations. Surgical guides fabricated using CBCT images will help to avoid possible root and maxillary sinuses damage. Finite element analysis constructed using CBCT will also guide the evaluation of mechanical advantages or disadvantages of the orthodontic appliances with TADs by simulating stress distribution.

There are several factors that affect the stability and success rate of TADs. If cortical bone thickness is less than 1 mm, primary stability may not be achieved, and the TAD may loosen during orthodontic treatment [58]. Evaluation of cortical bone quantity and quality is also critical for long-term stability. With finite element analysis, it has been shown that root contact is also one of the factors that can cause loss of miniscrew stability [59]. The information gathered from CBCT will be determinant for some of these factors, such as the dimension and insertion

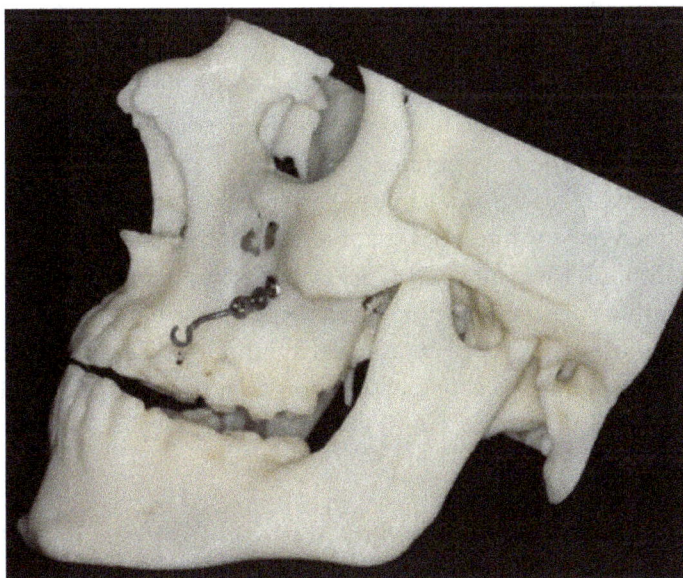

Figure 4. Planning and preparation of TAD (zygomatic skeletal anchorage) on a 3D model obtained from CBCT before surgery.

angle of the miniscrew, the insertion procedure, the depth of the screw insertion and insertion torque [38, 57, 60].

In some cases, routine panoramic, lateral and frontal cephalometric radiographs may not provide all information needed to optimize the location of a miniscrew placement. However, it should be kept in mind that in regions with a high bone quality, such as paramedian palate and palatal region, lateral cephalometric radiographs are usable to determine the location of TADs. Therefore, it is not necessary to take a CBCT in all cases [61].

It is recommended to use the smallest possible FOV unless the CBCT is needed for the diagnosis of another condition in which case a large FOV may be preferred [60].

3.11. Dentofacial deformities and craniofacial anomalies

Evaluation of changes in the craniofacial region during growth and with treatment using lateral cephalograms makes a great contribution to the science of orthodontics. However, in recent years, researches discussed the validity of evaluating a 3D craniofacial structure in a 2D plane. CBCT imaging can provide valuable information about dentofacial deformities and craniofacial anomalies, like facial asymmetry which affects three dimensions of the face, and it can be used to simulate virtual treatment plans for orthopedic corrections, orthognathic surgeries and distraction osteogenesis. By capturing images and analyzing the craniofacial hard and soft tissues and by generating virtual patient models, CBCT imaging permits the clinicians to reposition and reconstruct craniofacial structures (**Figure 5a, b**).

Several studies were conducted to determine reference planes, to develop cephalometric analysis, to evaluate the accuracy of these measurements, to establish the mean normality values and to assess the differences of gender and ethnic groups for 3D evaluations [62]. Besides morphological analysis, these images are used to evaluate the spatial relationship of the neighboring structures. CBCT technology enables carrying out the model surgery. So, computer assisted orthognathic surgery permits the design and fabrication of the occlusal surgical splints. By using virtual models, constructing anatomically grafts and correct replacement can be achieved (**Figure 6**). The data obtained from CBCT provide a better prediction of soft tissue response to the changes in the hard tissue after orthognathic surgery [63]. In the literature, CBCT is recommended for the assessment of preoperative orthodontic decompensation of maxillary and mandibular incisors [64]. This is an additional information from CBCT that is taken for orthognathic surgery planning, and it could not be one of the main purpose of using CBCT. Furthermore, CBCT proves a good method to assess TMJ after orthognathic surgery, particularly when there is considerable potential for resorption of the condyle [14].

3.12. Treatment outcomes

Taking CBCT at the end of orthodontic treatment is a controversial issue. However, it must be taken into consideration that studies on response to treatment can help elucidate clinical questions on variability of outcomes of treatment. There are studies assessing treatment

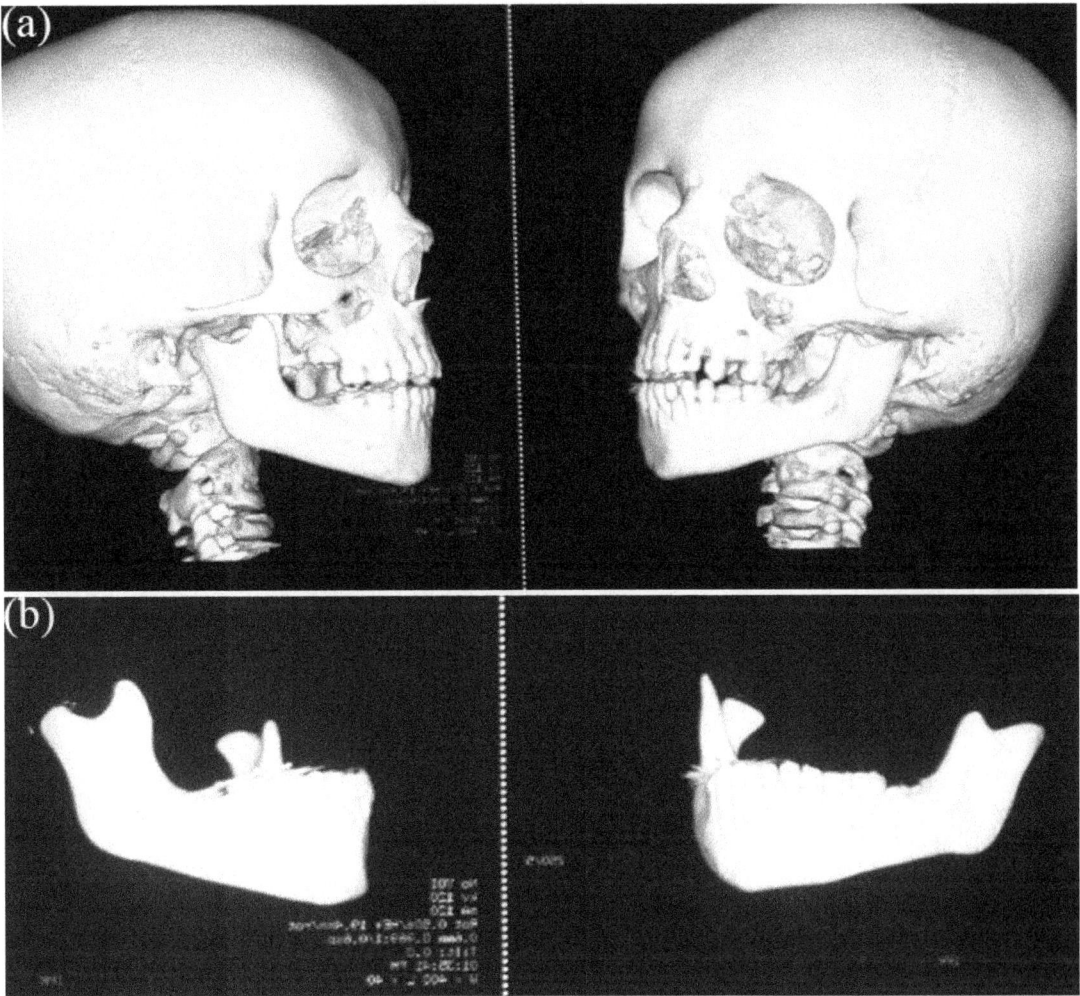

Figure 5. (a) 3D view of a case with Golden Haar syndrome. Note the asymmetric growth of left and right condyles. (b) 3D evaluation of mandible and condyles in this case.

outcomes of orthognathic surgery, maxillary expansion, bone grafting and several orthopedic appliances. A review of literature showed that jaw and teeth relationships, soft tissue, hyoid bone position, pharyngeal airway dimensions and morphology were evaluated after orthodontic and surgical treatments. To facilitate the evaluation of treatment outcomes, superimposition methods for CBCT images were also offered [28].

3.13. Evaluation of cervical vertebral maturation (CVM)

Skeletal maturation of patients is an important factor while planning orthodontic treatment. Hand-wrist and CVM methods were used for assessing the adolescent growth peak. It is suggested that the CBCT images may be useful for estimates of skeletal maturation, although they should not be used solely for that purpose [65]. Shim et al. [66] claimed that the esti-

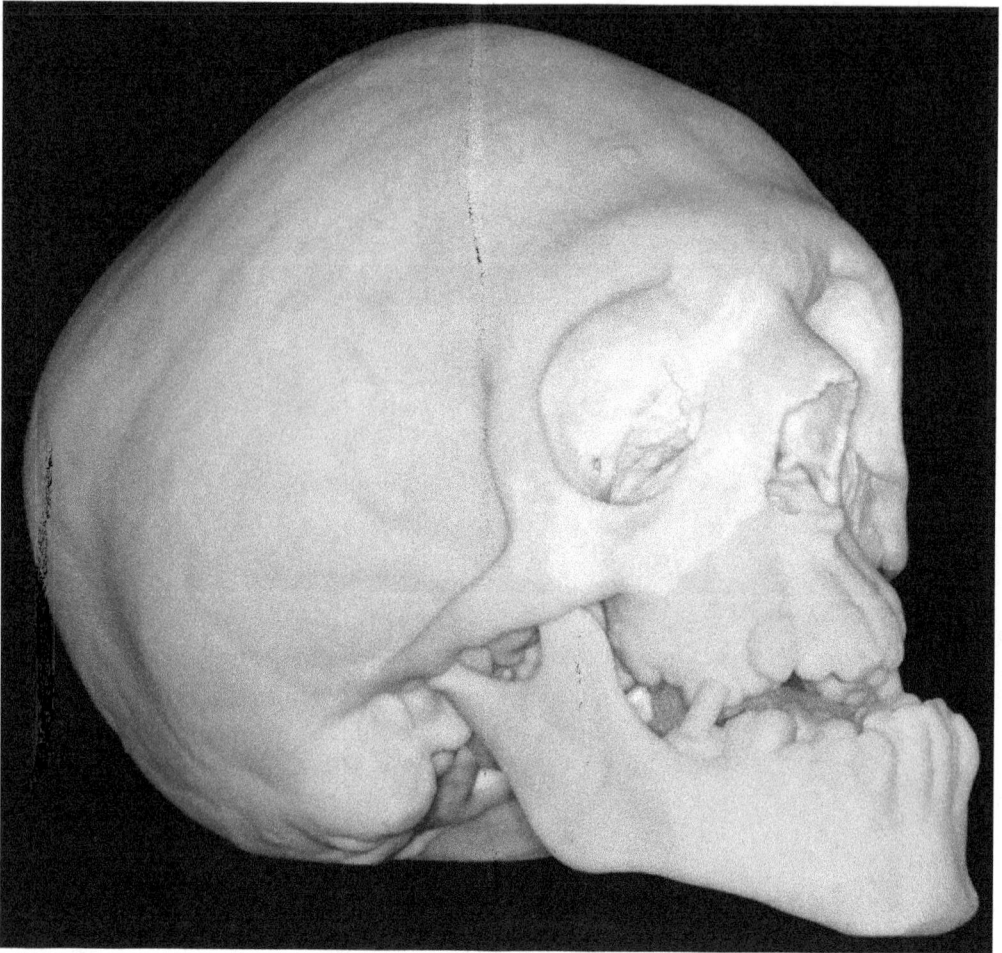

Figure 6. Presurgical 3D model of a case with Crouzon syndrome obtained from CBCT.

mate of maturation stages of the cervical vertebrae on CBCT provided a reliable evaluation of pubertal growth support and strongly positive correlations with lateral cephalograms and hand-wrist radiographs.

4. Radiation dose

Radiation dose depends on the CBCT scanner's specifications, milliampere setting, peak kilovoltage (kVp), voxel size, sensor sensitivity and number of images obtained, the time of scanning, and FOV. It is recommended to apply the 3D evaluation when the use of CBCT can be justified. Clinicians should always keep in mind that the radiation exposure to a human being should be kept "As Low As Reasonably Achievable" (ALARA) principle.

SEDENTEXCT project guidelines include a variety of topics, like justification, referral criteria, optimization, training, quality assurance and staff protection aspects [67]. Justification of using CBCT in dentistry can be considered if only a patient history and clinical information are available, if additional new information is expected, and if 2D radiographs are inadequate for diagnosis. The orthodontist should weigh the potential benefits of a CBCT against the chance of causing cancer for each patient. The chance may be small, but it is never negligible.

To reduce the patient dose, the smallest available volume size should be preferred. kVp and mAs of CBCT used in dental and maxillofacial region vary in a wide range and patients' doses varies considerably. It is recommended to standardize exposure parameters in dental and maxillofacial CBCT for each imaging task [68]. Gamache et al. [7] suggested that the total radiation exposure from CBCT scans can be reduced by while maintaining adequate image quality using low kV and moderate-to-high mA settings rather than the manufacturer-recommended settings.

Voxel size should be determined according to the purpose of the exam. When voxel dimension decreases, a better spatial resolution will be achieved, but the radiation dose will be increased [70]. Voxel sizes of 0.3–0.4 mm should be preferred if there is no need for a high level of detail [41].

Using child dose is offered because effective doses are higher compared with adults if exposure factors are not adapted. In a study on estimation of pediatric organ and effective doses from dental CBCT in 2012, it was reported that the average effective doses to the 10-year-old and adolescent phantoms were 116 and 79 mSv, respectively, which are similar to adult doses. So, the authors concluded that dental CBCT examinations on children should be fully justified over conventional X-ray imaging due to the higher radiosensitivity of children and that dose optimization by FOV collimation is particularly important in young children [69]. FOV should be restricted as much as possible [42]. So, the examination should include only the areas of interest in order to minimize radiation dose and ALARA principle must be followed. Repeated CBCT examinations should be avoided. The patient must be informed, and consent of the patient or parents must be obtained.

Technical properties of CBCT units were given inadequately in several studies. To make a comparison based on effective dose between studies, these properties must be reported and more evidence base studies on effective dose and image quality relation are still needed [70].

5. Future of CBCT in orthodontics

Further research-based technological developments are needed to achieve CBCT imaging, which is cost-effective, more precise on landmark identification and providing more accurate image quality with reduced radiation dose. By technological evolution and innovation of this technique, indications and the usage of CBCT in orthodontics will advance in the future. Future investigations are needed to investigate the dose levels for pediatric imaging protocols and to assess the use of a thyroid collar as a dose reduction technique.

6. Conclusions

In recent years, the use of CBCT in orthodontics has gained popularity and preferred as an imaging method by many clinicians for diagnosis and treatment planning. In this chapter, the indications and usage of CBCT in orthodontics are summarized. Clinicians should have comprehensive knowledge about advantages, disadvantages, limitations and potential risks due to increased radiation dose before deciding to use CBCT. Evidence-based studies are still needed whether using CBCT has any effect on clinical decision and lead to an improvement in treatment outcome.

Acknowledgements

We like to thank for their valuable contributions Dr. Sema Yuksel, Dr. Neslihan Ucuncu, Dr. Nilufer Darendeliler, Dr. Erdal Bozkaya, Dr.Secil Acar, Dr. Gülce Tosun who shared 3D views of their cases.

Author details

Emine Kaygısız* and Tuba Tortop

*Address all correspondence to: dt.emineulug@mynet.com

Faculty of Dentistry, Department of Orthodontics, Gazi University, Ankara, Turkey

References

[1] Palomo JM, Valiathan M, Hans MG. Orthodontic Diagnosis and Treatment Planning. Available from: http://pocketdentistry.com/11-3d-orthodontic-diagnosis-and-treatment-planning/3D

[2] Edwards R, Alsufyani N, Heo G, Flores-Mir C. Agreement among orthodontists experienced with cone-beam computed tomography on the need for follow-up and the clinical impact of craniofacial findings from multiplanar and 3-dimensional reconstructed views. American Journal of Orthodontics and Dentofacial Orthopedics. 2015;148(2):264-273

[3] Alqerban A, Jacobs R, Souza PC, Willems G. In-vitro comparison of 2 cone-beam computed tomography systems and panoramic imaging for detecting simulated canine impaction-induced external root resorption in maxillary lateral incisors. American Journal of Orthodontics and Dentofacial Orthopedics. 2009;136(6):764.e1-e11; discussion 764-5

[4] Alqerban A, Willems G, Bernaerts C, Vangastel J, Politis C, Jacobs R. Orthodontic treatment planning for impacted maxillary canines using conventional records versus 3D CBCT. European Journal of Orthodontics. 2014;36(6):698-707

[5] Ludlow JB, Gubler M, Cevidanes L, Mol A. Precision of cephalometric landmark iden-
      tification: Cone-beam computed tomography vs conventional cephalometric views.
      American Journal of Orthodontics and Dentofacial Orthopedics. 2009;**136**(3):312.e1-e10

[6] Ludlow JB, Laster WS, See M, Bailey LJ, Hershey HG. Accuracy of measurements of
      mandibular anatomy in cone beam computed tomography images. Oral Surgery, Oral
      Medicine, Oral Pathology, Oral Radiology, and Endodontology. 2007;**103**(4):534-542

[7] Gamache C, English JD, Salas-Lopez AM, Rong J, Akyalcin S. Assessment of image
      quality in maxillofacial cone-beam computed tomography imaging. Seminars in
      Orthodontics. 2015;**21**(4):248-253

[8] Seet KY, Barghi A, Yartsev S, Van Dyk J. The effects of field-of-view and patient size on
      CT numbers from cone-beam computed tomography. Physics in Medicine and Biology.
      2009;**54**(20):6251-6262

[9] Varghese S, Kailasam V, Padmanabhan S, Vikraman B, Chithranjan A. Evaluation of
      the accuracy of linear measurements on spiral computed tomography-derived three-
      dimensional images and its comparison with digital cephalometric radiography.
      Dentomaxillofacial Radiology. 2010;**39**:216-223

[10] Alqerban A, Jacobs R, Fieuws S, Nackaerts O, SEDENTEXCT Project Consortium,
       Willems G. Comparison of 6 cone-beam computed tomography systems for image qual-
       ity and detection of simulated canine impaction-induced external root resorption in max-
       illary lateral incisors. American Journal of Orthodontics and Dentofacial Orthopedics.
       2011;**140(3)**:129-139

[11] Larson BE. Cone-beam computed tomography is the imaging technique of choice
       for comprehensive orthodontic assessment. American Journal of Orthodontics and
       Dentofacial Orthopedics. 2012;**141**(4):402, 404, 406 passim

[12] Kusnoto B, Kaur P, Salem A, Zhang Z, Galang-Boquiren MT, Viana G, Evans CA, Robert
       Manasse, Monahan R, BeGole E, Abood A, Han X, Sidky E, Pan X. Implementation of
       ultra-low-dose CBCT for routine 2D orthodontic diagnostic radiographs: Cephalometric
       landmark identification and image quality assessment. Seminars in Orthodontics.
       2015;**21**(4):233-247

[13] Cevidanes LH, Bailey LJ, Tucker GR Jr, Styner MA, Mol A, Phillips CL, Proffit WR,
       Turvey T. Superimposition of 3D cone-beam CT models of orthognathic surgery patients.
       Dentomaxillofacial Radiology. 2005;**34**(6):369-375

[14] Cevidanes LH, Bailey LJ, Tucker SF, Styner MA, Mol A, Phillips CL, Proffit WR, Turvey
       T. Three-dimensional cone-beam computed tomography for assessment of mandibular
       changes after orthognathic surgery. American Journal of Orthodontics and Dentofacial
       Orthopedics. 2007;**131**(1):44-50

[15] Sawchuk D, Currie K, Vich ML, Palomo JM, Flores-Mir C. Diagnostic methods for
       assessing maxillary skeletal and dental transverse deficiencies: A systematic review. The
       Korean Journal of Orthodontics. 2016;**46**(5):331-342

[16] Baumrind S. The road to three-dimensional imaging in orthodontics. Seminars in Orthodontics. 2011;**17**(1):2-12

[17] Scholz R. The radiology decision. Seminars in Orthodontics. 2011;**17**:15-19

[18] Bayome M, Park JH, Kim Y, Kook Y. 3D analysis and clinical applications of CBCT images. Seminars in Orthodontics. 2015; 21: 254-262

[19] Valizadeh S, Tavakkoli MA, Karimi Vasigh H, Azizi Z, Zarrabian T. Evaluation of cone beam computed tomography (CBCT) system: Comparison with intraoral periapical radiography in proximal caries detection. Journal of Dental Research, Dental Clinics, Dental Prospects. 2012;**6**(1):1-5

[20] Chang ZC, Hu FC, Lai E, Yao CC, Chen MH, Chen YJ. Landmark identification errors on cone-beam computed tomography-derived cephalograms and conventional digital cephalograms. American Journal of Orthodontics and Dentofacial Orthopedics. 2011;**140**(6):e289-e297

[21] Alling CC, Helfrick JF, Alling RD. Impacted Teeth. Philadelphia, Pa: W.B. Saunders; 1993

[22] Oberoi S, Knueppel S. Three-dimensional assessment of impacted canines and root resorption using cone beam computed tomography. Oral Surgery, Oral Medicine, Oral Pathology, Oral Radiology. 2012;**113**(2):260-267

[23] Scarfe WC, Farman AG, Sukovic P. Clinical applications of cone beam computed tomography in dental practice. Journal - Canadian Dental Association. 2006;**72**(1):75-80

[24] Alqerban A, Jacobs R, Lambrechts P, Loozen G, Willems G. Root resorption of the maxillary lateral incisor caused by impacted canine: A literature review. Clinical Oral Investigations. 2009;**13**(3):247-255

[25] Walker L, Enciso R, Mah J. Three-dimensional localization of maxillary canines with cone-beam computed tomography. American Journal of Orthodontics and Dentofacial Orthopedics 2005;**128**(4):418-423

[26] Haney E, Gansky SA, Lee JS, Johnson E, Maki K, Miller AJ, Huang JC. Comparative analysis of traditional radiographs and cone-beam computed tomography volumetric images in the diagnosis and treatment planning of maxillary impacted canines. American Journal of Orthodontics and Dentofacial Orthopedics. 2010;**137**(5):590-597

[27] Kapila S, Nervina JM. 3D image-aided diagnosis and treatment of impacted and transposed teeth. In: Kapila S, editor. Cone Beam Computed Tomography in Orthodontics. John Wiley & Sons; 2014. pp. 349-382

[28] Kapila S, Conley RS, Harrell WE Jr. The current status of cone beam computed tomography imaging in orthodontics. Dentomaxillofacial Radiology. 2011;**40**(1):24-34

[29] Alqerban A, Hedesiu M, Baciut M, Nackaerts O, Jacobs R, Fieuws S; SedentexCT Consortium., Willems G. Pre-surgical treatment planning of maxillary canine impactions using panoramic vs cone beam CT imaging. Dentomaxillofacial Radiology. 2013;**42**(9):20130157

[30] Wriedt S, Jaklin J, Al-Nawas B, Wehrbein H. Impacted upper canines: Examination and treatment proposal based on 3D versus 2D diagnosis. Journal of Orofacial Orthopedics. 2012;**73**(1):28-40

[31] Becker A, Abramovitz I, Chaushu S. Failure of treatment of impacted canines associated with invasive cervical root resorption. The Angle Orthodontist. 2013;**83**(5):870-876

[32] Alqerban A, Jacobs R, Fieuws S, Willems G. Comparison of two cone beam computed tomographic systems versus panoramic imaging for localization of impacted maxillary canines and detection of root resorption. European Journal of Orthodontics. 2011;**33**:93-102

[33] Kapila SD, Nervina JM. CBCT in orthodontics: Assessment of treatment outcomes and indications for its use. Dentomaxillofacial Radiology. 2015;**44**(1):20140282

[34] Westphalen VP, Gomes de Moraes I, Westphalen FH, Martins WD, Souza PH. Conventional and digital radiographic methods in the detection of simulated external root resorptions: A comparative study. Dentomaxillofacial Radiology. 2004;**33**(4):233-235

[35] Ely NJ, Sherriff M, Cobourne MT. Dental transposition as a disorder of genetic origin. European Journal of Orthodontics. 2006;**28**(2):145-151

[36] Shafer WG, Hine MK, Levy BM. A Textbook of Oral Pathology. Philadelphia: WB Saunders Co; 1985

[37] Toureno L, Park JH, Cederberg RA, Hwang EH, Shin JW. Identification of supernumerary teeth in 2D and 3D: review of literature and a proposal. Journal of Dental Education. 2013;**77**(1):43-50

[38] Yi J, Sun Y, Li Y, Li C, Li X, Zhao Z. Cone-beam computed tomography versus periapical radiograph for diagnosing external root resorption: A systematic review and meta-analysis. The Angle Orthodontist. 2017;**87**(2):328-337

[39] Jawad Z, Carmichael F, Houghton N, Bates C. A review of cone beam computed tomography for the diagnosis of root resorption associated with impacted canines, introducing an innovative root resorption scale. Oral Surgery, Oral Medicine, Oral Pathology, Oral Radiology, and Endodontology. 2016;**122**(6):765-771

[40] Nervina JM, Kapila SD. Assessment of root position and morphology by Cone Beam Computed Tomography. In: Kapila S, editor. Cone Beam Computed Tomography in Orthodontics. John Wiley & Sons; 2014. pp. 319-348.

[41] Garib DG, Calil LR, Leal CR, Janson G. Is there a consensus for CBCT use in Orthodontics? Dental Press Journal of Orthodontics. 2014;**19**(5):136-149

[42] European Commission. Radiation protection no 172. Cone beam CT for dental and maxillofacial radiology (evidence based guidelines). 2012. Available: http://www.sedentexct.eu/files/radiation_protection_172.pdf. [Accessed 2014 Mar 16]

[43] Hamada Y, Kondoh T, Noguchi K, Iino M, Isono H, Ishii H, et al. Application of limited cone beam computed tomography to clinical assessment of alveolar bone grafting: a preliminary report. The Cleft Palate-Craniofacial Journal. 2005;**42**(2):128-137

[44] American Academy of Oral and Maxillofacial Radiology. Clinical recommendations regarding use of cone beam computed tomography in Orthodontics. Position statement by the American Academy of Oral and Maxillofacial Radiology. Oral Surgery, Oral Medicine, Oral Pathology, Oral Radiology, and Endodontology. 2013;**116**(2):238-257

[45] Scarfe WC, Farman AG. What is cone-beam CT and how does it work? Dental Clinics of North America. 2008;**52**(4):707-730

[46] Okeson JP. Management of Temporomandibular Disorders and Occlusion. Mosby Co.; 1998. pp. 281-303

[47] Honey OB, Scarfe WC, Hilgers MJ, Klueber K, Silveira AM, Haskell BS, et al. Accuracy of cone-beam computed tomography imaging of the temporomandibular joint: comparisons with panoramic radiology and linear tomography. American Journal of Orthodontics and Dentofacial Orthopedics. 2007;**132**(4):429-438

[48] Tuncer BB, Ataç MS, Yüksel S. A case report comparing 3-D evaluation in the diagnosis and treatment planning of hemimandibular hyperplasia with conventional radiography. Journal of Cranio-Maxillo-Facial Surgery. 2009;**37**(6):312-319

[49] Knappe SW, Bakke M, Svanholt P, Petersson A, Sonnesen L. Long-term side effects on the temporomandibular joints and orofacial function in patients with obstructive sleep apnoea treated with a mandibular advancement device. Journal of Oral Rehabilitation. 2017;44(5):354-362

[50] Alhammadi MS, Fayed MS, Labib A. Three-dimensional assessment of condylar position and joint spaces after maxillary first premolar extraction in skeletal Class II malocclusion. Orthodontics & Craniofacial Research. 2017. doi: 10.1111/ocr.12141

[51] Massie JP, Runyan CM, Stern MJ, Alperovich M, Rickert SM, Shetye PR, Staffenberg DA, Flores RL. Nasal septal anatomy in skeletally mature patients with cleft lip and palate. JAMA Facial Plastic Surgery. 2016;**18**(5):347-353

[52] Aboudara CA, Hatcher D, Neilsen IL, Miller A. A three-dimensional evaluation of the upper airway in adolescents. Orthodontics & Craniofacial Research. 2003;**6**(Suppl 1):173-175

[53] Lenza MG, Lenza MM, Dalstra M, Melsen B, Cattaneo PM. An analysis of different approaches to the assessment of upper airway morphology: A CBCT study. Orthodontics & Craniofacial Research. 2010;**13**(2):96-105

[54] Goldenberg DC, Alonso N, Goldenberg FC, Gebrin ES, Amaral TS, Scanavini MA, et al. Using computed tomography to evaluate maxillary changes after surgically assisted rapid palatal expansion. Journal of Craniofacial Surgery 2007;**18**:302-311

[55] Jang HI, Kim SC, Chae JM, Kang KH, Cho JW, Chang NY, Lee KY, Cho JH. Relationship between maturation indices and morphology of the midpalatal suture obtained using cone-beam computed tomography images. The Korean Journal of Orthodontics. 2016;**46** (6):345-355

[56] Koudstaal MJ, Wolvius EB, Schulten AJ, Hop WC, van der Wal KG. Stability, tipping and relapse of bone-borne versus tooth-borne surgically assisted rapid maxillary expansion: A prospective randomized patient trial. International Journal of Oral and Maxillofacial Surgery. 2009;**38**:308-315

[57] Holm M, Jost-Brinkmann PG, Mah J, Bumann A. Bone thickness of the anterior palate for orthodontic miniscrews. The Angle Orthodontist. 2016;**86**(5):826-831

[58] Motoyoshi M, Yoshida T, Ono A, Shimizu N. Effect of cortical bone thickness and implant placement torque on stability of orthodontic mini-implants. The International Journal of Oral & Maxillofacial Implants. 2007;**22**(5):779-784

[59] Motoyoshi M, Ueno S, Okazaki K, Shimizu N. Bone stress for a mini-implant close to the roots of adjacent teeth-3D finite element analysis. International Journal of Oral and Maxillofacial Surgery. 2009;**38**(4):363-368

[60] Baumgaertel S. Planning and placing temporary anchorage devices with the aid of cone beam computed tomography. In: Kapila S, editor. Cone Beam Computed Tomography in Orthodontics. John Wiley & Sons; 2014. pp. 411-426

[61] Baumgaertel S, Hans MG. Buccal cortical bone thickness for mini-implant placement. American Journal of Orthodontics and Dentofacial Orthopedics. 2009;**36**(2):230-235

[62] Porto OC, de Freitas JC, de Alencar AH, Estrela C. The use of three-dimensional cephalometric references in dentoskeletal symmetry diagnosis. Dental Press Journal of Orthodontics. 2014;**19**(6):78-85

[63] Schendel SA, Lane C, Harrell WE Jr. 3D Orthognathic surgery simulation using image fusion. Seminars in Orthodontics. 2009;**15**:48-56

[64] Sun B, Tang J, Xiao P, Ding Y. Presurgical orthodontic decompensation alters alveolar bone condition around mandibular incisors in adults with skeletal Class III malocclusion. International Journal of Clinical and Experimental Medicine. 2015;**8**(8):12866-12873

[65] Bonfim MA, Costa AL, Fuziy A, Ximenez ME, Cotrim-Ferreira FA, Ferreira-Santos RI. Cervical vertebrae maturation index estimates on cone beam CT: 3D reconstructions vs sagittal sections. Dentomaxillofacial Radiology. 2016;**45**(1):20150162

[66] Shim JJ, Heo G, Lagravère MO. Assessment of skeletal maturation based on cervical vertebrae in CBCT. International Orthodontics. 2012;**10**(4):351-362

[67] Menezes CC, Janson G, Cambiaghi L, Massaro C, Garib DG. Reproducibility of bone plate thickness measurements with cone-beam computed tomography using different image acquisition protocols. Dental Press Journal of Orthodontics. 2010;**15**(5):143-149

[68] ICRP. Radiological protection in Cone Beam Computed Tomography. ICRP Publication. 129. Annals of the ICRP. 2015;**44**(1)

[69] Theodorakou C, Walker A, Horner K, Pauwels R, Bogaerts R, Jacobs R. SEDENTEXCT Project Consortium. Estimation of paediatric organ and effective doses from dental cone beam CT using anthropomorphic phantoms. The British Journal of Radiology. 2012;**85**(1010):153-160

[70] Al-Okshi A, Lindh C, Sal'e H, Gunnarsson M, Rohlin M. Effective dose of cone beam CT (CBCT) of the facial skeleton: A systematic review. The British Journal of Radiology. 2015;**88**:20140658

4

Computed Tomography in Veterinary Medicine: Currently Published and Tomorrow's Vision

Matthew Keane, Emily Paul, Craig J Sturrock,
Cyril Rauch and Catrin Sian Rutland

Abstract

The utilisation of computed tomography (CT) in veterinary practise has been increasing rapidly in line with reduced cost, improved availability and the increase in expertise and technology. This review briefly examines the recent technological advancements in imaging in the veterinary sector, and explores how CT and micro-computed tomography (μCT) have furthered basic understanding and knowledge, and influenced clinical practise and medicine. The uses of CT technology in veterinary research, especially in relation to bone, vasculature and soft tissues are explored and compared in relation to the different species. CT is essential not only for the diagnosis and treatment of many disorders, but it is now being used to understand areas ranging from drug delivery and surgical advancements through to anatomical and educational uses throughout the world.

Keywords: veterinary, computed tomography, clinical, research, bone, vasculature

1. Overview of computed tomography in veterinary medicine

The introduction of computed tomography (CT) has provided one of the most important advancements in diagnostic imaging in the veterinary sector. In contrast to standard diagnostic radiography, CT produces an axial slice of the area under investigation and a resultant three-dimensional image. CT also allows greater differentiation between individual soft tissue structures than diagnostic radiography. This is due to the ability of CT to accurately measure the tissue absorption of X-ray beams as they pass through the patient [1].

Since the inception of CT, the technology has been developed to yield further improvements. The original first generation of CT scanners consisted of a single detector and an X-ray tube which produced a single narrow beam. The assembly of X-ray and detector linearly scanned the whole patient in the axial plane. Together, the X-ray beam and detector are rotated by 1° after each single line image. At the end of the process, each individual scan was then compiled to produce an image in a process known as reconstruction [1].

A pitfall of the first generation of CT scanners was the time taken to acquire an image, with a single slice taking up to 6 min [2]. The development of second generation CT scanners aimed to address this with the introduction of an X-ray tube which produced several narrow beams and generated a fan-shaped projection. The fan-shaped beam was directed at multiple detectors and together this system would rotate as a unit around 360° to generate an image. As fewer incremental steps were required whilst scanning the whole patient, this resulted in shorter scan times of up to 20 s for each slice [3, 4]. But even with this marked improvement in time taken to generate each slice, image quality was still affected by artefacts associated with the technology and movement blur [2, 5].

Further advancements of the technology resulted in third and fourth generation scanners which could acquire individual image slices considerable faster at a rate of one image per second from a patient. Third generation scanners consisted of an X-ray beam which spanned the entire width of the patient which was directed at an assembly of detectors. Both the X-ray tube and the assembly of detectors rotate 360° around the patient on a fixed frame (gantry) to produce a movement known as rotation-rotation. Fourth generation CT scanners are composed of an X-ray tube which rotates around the patient and directs its beam at a ring of fixed stationary detectors built into the machine housing [6].

2. Clinical uses of computed tomography in veterinary medicine

The use of CT in veterinary medicine in a clinical setting was first documented in the 1980s for the investigation of disease of the central nervous system and neoplasia in canines [7–10]. CT has become more common in veterinary medicine due to the technological advancements of CT and its increased availability in general practise. Another imaging modality which is becoming increasingly available in the veterinary sector is magnetic resonance imaging (MRI). The use of MRI is most commonly indicated in conditions that require differentiation between soft tissues, such as in the field of neurology, whereas CT is useful for imaging both bones and soft tissues [11].

In small animals, the use of CT is most commonly indicated in patients with thoracic and abdominal disease, intracranial and extracranial lesions, and disorders of the musculoskeletal system including the appendicular skeleton and spine [12–17]. As the generation of images in CT is so rapid, this diagnostic modality is important in cases where anaesthesia and sedation are not an option. CT is therefore useful in emergency critical cases or disorders which may be compromised by anaesthesia or sedation [18, 19].

In equine veterinary medicine, the use of CT is most appropriate in the assessment of structures with mixed tissue thickness and thus differing levels of tissue absorption of X-rays. Therefore, the structures most commonly assessed are the appendicular skeleton for diagnostic lameness work-ups, the dental arcade, paranasal sinuses and the skull [20–28]. In the clinic, patient positioning provides complications due to the size of the horse, although a hovercraft-design table alongside horse sedation (a technique revolutionised by the late Alastair Nelson) has enabled considerable development of scans involving the head [29].

The application of CT in a clinical setting to produce diagnostic images in cattle is not common. CT is often reserved for valuable cattle, primarily due to its expense but also due to the use of general anaesthetics and off-label drugs [30]. Unlike small animal and equine imaging, it is not often used for the appendicular skeleton or spine. The most common indications for its use are disease of the central nervous system, otitis media and dental disease.

3. The technical use of micro-computed tomography (μCT) in veterinary medicine and research

Recent technological advances are rendering the use of CT imaging as a diagnostic technique and preoperative tool increasingly common in veterinary medicine. These technological advances have, similarly, opened new possibilities in the field of research, which include the investigation of both hard and soft tissues, at and below the micrometre scale, providing physiological information non-destructively on the sample [31].

X-ray imaging is based around the principle of attenuation—the reduction of signal as the photons interact with electrons in the matter, known as the absorber, through which they are being passed [31]. The linear attenuation coefficient (μ), defined as the proportion of incident photon intensity reduction per unit length of absorber and expressed in cm^{-1}, is dictated by photon energy (E) and atomic number (Z). Photon intensity (I) decreases exponentially as a function of absorber thickness (t) in a homogenous absorber, as shown in the equation below [32, 33].

$$I = I_0 \exp(-\mu t) \tag{1}$$

I_0 is the incident radiation intensity, μ = linear attenuation coefficient, I = photon intensity, t = absorber thickness.

Attenuation principally arises from two processes: Compton scattering and photoelectric absorption [32]. Compton scattering involves the transfer of a proportion of the energy of the incident photon to an electron, resulting in the emission of a lower energy photon [34], and photoelectric absorption is the complete transfer of the incident photon energy [35]. Compton scattering is determined principally by Z, with the effect of E being only minimal, while photoelectric absorption is strongly dependent on both [32]. The attenuation of biological soft tissues, which display relative uniformity in their low-Z constituents [31], and bones is predominantly in the form of photoelectric absorption at low energy ranges (E = 30–50 keV) and Compton scattering and at higher energy levels (E = 200–1000 keV). With E ranging from 30 to 130 keV in X-ray radiographic imaging, attenuation in CT imaging usually results from a combination of photoelectric absorption and Compton scattering [32]. As CT detectors are not energy-discriminative and solely detect I, greater contrast is achieved at lower E levels where photoelectric absorption prevails [31, 32].

The X-rays used in μCT imaging may come from a laboratory X-ray generator or a synchrotron source. Synchrotron-source X-rays tend to be used monochromatically, with an E selected from a range, while laboratory-generated X-ray beams usually consist of peaks of characteristic X-rays with white (polychromatic) beams from breaking radiation (bremsstrahlung radiation). Thus voxel (volumetric pixel) values directly represent μ in synchrotron but not in laboratory CT [31].

4. Clinical and research investigations into bone tissue

CT has been used to investigate a number of bone and growth disorders. The key to CT scanning is that it can be used to visualise not only gross anatomy, such as fractures and general morphology, but can also show micro fractures, bone thickness, trabecular bone distortion and architecture, and bone curvature and angles in situ. When the variety of functions that can be applied to the normal body is considered, the uses for CT and μCT in diseases, disorders and in other studies are wide ranging. Cortical bone thickness and trabecular bone distortion can be used as indicators of localised mechanical strain [36] and it is likely that it is linked to many bone disorders in addition to fractures and trauma incidents.

Normal growth and development can be observed using CT scanning. As part of a study into human trabecular bone ontogeny, the femur trabecular number, thickness, and bone volume fraction were investigated from the foetus and youths up to 9 years of age [37]. These studies showed an increase in trabecular bone thickness and bone volume fraction, but a decrease in trabecular number at around a year old, coinciding with the onset of unaided walking and, as a consequence, load bearing was concluded to be causal of the changes observed. Similar observations have also been noted in nonhuman animals. An example is shown in the cat, where bone material density was used in the diagnosis of osteopenia and in order to quantify the benefits of the applied treatments [38]. μCT has shown the effectiveness of titanium lattice implants in relation to bone ingrowth and bone contact in rat, which has implications for not only veterinary but also human medicine [39]. Results from guinea pig have shown how bone research can help identify differences in bone development and structure. Despite adult weight being achieved at around 9–12 months of age, the study showed that bone development continued beyond 12 months [40]. The authors were also able to give detailed anatomical descriptions of the bones, show where weaker areas might occur, (which is useful in understanding fractures) and show that differing bones had different growth rates. Examples of the high quality of images and cortical bone thickness are shown in **Figure 1**. Using CT measurements has been shown to be more accurate than callipers in humans [41] and although the guinea pig study showed no significant differences between the two methods, the largest variation was observed within the smallest bones [40] indicating that for smaller measurements CT may be more applicable but more research needs to be undertaken in this area in differing measurement sizes to understand the limitations of each technique.

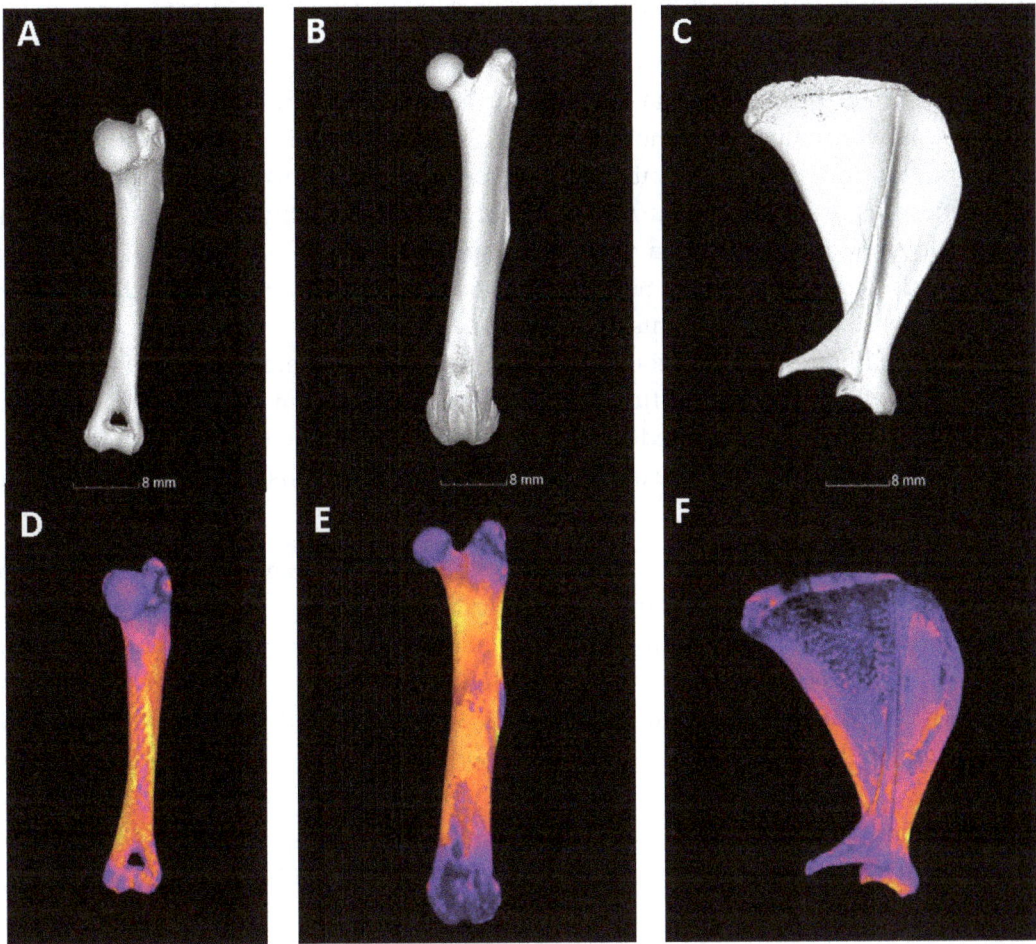

Figure 1. 3D rendered 4-year old guinea pig bones showing surface morphology (A, C, E) and cortical bone thickness (B, D, F) of the humerus (A, D), femur (B, E) and scapula (C, F). Bone thickness was mapped, where increasing brightness indicates thicker bone. BoneJ plugin for ImageJ [42] was utilised to calculate bone thickness.

CT for the assessment of equine disorders such as complex foot lameness cases is expanding [20]. Recent studies have shown visible thinning and fractures within bones of chronically laminitic horses, using μCT and histopathology in parallel [43]. μCT studies have also given enormous insights into bovine lameness. By combining clinical data with μCT images and measurements, direct correlations between bone damage, remodelling and growth were made, thus giving new insights into the mechanisms behind bovine lameness [44]. In addition to visualising bone measurements such as thickness, trabeculation and anatomical size, CT is an excellent platform for understanding bone angle and rotation, useful in understand deformities, dysplasia, neoplasia, osteopathies and degenerative diseases in addition to normal anatomy or in trauma situations. A good example of monitoring bone angles is some of the early imaging of the canine and feline temporomandibular joint, as this joint is particularly difficult to visualise using traditional radiographic techniques [45], and its use during/postsurgery to assess bone angle and healing, particularly in companion animals such as cats and dogs [46, 47].

CT is not restricted to small animal analysis and diagnosis. Although an elephant may be difficult to scan whilst alive, post-mortem tissue gives valuable insights into pathologies. An example was the work carried out into elephant foot pathology and anatomy. In this species, foot problems cause a substantial number of morbidity and mortality issues, and work undertaken to understand these showed a range of complications, from bone remodelling through to osteoarthritis and fractures [48]. Similar work has also been carried out in the rhinoceros [49]. Comparisons between elephants of differing ages, sexes and species (African vs. Asian) were made and, although captive (zoo) animals were used [48], there is potential for assessing and comparing wild animals in the future. Studies such as these can have beneficial outcomes on the way that animals are managed in captivity. Understanding what may influence disease and cause damage can help provide management mechanisms, thus enhancing animal health and welfare.

As a physiologically active tissue, bone's high adaptability to its environment can provide insight into the pathophysiological status of its surroundings [50]. While the osseous remodelling processes may be induced through a number of mechanisms such as trauma, ageing and disease, CT imaging can provide valuable insights into the bone's adaptive capabilities in terms of gross shape, cortical thickness, trabecular anisotropy and position within the body and in relation to other structures.

5. Clinical and research investigations into soft tissues

Visualising soft tissue and achieving contrast between the differing tissues can be a challenge [31]. Due to these difficulties there are numerous uses and techniques being developed in order to investigate soft tissue and liquids using CT. A separate section on vasculature CT is given below (Section 6).

The current method of staging canine appendicular osteosarcoma relies on radiography alongside scintigraphy, however work is being undertaken to try to use CT as an alternative. One such study showed that CT could effectively show malignancies in the thorax and abdomen, and lung lesions but it had a lower detection of appendicular osteosarcoma than the present methods [51]. It was suggested that diagnosis may be reduced due to reader fatigue, as shown in human radiology, but that slice thickness and lesion size may also play important roles. More development is needed in this area before CT can be used as a standalone tool for diagnosis. In other tumour types, CT is more successful. In the case of canine thyroid tumours, CT is recommended for both preoperative diagnosis and for staging [52, 53]. It has also been recommended that any middle aged dog that has a body CT should be checked for incidental thyroid nodules as, although rare, they are identifiable [54]. CT is already regularly used for staging cancers, and each tumour type must be individually assessed as to which method is most appropriate for this vital process.

Significant improvements in dogs with nasal neoplasia are observed when CT is utilised to stage tumours [55] and whereas the World Health Organisation staging guidance was originally based around radiography, this has since been updated to include CT [56, 57].

CT can reduce the number of surgical procedures undertaken or enable keyhole surgeries. Thoracic duct lymphography has been undertaken under research conditions and in canine patients with chylothorax, using CT and iodine as a contrasting agent. Furthermore, the technique was demonstrated to be beneficial when used post-surgery to check for recurrence [58, 59] as it was described as minimally invasive and easy to perform. A similar technique was used to look at feline lymphography. CT was able to show the small mammary lymphatic vessels and lymph nodes with minimal side effects [60].

CT has shown considerable promise for study of lesions such as cysts, abscesses, hydrocephalus and coenurosis lesions in ruminants, including sheep, cattle and the alpaca [61–64]. Ruminant brain disorders and malformations have been observed [61, 65]. These are increasingly used as the lower cost and reduced anaesthesia required in comparison to MRI is seen as favourable, especially in small ruminants and calves [66]. CT is presently used for assessing muscle mass, and is considered as the 'gold standard' alongside MRI. The technique is able to successfully differentiate between differing soft tissues such as skin and muscle. Muscle mass is critical in a number of situations including injury, chronic wasting, malnourishment, and during hospital and rest phases. In an interesting study, urine was examined rather than soft tissues. CT was used in a non-invasive manner to gauge whether urine concentration could be assessed in canine patients undergoing abdominal imaging [67]. The work even showed that the X-ray attenuation of urine could be measured. This has significant implications not only for measuring urine in differing species, but holds the potential for measuring other types of biological fluids.

Echocardiograms are frequently used for cardiovascular disorders, but CT is increasingly being utilised in research and in the clinical setting. One of the attractions of using CT is that second or third generation dual source scanner can scan animals at high speed and therefore within a heartbeat—if the heart is not beating too quickly [68]. Frequently CT is used to locate physical deformities such as atrial and ventricular septal defects, following device placement and surgery. It can also be used to look at general heart morphology and development in models of disease, and in animals with abnormalities such as endocarditis and regurgitation, to look at narrowing of the blood vessels such as the aorta, and to look for occlusions, seromas and abscesses [69].

6. Clinical and research investigations into vasculature

Vascular disturbances have long been associated to the pathologenesis of differing disorders [70], and digital venography is a commonly employed technique providing vital information for treatment options and for monitoring their progress [71]. CT images provide higher levels of quantitative information than venograms, enabling the visualisation of discrete areas rather than an overall impression of perfusion rate based on X-ray attenuation of contrast agents in numerous vessels simultaneously. Naturally, in the case of μCT, the post-mortem nature of the samples renders speculation on vasoactivity impossible, but this technique can still provide insights into vascularisation.

A number of different functions can now be investigated in relation to vasculature using CT. Complex 3D models of whole or partial organism vasculature can show areas of angiogenesis and neovascularisation. This technique can also show network interactions, show where vascular junctions and branching occurs, and indicate lumen diameter within a given area. There is an added complexity with blood vessels in that once blood flow ceases, the vascular morphology is altered. In order to preserve the tissues and permit a good visibility of the vasculature once scanned, tissues can be perfused and fixed while fresh. The aim of fixation is to maintain tissues in a life-like state, and perfusion fixation provides the optimal route for the fixative to reach the tissues upon which it can quickly act [72], while fixing the blood vessels in such a way to prevent their collapse and allow them to fill with air, providing the contrast between vessel lumen and the surrounding tissues. Achieving a balance in contrast between soft tissues, vasculature and hard tissue such as bone is complex. Previous studies have indicated that the perfusion of a high-Z contrast agent resulted in images where vasculature and bone were indistinguishable [73]. In one of our studies, the vasculature of the equine foot was flushed and fixed with para-formaldehyde (PFA). As the PFA was absorbed into the surrounding tissues, the empty vascular lumen filled with air. This air acted as the perfect contrast medium, allowing the vasculature not only to be distinguished from the surrounding soft tissues, but also from the bone (**Figures 2–4**).

One criticism of any vascular fixation method is that it could be argued that manually pres-surising the vessels is subjective and could lead to a degree of variability in visible vessel diameter. This method may therefore be useful when comparing similarly fixed tissues, but its variable nature should be kept in mind when direct measurements are being taken The system is not being visualised *in vivo*, but this does reflect observations made under histopa-thology conditions for example.

In vivo CT scanning is advancing rapidly and the use of single photon emission computed tomography (SPECT) that utilises a radiolabelled tracer has shown that the technique works well in animals. Following its use in humans, SPECT was used to assess cerebral blood flow in canine hepatic encephalopathy patients [74]. Comparing both healthy and hepatic encephalopathy canine patients, hypoperfusion was observed for the first time in the temporal cortex subcortical region. Not only was this condition comparable to humans, but also showed that the scanning method was well tolerated by the animals and that the technique itself was comparable to human studies [74]. In addition to the use of tracers and air to differentiate vasculature, a number of researchers have used corro-sions casting in order to understand vascularisation in a number of disorders and systems, ranging from kidney development to ocular disorders in species from mice through to sheep [75–77].

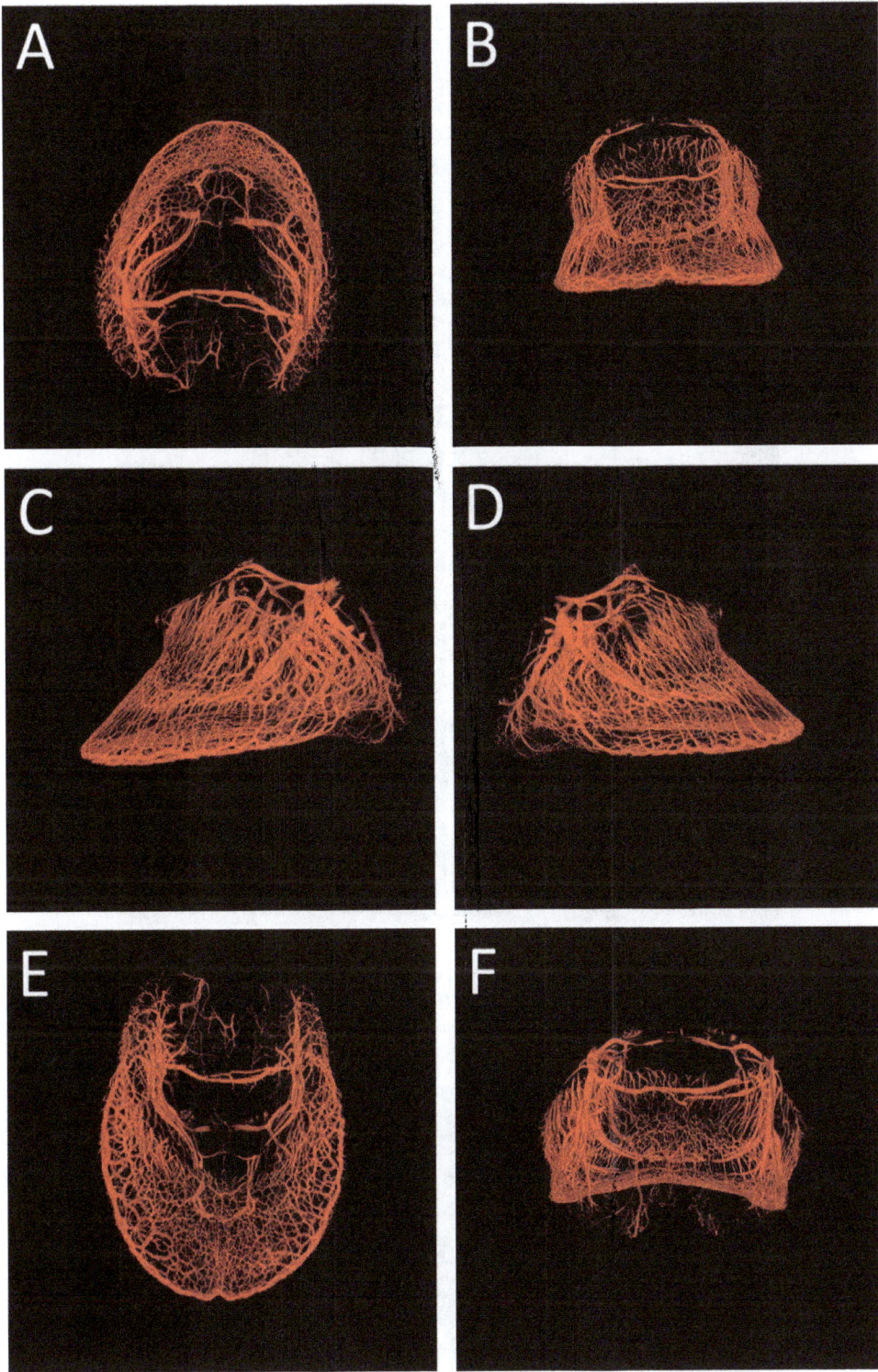

Figure 2. Vasculature of the equine foot. (A) Dorsally, (B) cranially, (C) laterally/medially, (D) laterally/medially, (E) ventrally, and (F) caudally. Scan spatial resolution = 120 μm.

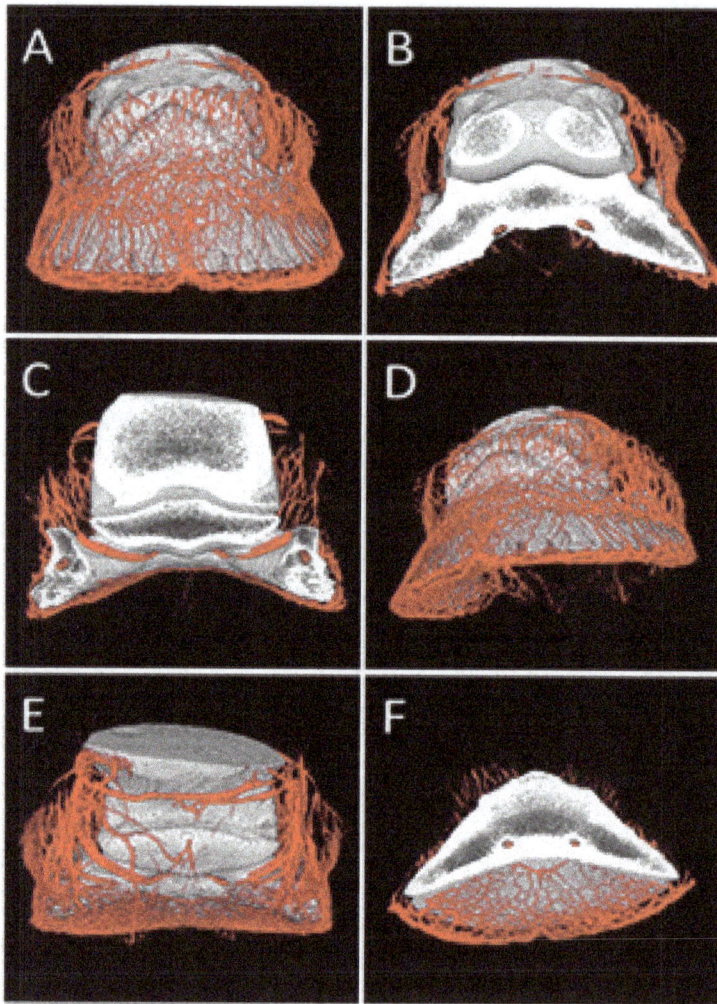

Figure 3. Cranial and caudal views of equine hoof bones and vasculature. (A) Cranially as a whole, (B) cranially as a mid-P3 coronal cut, (C) caudally as a mid-navicular coronal cut, (D) cranolaterally/cranomedially as a whole, (E) caudally as a whole, and (F) ventrocaudally as a coronal cut just cranial of P2 to include only P3. Scan spatial resolution = 120 μm.

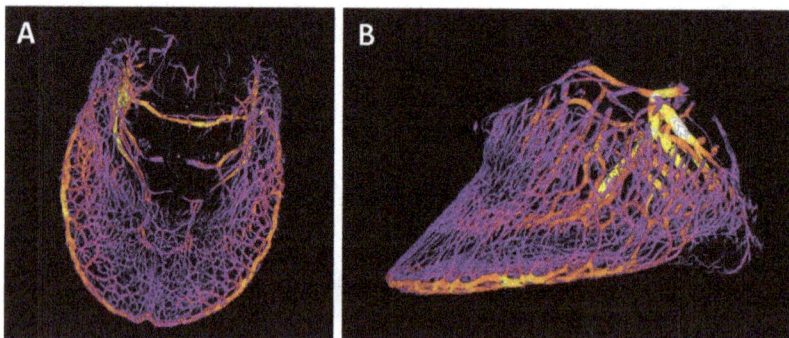

Figure 4. Blood vessel lumen rendered CT images. (A) Entire equine foot from a palmar/plantar perspective, and (B) from a lateral perspective. Lumen size was mapped, where increasing brightness indicates thicker vessels using BoneJ plugin for ImageJ [42]. Scan spatial resolution = 120 μm.

7. The future of CT in veterinary medicine and research

This chapter has explored the development of CT techniques and their uses, and has shown some of the present research in both the clinical and laboratory setting. Many of the examples shown throughout present ideas for uses in veterinary medicine and science, in addition to indications about where further research is required. Further advancements of CT in the clinic have frequently been directed at using the technology available alongside movement-restricting devices to produce images without general anaesthesia. This is important in patients who may be compromised by the use of anaesthetic drugs. The use of movement-restricting devices with or without sedation can be used to produce diagnostic CT images, and can thus be used to decrease the morbidity rates associated with the use of general anaesthetics [78].

Dynamic imaging, using contrast-enhanced CT and MRI, for the exploration of cerebral and tumour microvasculature is an ever-expanding area of interest [79]. As it stands, such dynamic imaging techniques have not been employed in all disorders but would be of benefit, especially in other highly vascularised structures which can undergo extreme pathogenic changes. The utilisation of such techniques could revolutionise our understanding of the complex pathologies of many areas of the body and differing pathological situations.

Exploitation of the unique characteristics of a synchrotron radiation based μCT facilities could render dynamic experimentation possible, enabling the full elucidation the pathogenic mechanisms involved in differing diseases and disorders in addition to understanding basic anatomical structures. This might involve the visualisation of cellular changes, in addition to tissue alterations. One significant advancement would be to keep tissues metabolically alive and submit them to a variety of physical and chemical stressors, measuring cellular response with the aid of antibody-conjugated high-Z nanoparticles in conjunction with synchrotron-sourced X-ray CT. Synchrotron-based μCT offers high spatial resolution which, when wishing to view microscopic components of large, intact specimens, could very rapidly become a limiting factor. It is this feature that would render dynamic imaging of constantly evolving structures possible. Studies in live blowfly showed the mechanisms behind their flight motors however it also caused damage to the organisms which died shortly after the experiments [80]. A study designed to show the effects of synchrotron-sourced X-ray CT in ants, grasshoppers, beetles and fruit flies indicated that differing protocols could attenuate cell and system damage, thus making it a more viable imaging source if the protocols were carefully developed [81]. μCT has been utilised to study insects such as the Painted Lady chrysalis, many of the pupae hatched despite multiple scans, but the samples were also immobile thus making μCT scans possible [82]. It should also be highlighted that insects generally tolerate radiation much better than mammalian cells [83]. Naturally the expense and space requirement needed for such high calibre machines and experimental set up restricts these possibilities in the normal clinical setting but is increasingly possible under research conditions.

An equally important and expanding use of CT in veterinary medicine and research is the use of images in order to create 3D reconstructions. This may assist the surgeon prior to surgery or during the recovery period. In addition, the images and 3D reconstructions can be an invaluable teaching tool. Whether teaching young children, undergraduates or surgeons, they are a reusable and valuable addition to the mechanisms available. The uses range from teaching anatomy and physiology using 2D pictures, 3D videos, in virtual museums or even 3D printed examples and providing virtual dissection experiences through to their use as moulds for creating devices and as practise for surgery [84]. The use of CT in forensics and archaeology has also risen in line with the technologies available, although in many cases it would be suggested that this field is still 'emerging'. To date in forensics, this has included identifying tool marks on bones, age determination, assessing gunshot wounds, analysing teeth, understanding the pathology of bones and estimating post-mortem intervals [85, 86]. These and the use of CT in many other situations are essential in the development of the veterinary profession and research. A high profile human example was the use of CT and μCT in establishing the cause of death, and injuries sustained by King Richard III who died in the Battle of Bosworth, England in 1485 [87]. His skeleton was excavated in 2012 and thereafter researchers sought to identify the body and to understand the skeleton and injuries. The information from the CT analysis, alongside DNA evidence [88] was used to help unravel the story behind the royal skeleton.

The laboratory CT, synchrotron imaging and software developed, is increasingly utilised to investigate areas previously imaged using histological and gross anatomical techniques, such as measuring vasculature and angiogenesis, bone morphology, assessing cell proliferation and identifying soft tissue structure and morphology. A number of studies use a variety of these techniques simultaneously to achieve insights into veterinary medicine and science. Many of the techniques discussed in this chapter have been used in the research and/or university setting. A challenge to the frequency of use and to use in the clinical setting of these techniques is the availability of equipment and expertise in these very challenging methodologies. The research does enable studies to be carried out to show proof of concept and to develop protocols, which can then be used within the clinical setting. With increasing levels of sophistication of both CT scanning units and associated software, this field presents an ever changing and dynamic field. The next generation of imaging techniques includes nano-CT, which can already achieve resolutions of 400 nm [89], and new software and algorithms that are frequently being designed and advance the present uses of available hardware. Nano-CT has been used in a number of animal based studies ranging from morphological features of osteocyte lacunae in murine bones [90] and comprehending cephalopod chamber formation, morphology and evolution [91], through to musculoskeletal and vascular research in the rat [92, 93]. As always, the key to advancing clinical techniques is the sharing of world class research alongside the financial ability to provide a service according to the needs of the patient.

Acknowledgements

This work was supported by the Biotechnology and Biological Sciences Research Council [grant number BB/I024291/1], by generous funding to Catrin S. Rutland and from the School of Veterinary Medicine and Science, University of Nottingham. This work was also supported by The Weston Scholarship to Catrin S. Rutland and Cyril Rauch to fund Emily Paul.

All scanning was carried out on a GE phoenix v|tome|x m (General Electric, Germany, 2013) at The Hounsfield Facility, School of Biosciences, University of Nottingham. The Hounsfield Facility is supported by funding from European Research Council (Futureroots Project), the BBSRC and The Wolfson Foundation.

The Authors would like to thank Dr Agata Witkowska and Dr Ramzi Al-Agele for collecting and preparing CT samples. Ethical permission was given by The University of Nottingham Ethical Committee to collect the naturally deceased guinea pigs and slaughterhouse equine cadavers used to create the figures presented in this chapter.

Author details

Matthew Keane[1†], Emily Paul[1†], Craig J Sturrock[2], Cyril Rauch[1] and Catrin Sian Rutland[1*]

*Address all correspondence to: Catrin.rutland@nottingham.ac.uk

1 School of Veterinary Medicine and Science, University of Nottingham, Nottingham, UK

2 The Hounsfield Facility, School of Biosciences, University of Nottingham, Nottingham, UK

† Joint first authors

References

[1] Hounsfield GN. Computerized transverse axial scanning (tomography). 1. Description of system. British Journal of Radiology. 1973;**46**(552):1016-1022

[2] Goldman LW. Principles of CT and CT technology. Journal of Nuclear Medicine Technology. 2007;**35**(3):115-128

[3] Bushberg JT, Seibert, Leidholdt EM. Essential Physics of Medical Imaging. Philadelphia, United States: Wolters Kluwer Health; 2011

[4] Ketteringham J, Gempel P. History of computed tomography: 1967-1978—excerpts from an ongoing study for the National Science Foundation. Cambridge, MA: Arthur D. Little, Inc; 1978

[5] Ohlerth S, Scharf G. Computed tomography in small animals–Basic principles and state of the art applications. The Veterinary Journal. 2007;**173**(2):254-271

[6] Brooker MJ. Computed Tomography for Radiographers. MTP Press, Netherlands; 1986

[7] Fike J, LeCouteur R, Cann C. Anatomy of the canine brain using high resolution computed tomography. Veterinary Radiology & Ultrasound. 1981;**22**(6):236-243

[8] Fike JR, et al. Computerized tomography of brain tumors of the rostral and middle fossas in the dog. American Journal of Veterinary Research. 1981;**42**(2): 275-281

[9]   LeCouteur R, et al. Computed tomography of brain tumors in the caudal fossa of the dog. Veterinary Radiology. 1981;**22**(6): 244-251

[10] Marincek B, Young SW.Computed tomography of spontaneous canine neoplasms. Veterinary Radiology. 1980;**21**(4): 181-184

[11] Marolf AJ. Computed tomography and MRI of the hepatobiliary system and pancreas. The Veterinary Clinics of North America. Small Animal Practice. 2016;**46**(3):481-497, vi

[12] De Rycke LM, et al. Computed tomography and cross-sectional anatomy of the thorax in clinically normal dogs. American Journal of Veterinary Research. 2005;**66**(3):512-524

[13] Henninger W. Use of computed tomography in the diseased feline thorax. The Journal of Small Animal Practice. 2003;**44**(2):56-64

[14] Kuehn NF. Nasal computed tomography. Clinical Techniques in Small Animal Practice. 2006;**21**(2):55-59

[15] Kraft SL, Gavin PR. Intracranial neoplasia. Clinical Techniques in Small Animal Practice. 1999;**14**(2):112-123

[16] Ballegeer EA. Computed tomography of the musculoskeletal system. Veterinary Clinics of North America: Small Animal Practice. 2016;**46**(3):373-420

[17] da Costa RC, Samii VF.Advanced imaging of the spine in small animals. Veterinary Clinics of North America: Small Animal Practice. 2010;**40**(5):765-790

[18] Stadler K, et al. Computed tomographic imaging of dogs with primary laryngeal or tracheal airway obstruction. Veterinary Radiology & Ultrasound. 2011;**52**(4):377-384

[19] Stadler K, O'Brien R. Computed tomography of nonanesthetized cats with upper airway obstruction. Veterinary Radiology & Ultrasound. 2013;**54**(3):231-236

[20] Puchalski SM. Advances in equine computed tomography and use of contrast media. Veterinary Clinics of North America. Equine Practice. 2012;**28**(3): 563-581

[21] Puchalski SM, et al. Use of contrast-enhanced computed tomography to assess angiogenesis in deep digital flexor tendonopathy in a horse. Veterinary Radiology & Ultrasound. 2009;**50**(3):292-297

[22] Puchalski SM, et al. Intraarterial contrast-enhanced computed tomography of the equine distal extremity. Veterinary Radiology & Ultrasound. 2007;**48**(1):21-29

[23] Claerhoudt S, et al. Differences in the morphology of distal border synovial invaginations of the distal sesamoid bone in the horse as evaluated by computed tomography compared with radiography. Equine Veterinary Journal. 2012;**44**(6):679-683

[24] Raes EV, et al. Comparison of cross-sectional anatomy and computed tomography of the tarsus in horses. American Journal of Veterinary Research. 2011;**72**(9):1209-1221

[25] Windley Z, et al. Two- and three-dimensional computed tomographic anatomy of the enamel, infundibulae and pulp of 126 equine cheek teeth. Part 1: Findings in teeth

without macroscopic occlusal or computed tomographic lesions. Equine Veterinary Journal. 2009;**41**(5):433-440

[26] Windley Z, et al. Two- and three-dimensional computed tomographic anatomy of the enamel, infundibulae and pulp of 126 equine cheek teeth. Part 2: Findings in teeth with macroscopic occlusal or computed tomographic lesions. Equine Veterinary Journal. 2009;**41**(5):441-447

[27] Probst A, Henninger W, Willmann M. Communications of normal nasal and paranasal cavities in computed tomography of horses. Veterinary Radiology & Ultrasound. 2005;**46**(1):44-48

[28] Lacombe VA, Sogaro-Robinson C, Reed SM. Diagnostic utility of computed tomography imaging in equine intracranial conditions. Equine Veterinary Journal. 2010;**42**(5):393-399

[29] Dakin SG, et al. Technical set-up and radiation exposure for standing computed tomography of the equine head. Equine Veterinary Education. 2014;**26**(4):208-215

[30] Nuss K, et al. Klinische Anwendung der Computertomographie beim Rind. Tierärztliche Praxis Großtiere. 2011;**39**(5):317-324

[31] Mizutani R, Suzuki Y. X-ray microtomography in biology. Micron. 2012;**43**(2-3):104-115

[32] Kinahan PE, Hasegawa BH, Beyer T. X-ray-based attenuation correction for positron emission tomography/computed tomography scanners. Seminars in Nuclear Medicine. 2003;**33**(3):166-179

[33] Rennie R. ed. A Dictionary of Physics. 7th ed. 2015. Oxford: Oxford University Press. 299

[34] Willmott P. An introduction to synchrotron radiation: Techniques and applications. Chichester: John Wiley and Sons; 2011

[35] Franklin K, et al. Introduction to Biological Physics for the Health and Life Sciences. Chichester: Wiley; 2010

[36] Cornette R, Tresset A, Herrel A. The shrew tamed by Wolff's law: Do functional constraints shape the skull through muscle and bone covariation?. Journal of Morphology. 2015;**276**(3):301-309

[37] Ryan TM, Krovitz GE. Trabecular bone ontogeny in the human proximal femur. Journal of Human Evolution. 2006;**51**(6):591-602

[38] Won S, Chung WJ, Yoon J. Clinical application of quantitative computed tomography in osteogenesis imperfecta suspected cat. Journal of Veterinary Science. 2017

[39] Geng H, et al. A correlative imaging based methodology for accurate quantitative assessment of bone formation in additive manufactured implants. Journal of Materials Science. Materials in Medicine. 2016;**27**(6):112

[40] Witkowska A, et al. Computed tomography analysis of guinea pig bone: Architecture, bone thickness and dimensions throughout development. PeerJ. 2014;**2**

[41] Citardi MJ, et al. Comparison of scientific calipers and computer-enabled CT review for the measurement of skull base and craniomaxillofacial dimensions. Skull Base-an Interdisciplinary Approach. 2001;**11**(1):5-11

[42] Doube M, et al. BoneJ free and extensible bone image analysis in ImageJ. Bone. 2010;**47**(6):1076-1079

[43] Engiles JB, et al. Osteopathology in the equine distal phalanx associated with the development and progression of laminitis. Veterinary Pathology. 2015;**52**(5):928-944

[44] Newsome R, et al. Linking bone development on the caudal aspect of the distal phalanx with lameness during life. Journal of Dairy Science. 2016;**99**(6):4512-4525

[45] Schwarz T, et al. Imaging of the canine and feline temporomandibular joint: A review. Veterinary Radiology & Ultrasound. 2002;**43**(2):85-97

[46] Crosse KR, Worth AJ. Computer-assisted surgical correction of an antebrachial deformity in a dog. Veterinary and Comparative Orthopaedics and Traumatology. 2010;**23**(5): 354-361

[47] Santoro D, et al. Diaphyseal osteotomy after post-traumatic malalignment. Current Reviews in Musculoskeletal Medicine. 2014;**7**(4):312-322

[48] Regnault S, et al. Skeletal pathology and variable anatomy in elephant feet assessed using computed tomography. PeerJ. 2017;**5**:e2877

[49] Regnault S, et al. Osteopathology in the feet of rhinoceroses: Lesion type and distribution. Journal of Zoo and Wildlife Medicine. 2013;**44**(4):918-927

[50] Clarke B. Normal bone anatomy and physiology. Clinical Journal of the American Society of Nephrology. 2008;**3**(Suppl 3):S131-S139

[51] Talbott JL, et al. Retrospective evaluation of whole body computed tomography for tumor staging in dogs with primary appendicular osteosarcoma. Veterinary Surgery. 2017;**46**(1):75-80

[52] Deitz K, et al. Computed tomographic appearance of canine thyroid tumours. The Journal of Small Animal Practice. 2014;**55**(6):323-329

[53] Taeymans O, Penninck DG, Peters RM. Comparison between clinical, ultrasound, CT, MRI, and pathology findings in dogs presented for suspected thyroid carcinoma. Veterinary Radiology & Ultrasound. 2013;**54**(1):61-70

[54] Bertolini G, et al. Incidental and nonincidental canine thyroid tumors assessed by multi-detector row computed tomography: A single-centre cross sectional study in 4520 dogs. Veterinary Radiology & Ultrasound. 2017. PubMed: 28185344 DOI: 10.1111/vru.12477

[55] Adams WM, et al. Prognostic significance of tumor histology and computed tomographic staging for radiation treatment response of canine nasal tumors. Veterinary Radiology & Ultrasound. 2009;**50**(3):330-335

[56] Kondo Y, et al. Prognosis of canine patients with nasal tumors according to modi-fied clinical stages based on computed tomography: A retrospective study. Journal of Veterinary Medical Science. 2008;**70**(3):207-212

[57] Elliot KM, Mayer MN. Radiation therapy for tumors of the nasal cavity and parana-sal sinuses in dogs. Canadian Veterinary Journal-Revue Veterinaire Canadienne. 2009;**50**(3):309-312

[58] Iwanaga T, Tokunaga S, Momoi Y. Thoracic duct lymphography by subcutaneous con-trast agent injection in a dog with chylothorax. Open Veterinary Journal. 2016;**6**(3):238-241

[59] Ando K, et al. Computed Tomography and Radiographic Lymphography of the Thoracic Duct by Subcutaneous or Submucosal Injection. Journal of Veterinary Medical Science. 2012;**74**(1):135-140

[60] Patsikas MN, et al. Computed Tomography and Radiographic Indirect Lymphography for Visualization of Mammary Lymphatic Vessels and the Sentinel Lymph Node in Normal Cats. Veterinary Radiology & Ultrasound. 2010;**51**(3):299-304

[61] Lee K, et al. Clinical experience of using multicletector-row CT for the diagnosis of disorders in cattle. Veterinary Record. 2009;**165**(19):559-562

[62] El-Khodery S, et al. Brain abscess in a Japanese black calf: Utility of computed tomography (CT). Journal of Veterinary Medical Science. 2008;**70**(7):727-730

[63] Gonzalo-Orden JM, et al. Computed tomographic findings in ovine coenurosis. Veterinary Radiology & Ultrasound. 1999;**40**(5):441-444

[64] Hardefeldt LA, et al. Diagnosis and surgical treatment of an intracranial cyst in an alpaca cria. Javma-Journal of the American Veterinary Medical Association. 2012;**240**(12): 1501-1506

[65] Ohba Y, et al. Computer tomography diagnosis of meningoencephalocele in a calf. Journal of Veterinary Medical Science. 2008;**70**(8):829-831

[66] Nagy DW. Diagnostics and Ancillary Tests of Neurologic Dysfunction in the Ruminant. The Veterinary Clinics of North America. Food Animal Practice. 2017;**33**(1):9-18

[67] Zwingenberger AL, Carrade Holt DD. Computed tomographic measurement of canine urine concentration. The Canadian Veterinary Journal. 2017;**58**(2):180-182

[68] Halliburton S, et al. State-of-the-art in CT hardware and scan modes for cardiovascular CT. Journal of Cardiovascular Computed Tomography. 2012;**6**(3):154-163

[69] Rajiah P, Saboo SS, Abbara S. Role of CT in Congenital Heart Disease. Current Treatment Options in Cardiovascular Medicine. 2017;**19**(1):6

[70] Heymering HW. 80 causes, predispositions, and pathways of laminitis. The Veterinary Clinics of North America. Equine Practice. 2010;**26**(1):13-19

[71] Rucker A. Equine venography and its clinical application in North America. The Veterinary Clinics of North America. Equine Practice. 2010;**26**(1):167-177

[72] Gage GJ, Kipke DR, Shain W. Whole animal perfusion fixation for rodents. Journal of Visualized Experiments. 2012**65**

[73] Pollitt CC. The anatomy and physiology of the suspensory apparatus of the distal phalanx. The Veterinary Clinics of North America. Equine Practice. 2010;**26**(1):29-49

[74] Or M, et al. Regional cerebral blood flow assessed by single photon emission computed tomography (SPECT) in dogs with congenital portosystemic shunt and hepatic encephalopathy. The Veterinary Journal. 2017;**220**:40-42

[75] Atwood RC, et al. Quantitation of microcomputed tomography-imaged ocular microvasculature. Microcirculation. 2010;**17**(1):59-68

[76] Lee PD, et al. A comparison of three different micro-tomography systems for accurate determination of microvascular parameters. Developments in X-Ray Tomography VI. 2008;**7078**

[77] Dunford LJ, et al. Maternal protein-energy malnutrition during early pregnancy in sheep impacts the fetal ornithine cycle to reduce fetal kidney microvascular development. Faseb Journal. 2014;**28**(11):4880-4892

[78] O'Brien B. The future of CT imaging (… as I see it!). The Journal of Small Animal Practice. 2011;**52**(5):229-230

[79] O'Connor JP, et al. Dynamic contrast-enhanced imaging techniques: CT and MRI. British Journal of Radiology. 2011;**84** Spec No 2:S112-S120

[80] Mokso R, et al. Four-dimensional *in vivo* X-ray microscopy with projection-guided gating. Scientific Reports. 2015;**5**:8727

[81] Socha JJ, et al. Real-time phase-contrast X-ray imaging: A new technique for the study of animal form and function. BMC Biology. 2007;**5**:6

[82] Lowe T, et al. Metamorphosis revealed: Time-lapse three-dimensional imaging inside a living chrysalis. Journal of the Royal Society Interface. 2013;**10**(84):20130304

[83] Koval TM. Intrinsic resistance to the lethal effects of x-irradiation in insect and arachnid cells. Proceedings of the National Academy of Sciences of the United States of America. 1983;**80**(15):4752-4755

[84] Dundie A, et al. Use of 3D printer technology to facilitate surgical correction of a complex vascular anomaly with esophageal entrapment in a dog. Journal of Veterinary cardiology. 2017

[85] Hughes S. CT scanning in archaeology, in Computed Tomography - Special Applications. Saba L, Editor. 2011, InTechOpen, Croatia

[86] Rutty GN, et al. The role of micro-computed tomography in forensic investigations. Forensic Science International. 2013;**225**(1-3):60-66

[87] Appleby J, et al. Perimortem trauma in King Richard III: A skeletal analysis. Lancet. 2015;**385**(9964):253-259

[88] King TE, et al. Identification of the remains of King Richard III. Nature Communications. 2014;**5**

[89] Kampschulte M, et al. Nano-Computed Tomography: Technique and Applications. Röfo. 2016;**188**(2):146-154

[90] Vatsa A, et al. Osteocyte morphology in fibula and calvaria–Is there a role for mechano-sensing? Bone. 2008;**43**(3):452-458

[91] Lemanis R, et al. The Evolution and Development of Cephalopod Chambers and Their Shape. PLoS One. 2016;**11**(3):e0151404

[92] Khoury BM, et al. The use of nano-computed tomography to enhance musculoskeletal research. Connective Tissue Research. 2015;**56**(2):106-19

[93] Langheinrich AC, et al. Evaluation of the middle cerebral artery occlusion techniques in the rat by *in-vitro* 3-dimensional micro- and nano computed tomography. BMC Neurology. 2010;**10**:36

5

Computed Tomography: Role in Femoroacetabular Impingement

Maximiliano Barahona, Jaime Hinzpeter and
Cristian Barrientos

Abstract

Femoroacetabular impingement (FAI) physiopathology is still unclear; however, there is a consensus that a pathological mechanical contact between the femoral neck-head junction and the acetabulum leads to pain and cartilage damage. Computed tomography (CT) is useful in FAI diagnosis and surgical planning. In the present chapter, we will analyze the role of CT in FAI, with special emphasis on alignment and comparison of measurements related to epidemiological variables. We analyzed 101 CT of patients that consulted in our institution for a non-joint-or-bone-related reason. Prior to the measurement of acetabular variables, CT image must be corrected in three planes. Acetabular version is a gender- and age-related measurement. As age increased, acetabular version increased, and the same impact age has on Wiberg angle. Femoral FAI-related measurement is not related to epidemiological variables. CT has a very important role for a better understanding of hip anatomy, and further research using CT images should be encouraged.

Keywords: femoroacetabular impingement, computed tomography, femoral alpha angle, acetabular version angle, Wiberg angle

1. Introduction

Femoroacetabular impingement (FAI) is a relatively new pathology, described in the early 1990s. FAI physiopathology is still unclear; however, there is a consensus that a pathological mechanical contact between the femoral neck-head junction and the acetabulum leads to pain, microinstability, joint cartilage damage and labrum tear. FAI diagnosis should be based on clinical evaluation and subsequent appropriate radiological confirmation that aim to detect excessive femoral head coverage (pincer-type) and/or insufficient femoral head-neck offset hip (cam-type) [1–3].

Computed tomography (CT) is a very useful tool in the diagnosis and surgical planning for FAI; however, normal values have not been still defined and lesser is the relation of these measurements according to gender, age weight and height [4–6].

In the present chapter, we will analyze the role of CT in FAI, with special emphasis on alignment and comparison of measurements related to gender, weight, height and age.

2. Methods

We analyzed 101 CT of patients that consulted in our institution for a non-joint-or-bone-related reason and who required an abdominal and pelvic CT for diagnosis. Before enrollment, volunteers completed a questionnaire, which included asking for current or historic hip-related pain and hip surgery. Positive answers led to the volunteers being excluded from the study.

In this population of 101 patients, we will perform an analysis regarding different situations related to femoroacetabular impingement in which CT has a fundamental role.

The images were obtained using a Siemens Multicut Computerized Tomography Machine, a model of Somaton Sensation 64®. In the study, a protocol of 1.5-mm cuts for every 0.3 mm was used, information that was later processed to 3-mm multiplanar reconstructions in bone window and 3D reconstructions, processed with 3D and INSPACE®, respectively.

3. CT radiological measures related to FAI

3.1. Acetabular version

The acetabular version is described as the acetabular orientation regarding the sagittal plane. It is considered normal that the acetabulum has an anterior orientation called anteversion [7].

The measurement is performed in an image obtained in CT in axial reconstruction. The angle is measured by drawing a line from the anterior border to the posterior border of the ipsilateral acetabulum and another vertical line which runs from the posterior edge of the acetabulum and is tangential to a horizontal line joining the posterior edges of the acetabulum (**Figure 1**). The measurement taken at the height where the acetabulum is deeper or in which the medial wall of the acetabulum is deeper corresponds to the "classic" measurement described for the diagnosis of acetabular dysplasia. It's considered retroversion when the angle is ≤15° [8, 9].

3.2. Crossover sign

In a regular pelvis, the acetabulum is in anteversion so in an anterior-posterior (AP) X-ray and in a transparent reconstruction of a CT that simulates an AP X-ray, the anterior wall of the

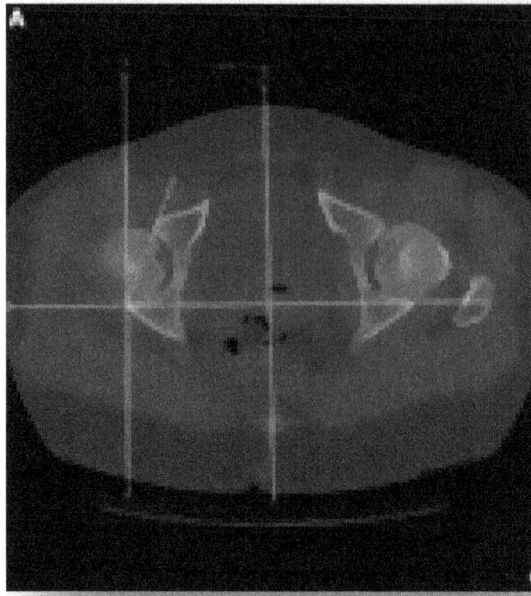

Figure 1. It shows acetabular version angle measurement. It is measured by drawing a line from the anterior border to the posterior border of the ipsilateral acetabulum and another vertical line, which runs from the posterior edge of the acetabulum and is tangential to a horizontal line joining the posterior edges of the acetabulum.

acetabulum is always medial to the edge of the posterior wall. The sign is positive if in some portion the anterior border becomes lateral to the posterior border (**Figure 2**). This translates into an acetabular retroversion at the height where the crossover occurs and is associated with anterior focal over-coverage [9].

3.3. Center edge or Wiberg angle

The acetabular center-border angle is measured on an anteroposterior X-ray or in the reconstruction of a CT that simulates an AP X-ray.

From the center of the femoral head, a line is drawn that goes to the edge of the acetabulum. The other line is a vertical line from the center of the femoral head, which is perpendicular to a horizontal line passing between the ischial tuberosities (**Figure 3**). A Wiberg angle is considered normal between 20 and 40°; angles less than 20° are associated with hip dysplasia. Angles greater than 40° are associated with deep thigh and therefore there is global overcoverage [8].

3.4. Femoral alpha angle

It is an angle formed at the intersection of a line that goes from the axis of the femoral neck and another line extending from the center of the femoral head to the point where a circumference, imagined on the femoral head, is intercepted with the anterior perimeter of the femoral neck (**Figure 4**) [10].

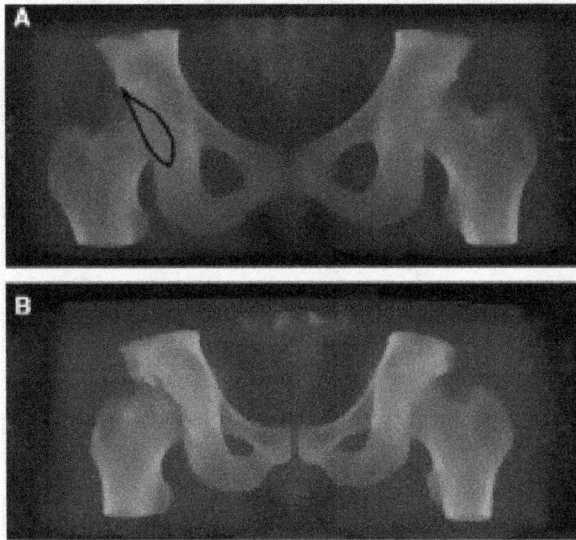

Figure 2. It shows a crossover sign. In a normal AP view of the pelvis, the anterior wall of the acetabulum is always medial to the edge of the posterior wall (A). It is positive when the posterior wall becomes medial to the anterior wall of the acetabulum (B).

The normal value of this angle is controversial, even more controversial than the value that must be considered pathological. Notzli et al. [11], in a paper from 2002, suggests 50% as a pathological value in a study that was performed by measuring the alpha angle in magnetic resonance imaging (MRI) and in which only the average difference test was applied between the groups. Tannast et al. [9], in a review published in 2007, uses the same value but now in CT.

Beaulé et al. [4] proposed a 50.5° CT cutoff value in a study in which they compared symptomatic and asymptomatic patients. Five years later, he published an article in which he points

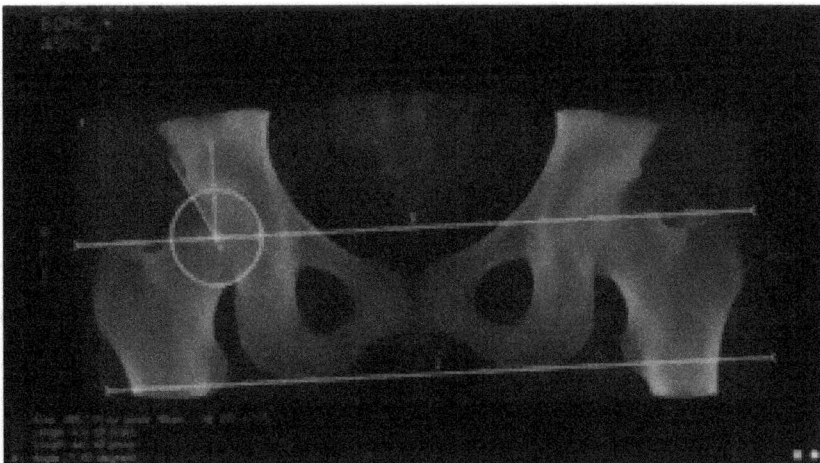

Figure 3. It shows Wiberg angle measurement. It is considered normal between 20 and 40°.

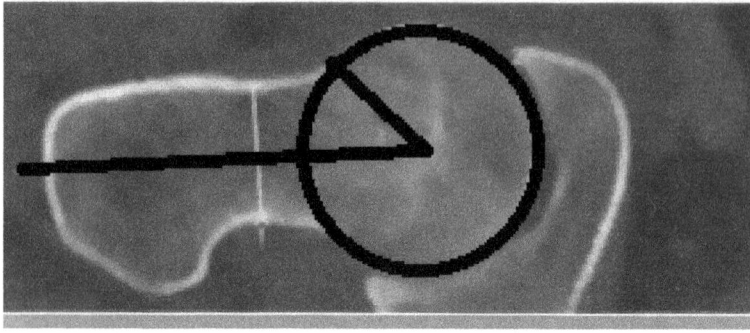

Figure 4. The alpha angle was measured in an axial oblique cut of the neck. The normal value of this angle is controversial.

out that in MRI the average alpha angle in asymptomatic patients is 50.15° [12]. Allen et al., on X-rays and Kang et al., in CT, arbitrarily define the angle value at 55.5 and 55°, respectively, as pathological, arguing the findings in asymptomatic and inter-intraobserver measurement variability [8, 13].

In a study carried out by our working group, it was determined that if the cutoff value was 50° in CT, 28% of the asymptomatic population should be classified with a pathological alpha value [14]. Finally, Pollard et al. [15], in 2010, in a study carried out on X-rays, establishes that the normal average value of the alpha angle is 95% between 46 and 49°, that is, very close to the 50° proposed.

The initial studies that established pathological cutoff values between 50 and 55° for the alpha angle have been invalidated by subsequent studies in healthy populations in which higher values have been found for the angle described by Notzli; in addition, they lack the methodology suitable for setting cut values in diagnostic tests [11].

We conducted an investigation in which our cohort of 101 asymptomatic patients was compared to a cohort of patients who were operated on with femoroacetabular impingement. This cohort presented hip pain referred to the inguinal region, positive flexion adduction internal rotation (FADIR) on physical examination and positive lidocaine test. In our center, the lidocaine test is performed by a radiologist specialized in the musculoskeletal region, who, under ultrasound, infiltrates intra-articular lidocaine. Before and after infiltration, a FADIR test is performed and the test is considered positive when the patient subjectively reported a decrease of more than 50% of the pain. In addition, it was considered as an inclusion requirement, the presence of intraoperative bump. Patients with previous hip surgeries, with a history of hip dysplasia, and in whom only acetabular surgical gestures were performed, were excluded.

The alpha angle was measured in an axial oblique cut of the neck, determining three levels, cephalic third, middle and caudal femoral neck, and measurements were made in the center of these levels. The measurement performed in the middle third was compared for the purposes of this study. In the case of controls, the measurement was performed on both hips and the average between right and left was registered. Regarding the cases, the value of the angle of the operated hip was registered.

A logistic regression model was estimated, in which the presence of FAI (case/control) was used as the dependent variable and the alpha angle measurement as the independent variable. A Hosmer-Lemeshow goodness-of-fit test was done to test logistic regression assumptions (this is considered appropriate if $p > 0.15$) [16]. The receiver operating characteristics (ROC) curve was calculated and interpreted according to Hosmer and Lemeshow recommendations [17, 18]. A significance level of 0.05 was established and 95% confidence interval is reported. All analyses were performed using Stata v11.2 (StataCorp LP, College Station, Texas, USA).

Nearly, 38 patients with femoroacetabular impingement were recruited, who had an alpha angle of 66.78° (±12.23°), while the cohort of 101 asymptomatic patients had an average alpha angle of 47.81° (±5.30°). The relationship between controls and cases is 3:1.

When estimating a logistic regression model, an odds ratio of 1.28 [1.18–1.39] was obtained, which implies that as the alpha angle measurement increases 1°, the risk of having FAI type cam increases by 28% compared to having 1° less.

The ROC curve has an area under the curve of 0.96 [0.93–0.99], which gives an excellent level of discrimination. The angle of 57° is the value that maximizes the sensitivity 92.11% and the specificity 95.05%, correctly classifying 94% of our sample.

The study by Sutter et al. [19] included 53 healthy individuals and 53 pathological patients, measuring the alpha angle in different time radii, finding a sensitivity between 72 and 76% and specificity between 73 and 80%, with an angle of 60° as the cut in the anterosuperior region. This finding is similar to that found in our work in which the cut value is higher than the 50–55° angle proposed initially and uses a similar methodology. However, the measurement of the alpha angle in radians is not the measurement that is used daily in clinical practice; it is more commonly used for research purposes, and in the relation, they used one control for each case.

The value of the alpha angle measured in an axial oblique femoral neck reconstruction has a high discriminative power for the diagnosis of symptomatic FAI type cam. The finding of an alpha angle value above 57° is suggestive of symptomatic FAI type cam.

3.5. Femoral offset

The femoral head-neck offset is the distance between the anterior margin of the femoral neck and the anterior margin of the femoral head (**Figure 5**). As the sphere shape of the femoral head is lost, the offset decreases, and so it is a measure related to FAI type cam. Kang et al. [8] report that an offset smaller than 8 mm is considered pathological, whereas Tannast et al. [9] mention that a distance less than 10 mm is related to FAI.

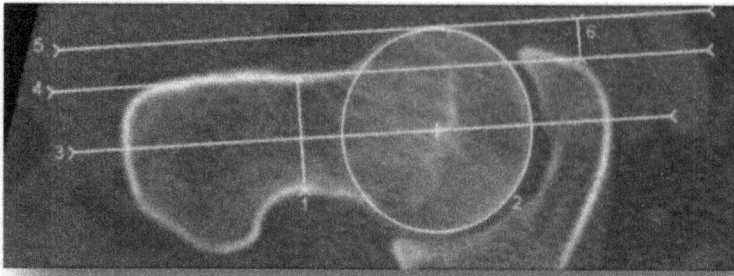

Figure 5. It shows femoral offset measurement. The distance between the anterior margin of the femoral neck and the anterior margin of the femoral head is shown.

4. Measurement analysis in CT by image correction in two or three planes

The multiplanar reconstructions of the 101 asymptomatic individuals included the axial planes to the pelvis and axial slants to the femoral neck. Since the pelvis has a spatial arrangement in three dimensions and considering the deviations by the position of the pelvis in relation to the table of the tomographer, the axial reconstructions and in the three dimensions were corrected in three planes [20, 21], that is to say corrected the rotation, the lateral inclination and the tilting of the pelvis. For the latter, differences between genders were considered, setting a distance of 3 cm between the sacrococcygeal junction and upper border of the pubis in men and 6 cm in women [22]. The evaluation of the images and the measurements were made by radiologists and orthopedic surgeons, using the software Osirix® v4.0.

Our hypothesis is that if acetabular measurements, like Wiberg angle and acetabular version angle, are performed without correction in three planes, the retroversion measures of the pelvis are significantly different, which can lead to misdiagnosis of acetabular overcoverage, meaning pincer-type impingement.

Non-parametric median test was used to compare both groups. A significance level of 0.05 was established and 95% confidence interval was reported. All analyses were performed using Stata v11.2 (StataCorp LP, College Station, Texas, USA).

When analyzing the Wiberg angle, the average value without correction is 38.8° (±7.54), while when correcting in three planes, the average value of the angle increases to 39.4 (±7.59). Although the average difference between the two measurements is 0.6° (±2.9° and range: −6.9–14), this is significant when applying a comparison test for medians (p = 0.01).

Secondly, acetabular retroversion measures were analyzed. Acetabular version angle was measured in six levels of cephalic to caudal, every 3 mm from the upper edge of the acetabular to distal. The sixth measurement coincides with the classic measure of acetabular version, which is performed where the acetabulum is deeper. The measurement was performed as proposed by Kang et al. [8].

The average value of acetabular version angle is shown in **Table 1**. It is evident that the angle value is consistently lower in the measurements made with the pelvis corrected in three planes. The average difference is $-07.6°$ ($\pm 08.0°$), this difference being significant (test, $p < 0.00$). The detail of the differences for each level is shown in **Table 1**.

In conclusion, the correction in three planes is important to standardize the measures. Failure to correct the spatial position of the pelvis in the patient overestimates the anteversion and decreases the lateral coverage angle. This is important because it can modify the diagnosis and/or surgical planning.

Level	Not corrected	Three-plane corrected	Average difference
1	11.4° (−15.0 to 45.7°)	02.7° (−25.8 to 35.9°)	−08.8° (−15.0 to 45.7°)
2	17.4° (−12.1 to 45.9°)	07.8° (−24.3 to 37.2°)	−09.7° (−12.1 to 45.9°)
3	20.9° (−0.64 to 20.9°)	13.5° (−15.3 to 31.6°)	−08.6° (−0.64 to20.9°)
4	21.2° (00.1 to 38.0°)	15.2° (−12.8 to 31.3°)	−06.4° (00.1 to38.0°)
5	20.7° (30.9 to 35.5°)	15.8° (−06.9 to 30.7°)	−05.0° (30.9 to 35.5°)
6	20.0° (05.6 to 34.8°)	15.5° (00.8 to 30.1°)	−04.1° (05.6 to 34.8°)

Three-plane corrected CT shows lower angle value in each level.

Table 1. It shows median and range of the acetabular version angle by level. Acetabular version angle increased from proximal to distal.

5. Measurement analysis related to impingement according to epidemiological variables

There are physiological differences in the anatomy of the hip according to epidemiological characteristics. It is known that women have greater acetabular anteversion, greater acetabular inclination and greater femoral anteversion. It is therefore presumed that normal values in FAI-related measurements vary between genders [23]. On the other hand, Dudda et al. [24] found that white women had a significantly lower mean alpha angle and a higher average value at the center edge angle as compared to women born in China. This finding suggests that the measures vary between different races, so it is also a variable to consider [24]. Finally, we found a directly proportional increase between the measurement of the acetabular edge center angle and age [25].

In this section, the relationship between three FAI-related variables (acetabular version angle, Wiberg angle and alpha angle) and the epidemiological variables, gender, age, height and weight will be analyzed. A multivariate analysis is applied using Wards's linkage cluster analysis. After clustering, groups will be compared using regression models and non-parametric median test. A significance level of 0.05 was established and 95% confidence interval is reported. All analyses were performed using Stata v11.2 (StataCorp LP, College Station, Texas, USA).

5.1. Acetabular version angle

5.1.1. Results

The variables used in this analysis are the acetabular version angles measured from level one to six bilateral in the three-plane correction.

Ninety-nine patients were included. Cluster analysis separated two groups of patients (see **Figure 6**). In group 2, 19 patients were assigned; this group presented lower values of acetabular version (acetabulum plus retroversion) with statistical significance in the 14 measured levels (see **Table 2**).

When observing the epidemiological variables, group 2 presents an average age lower than group 1, which is statistically significant and with high power (α = 0.02 and 1-β = 0.86). The age distribution by the group is shown in **Figure 7**. The differences in weight (α = 0.03 and 1-β = 0.59) and height (α = 0.05, 1-β = 0.64) are statistically significant but the power is moderate. Differences in BMI were not significant (α = 0.13 and 1-β = 0.35). Regarding gender, it is observed that there are more women in group 2, this association being significant (α = 0.01 and 1-β = 0.74) (see **Tables 3** and **4**).

When estimating a multivariate logistic regression model with the variables age and sex as independent variables, age has an OR of 1.06 [1.01–1.11] (goodness of fit test = 0.62) and being male has an OR of 4.80 [1.58–14.64] to belong to group 1. The area under the ROC curve is of 0.76 [0.63–0.89].

When estimating a logistic regression model using age as an independent variable, we obtain an OR of 1.06 [1.01–1.11]. The area under the curve is 0.68 [0.55–0.80]. The cut value that maximizes sensitivity and specificity is 34 years, being 58.75 and 73.68%, respectively, correctly

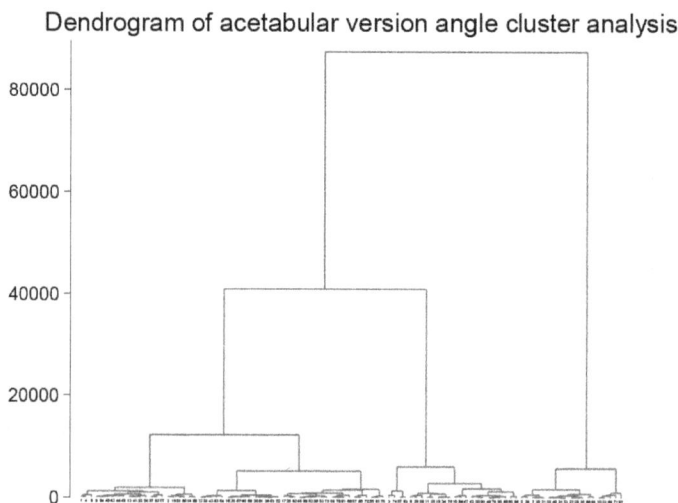

Figure 6. A dendrogram showing cluster analysis of acetabular version angle, and two groups are identified.

Variable	Group 1	Group 2	Total	P
N	80 (80.81%)	19 (19.19%)	99	0.00
VERSION 3P L1 R.	5.80(±9.26)	−11.48(±4.80)	2.48(±10.96)	0.00
VERSION 3P L1 L.	7.17(±9.74)	−14.22(±5.58)	3.06(±12.40)	0.00
VERSION 3P L2 R.	10.25(±8.02)	−6.98(±4.97)	6.94(±10.14)	0.00
VERSION 3P L2 L.	10.78(±8.49)	−8.68(±5.60)	7.04(±11.10)	0.00
VERSION 3P L3 R.	14.72(±7.58)	−1.39(±6.00)	11.62(±9.67)	0.00
VERSION 3P L3 L.	15.26(±6.77)	−3.48(±6.36)	11.66(±9.97)	0.00
VERSION 3P L4 R.	16.76(±6.11)	3.05(±6.08)	14.13(±8.14)	0.00
VERSION 3P L4 L.	17.30(±4.96)	1.9(±7.09)	14.34(±8.14)	0.00
VERSION 3P L5 R.	17.29(±5.26)	8.12(±4.49)	15.53(±6.26)	0.00
VERSION 3P L5 L.	17.67(±4.33)	7.74(±3.57)	15.77(±5.73)	0.00
VERSION 3P L6 R.	17.08(±4.87)	9.58(±3.88)	15.64(±5.54)	0.00
VERSION 3P L6 L.	17.43(±4.10)	9.99(±3.26)	16.00(±4.92)	0.00
VERSION 3P L7 R.	16.80(±5.16)	10.51(±3.38)	15.59(±5.46)	0.00
VERSION 3P L7 L.	17.04(±4.05)	10.51(±3.42)	15.78(±4.69)	0.00

The probability obtained in the test of median comparison is shown in the last column, and at each level the differences reach statistical significance. R= right, L = left, 3p = 3-plane corrected CT and L = level.

Table 2. It shows the mean and standard deviation of acetabular version angle by the group that results from the cluster analysis.

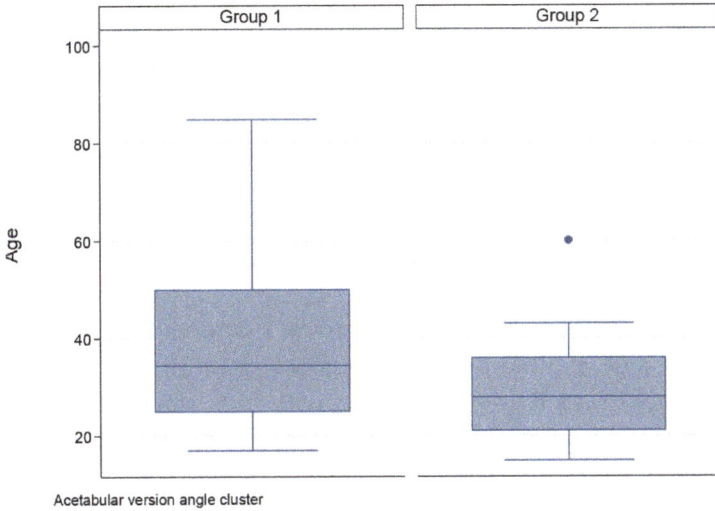

Figure 7. It shows age distribution among both groups resulting from cluster analysis of the acetabular version angle.

	Group 1	Group 2	Total
Age	38.36 (±14.84)	29.42 (±10.46)	36.65 (±14.50)
Weight (kg)	73.09 (±12.96)	65.58 (±12.58)	71.66 (±13.16)
Height (Mts.)	1.69 (±0.09)	1.64 (±0.09)	1.68 (±0.09)
BMI	25.59 (±3.33)	24.24 (±3.44)	25.33 (±3.38)

BMI= body mass index, kg = kilograms and mts = meters.

Table 3. It shows mean and standard deviation of epidemiological variables by the group that results from the cluster analysis of acetabular version angle.

Group	Female	Male	Total
1	26 (32.50%)	54 (67.50%)	80
2	13 (68.42%)	6 (31.58%)	19

Table 4. It shows gender distribution among both groups that results from the cluster analysis of acetabular version angle .

classifying 70.31% of the sample. In the case of 40 years, the sensitivity decreases to 54.05% and the specificity increases to 77.78%, so having 40 years or more gives you an OR of 6.28 [1.36–29.04] belonging in group 1.

In the estimation of a multinomial regression model, it was observed that the relative risk of having a unilateral positive crossover sign given that the individual belongs to group 2 is 1.05 [0.11–9.72] and bilateral is 7.13 [2.32–21.90].

When estimating a multivariate logistic regression model, including the dichotomized age of 40 years and the presence of a sign of crossover (positive, unilateral and bilateral), it appears that being under 40 years old has an OR of 4.90 [1.02–23.68] and the sign of positive crossover has an OR of 2.40 [1.34–4.30] belonging in group 2. This model presents an area under the curve of 0.77 [0.67–0.87].

5.1.2. Discussion

In the acetabular version, it was observed that group 1 consistently presented in each level measured medians of angle in a more forward position than group 2. Group 2 presented an average age significantly lower than group 1 and with high statistical power. This suggests that the acetabular orientation varies with age. The calculated OR shows that for each year you grow older, there is a 6% chance of belonging to the group with more predatory acetabulum. Interestingly, the cut point was found at age 34, since the disease is generally described in women who are about 40 years old; therefore, it is possible that the acetabulum that remained retroverted after the age of 30 years is the one that eventually causes the symptomatology.

Likewise, the resulting groups differ in the proportion of individuals by gender, with the number of men in group 1 being more significant, with statistical significance and high power. This suggests that there are differences in acetabular orientation by gender. The individuals included in group 1 are in greater proportion in men, that is to say, male individuals have more anteverse acetabulum than women, which agrees with the literature described for FAI, where the majority of the patients with pincer impingement are women [9, 26].

Ito et al. [27] reports in a cross-sectional study that there is no difference in the version angle regarding age or sex. The number of individuals recruited for the study was 24 symptomatic and 24 healthy. The comparison was performed by ANOVA test, grouping sex and age dichotomized at 40 years old. The difference of their results with respect to this report may be due to the size of the sample used since each group studied contains a maximum of eight individuals.

On the other hand, the estimation of the multinomial regression model shows that there is an association between the clusters formed and the presence of crossover sign. Thus, belonging to group 2 (retroverted acetabulum) increases the relative risk for the presence of both bilateral and unilateral positive crossover sign. This finding suggests that there may be "physiological" crossover at an early age so it is not always pathological. Thus, the development of the pathology will depend on the load applied by each individual in this overcoverage and on how it evolves as it reaches the age, that is, if the acetabulum is oriented anteriorly.

5.2. Wiberg angle

5.2.1. Results

The variables used in this analysis are the Wiberg angle measured in coronal CT in bilateral form and corrected in three planes.

The result of the analysis is presented in the dendrogram (see **Figure 8**), where the presence of two groups with greater distances is observed. When creating these two groups, it is observed that group 1 has average values of acetabular version angle significantly larger than group 2 (see **Table 5**).

When observing the epidemiological variables, it is observed that group 2 presents an average age lower than group 1; this finding is significant and has a high power ($\alpha = 0.00$ and $1-\beta = 0.99$). The distribution of age is shown in **Figure 9**. The differences found in weight and BMI are also significant however the power is moderate, with $\alpha = 0.05$ $1-\beta = 0.52$ and $\alpha = 0.02$ and $\beta = 0.64$, respectively. Finally, the differences found in size are not statistically significant ($\alpha = 0.52$, $\beta = 0.09$); the same occurs with the higher proportion of males in group 1 ($\alpha = 0.99$, $\beta = 0.09$) (see **Tables 6** and **7**).

When estimating a logistic regression model, age has an OR of 1.08 [1.04–1.12] (goodness of fit test = 0.30) belonging to group 1, with an area under the ROC curve of 0.74 [0.64–0.84]. The cut value that maximizes sensitivity and specificity is 38 years, being 64.58 and 83.02%,

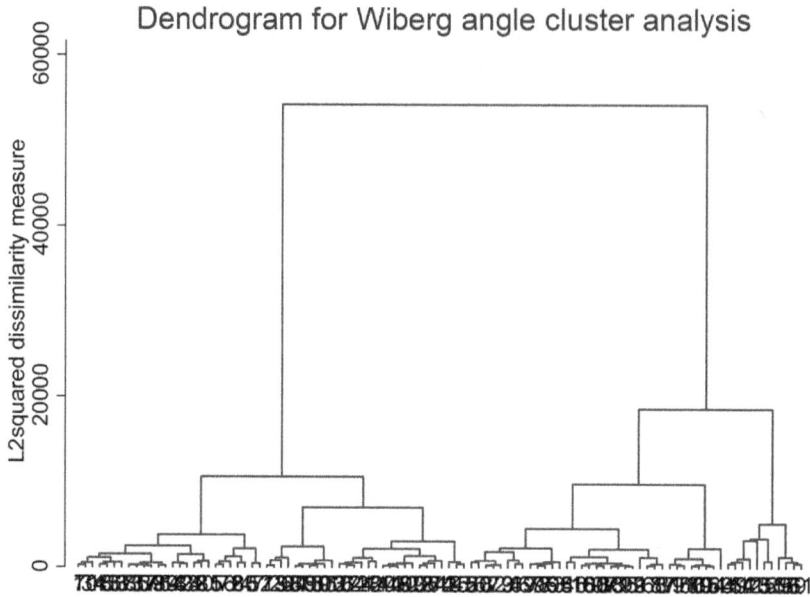

Figure 8. A dendrogram showing cluster analysis of Wiberg angle, and two groups are identified.

respectively, correctly ranking 74.26% of the sample. In the case of the 40 years, the sensitivity remains at 60.42% and the specificity decreases to 83.02%, whereby being 40 years or older has an OR of 7.46 [2.97–18.75] belonging to group 1.

5.2.2. Discussion

In the conglomerate analysis of the Wiberg angle, a correlation with age is also observed, showing that as the age increases the average value of the Wiberg angle does as well. For each completed year, the probability of belonging to the group with higher Wiberg angle increases by 6%. The cut value found is 6 years longer than in the case of the acetabular version angle,

Wiberg angle	Group 1	Group 2	Total	P
N	48 (47.52%)	53 (52.48%)	101	
3-P corrected R.	45.18 (±6.00)	33.70 (±4.14)	39.16 (±7.68)	0.00
3-P Corrected L.	46.36 (±4.94)	33.89 (±3.41)	39.82 (±7.53)	0.00
Coronal R.	44.47 (±5.62)	33.73 (±4.65)	38.83 (±7.43)	0.00
Coronal L.	45.09 (±5.78)	33.22 (±3.92)	38.86 (±7.69)	0.00

The probability obtained in the test of median comparison is shown in the last column, and at each level the differences reach statistical significance. R = right, L = left and 3-p = 3-plane corrected.

Table 5. It shows mean and standard deviation of Wiberg angle by the group that results from the cluster analysis.

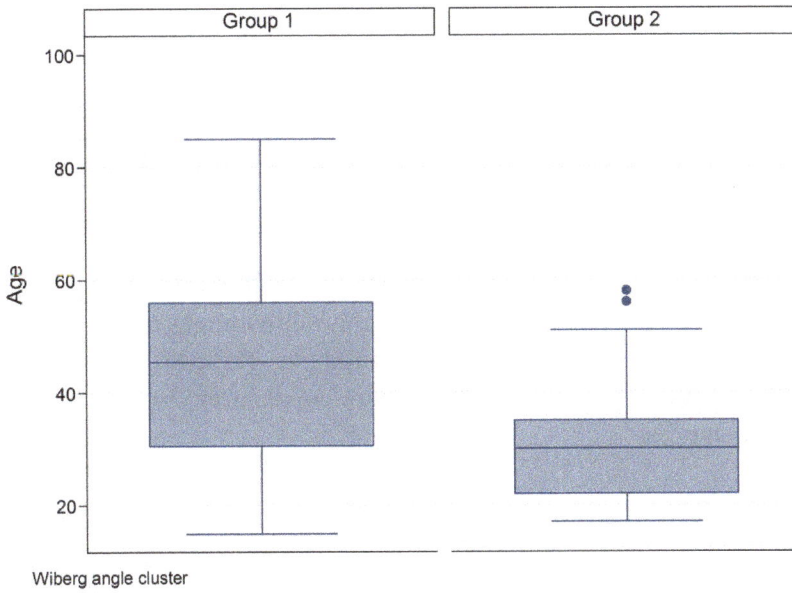

Figure 9. It shows age distribution among both groups, resulting from cluster analysis of Wiberg angle.

	Group 1	Group 2	Total
Age	43.54 (±15.81)	30.74 (±9.76)	36.82 (±14.43)
Weight (kg)	74.23 (±13.14)	69.09 (±12.58)	71.56 (±13.04)
Height (mts)	1.68 (±0.09)	1.67 (±0.08)	1.68 (±0.09)
BMI	26.14 (±3.36)	24.63 (±3.20)	25.35 (±3.35)

BMI = body mass index, kg = kilograms and mts = meters.

Table 6. It shows mean and standard deviation of epidemiological variables by the group that results from the cluster analysis of Wiberg angle.

Wiberg cluster	Female	Male
1	19 (39.58%)	29 (60.42%)
2	22 (41.51%)	31 (58.49%)
TOTAL	41 (40.69%)	60 (59.41%)

Table 7. It shows gender distribution among both groups that result from the cluster analysis of Wiberg angle.

which implies that the acetabular coverage increases later. This finding is consistent with what was described by Konishi et al. [28], where it is mentioned that the angle increases with age.

5.3. Alpha angle

5.3.1. Results

The variables used in this analysis correspond to alpha femoral angle measurements. In an axial oblique cut of the femoral neck, it was divided into thirds from chepalic to caudal. The measurement was made at the second third in the anterosuperior region, that is to say, using the clock handle form, from 1:00 to 3:00. This measurement was made in both hips.

Hundred patients were included. Cluster analysis separated two groups of patients. In group 2, 13 patients were assigned, which presented higher alpha angle values with statistical significance in 16 of the 18 measurement levels analyzed (see **Table 8**). The result of the analysis is presented in the dendrogram (**Figure 10**), where we observe the presence of two groups that have greater distances.

Variable	Group 1	Group 2	Total	P (ranksum)
N	87 (87.00%)	13 (13.00%)	100	0.00
ALPHA N1 R.	48.14 (±8.78)	65.00 (±6.43)	50.33 (±10.22)	0.00
ALPHA N1 L.	47.12 (±7.19)	61.57 (±7.64)	49.00 (±8.71)	0.00
ALPHA N2 R.	46.45 (±5.90)	53.64 (±9.05)	47.39 (±6.78)	0.00
ALPHA N2 L.	47.14 (±4.93)	56.08 (±7.56)	48.30 (±6.10)	0.00
ALPHA N3 R.	37.73 (±5.27)	40.12 (±3.91)	38.04 (±5.16)	0.13
ALPHA N3 L.	39.57 (±4.86)	40.93 (±3.44)	39.74 (±4.71)	0.19
ALPHA 1:00 R.	50.28 (±6.92)	64.46 (±9.63)	52.12 (±8.71)	0.00
ALPHA 1:00 L.	50.77 (±6.16)	67.31 (±7.55)	52.92 (±8.43)	0.00
ALPHA 1:30 R.	51.68 (±7.14)	66.62 (±5.16)	53.62 (±8.54)	0.00
ALPHA 1:30 L.	52.85 (±6.34)	65.77 (±6.62)	54.53 (±7.70)	0.00
ALPHA 2:00 R.	50.51 (±6.44)	61.62 (±4.87)	51.95 (±7.27)	0.00
ALPHA 2:00 L.	50.74 (±5.45)	60.85 (±8.23)	52.05 (±6.76)	0.00
ALPHA 2:30 R.	48.20 (±5.54)	59.92 (±6.87)	49.72 (±6.93)	0.00
ALPHA 2:30 L.	47.28 (±4.53)	56.38 (±9.70)	48.46 (±6.22)	0.00
ALPHA 3:00 R.	46.02 (±5.09)	56.93 (±7.86)	47.44 (±6.60)	0.00
ALPHA 3:00 L.	45.34 (±5.75)	52.38 (±9.20)	46.26 (±6.68)	0.01
ALPHA 3:30 R.	44.74 (±5.29)	51.15 (±9.33)	45.57 (±6.29)	0.02
ALPHA 3:30 L.	44.43 (±4.34)	48.08 (±6.05)	44.90 (±4.72)	0.0

The probability obtained in the test of median comparison is shown in the last column, and at each level the differences reach statistical significance. R = right and L = left.

Table 8. It shows mean and standard deviation of alpha angle by a group that results from the cluster analysis.

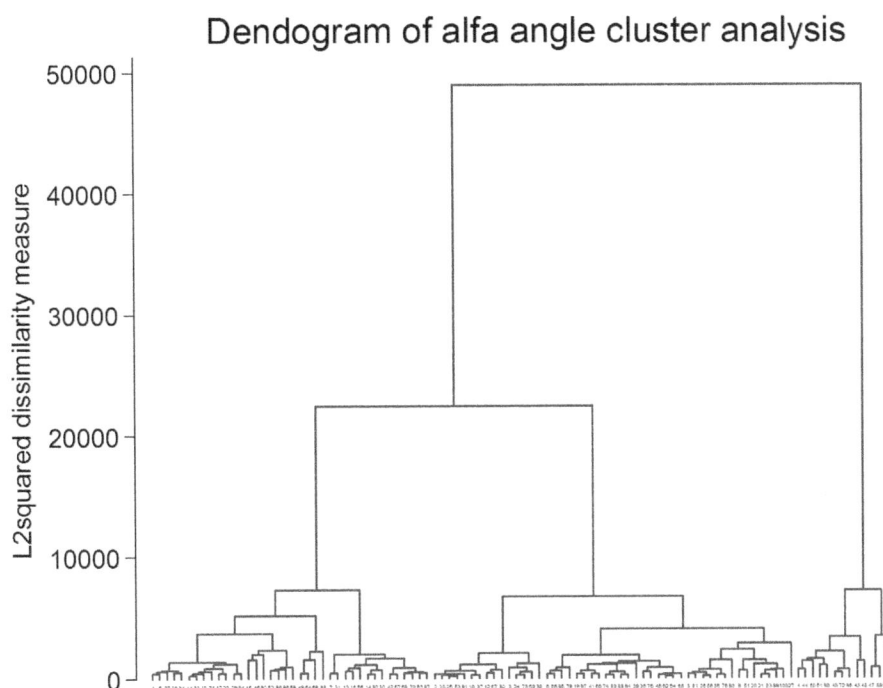

Figure 10. A dendrogram showing cluster analysis of femoral alpha angle, and two groups are identified.

In the measurements of the alpha angle by levels, the difference was significantly greater in group 2 in levels 1 and 2 bilaterally. However, although the average value in group 2 was higher, the difference in level 3 was not significant, either to the right or to the left. In the measurements of the alpha angle by radians, the difference in all hourly radii was significant bilaterally, the average being consistently higher in group 2.

Observing the epidemiological variables, it is observed that group 2 has a higher average age, but the difference is not significant ($\alpha = 0.22$, $1-\beta = 0.44$). The differences in size, weight and BMI are minimal and therefore are not statistically significant [(height, $\alpha = 0.36$, $1-\beta = 0.46$), weight, $\alpha = 0.19$, $1-\beta = 0.52$ and BMI, $\alpha = 0.29$; $1-\beta = 0.99$)]. The distributions of these variables by groups can be observed in graphs 17, 18, 19 and 20. As for gender, it is observed that in

	Group 1	Group 2	Total
Age	36.40 (±14.89)	40.15 (±11.33)	36.89 (±14.49)
Weight (kg)	70.87 (±13.42)	75.00 (±09.72)	71.41 (±13.03)
Height (Mts)	1.67 (±0.09)	1.70 (±0.10)	1.67 (±0.09)
BMI	25.23 (±3.51)	25.98 (±2.06)	25.33 (±3.36)

BMI = body mass index, Kg = kilograms and mts = meters.

Table 9. It shows mean and standard deviation of epidemiological variables by a group that results from the cluster analysis of Wiberg angle.

Group	Female	Male	Total
1	39 (44.83%)	48 (55.17%)	87
2	2 (15.83%)	11 (84.62%)	13

Table 10. It shows gender distribution among both groups that result from the cluster analysis of the alpha angle.

group 2, there is a greater proportion of men than in group 1, however, this is not significant (p = 0.07) (see **Tables 9** and **10**).

5.3.2. Discussion

The variables measured in the femur are not related to the epidemiological variables analyzed: age, gender, height, weight and body mass index, which is consistent with the literature reviewed [29, 30].

6. Conclusions

- CT is an important tool for FAI diagnosis and surgical planning.

- CT has a very important role for a better understanding of hip anatomy; further research using CT images should be encouraged.

- The pathological value of the alpha value is controversial. We think that over 57° should be considered pathological. Cases between 50 and 57° should be analyzed with caution.

- To overlook the correction in three planes overestimates the acetabular anteversion and underestimates the lateral coverage in a significant way.

- Acetabular version is a gender- and age-related measurement. As age increases, acetabular version increases. Women have lesser acetabular version angle.

- Wiberg angle is an age-related measurement. As age increased, the Wiberg angle increased.

- Femoral FAI-related measurement is not related to gender, age, weight and height.

- FAI measurement is not related to weight and height.

Author details

Maximiliano Barahona*, Jaime Hinzpeter and Cristian Barrientos

*Address all correspondence to: maxbarahonavasquez@gmail.com

Orthopedic Surgery Department, Hospital Clinico Universidad de Chile, Chile

References

[1] Canham CD, Domb BG, Giordano BD. Atraumatic hip instability. JBJS Reviews. 2016;**4**(5):e3

[2] Lee A, Emmett L, Van der Wall H, Kannangara S, Mansberg R, Fogelman I. SPECT/CT of femeroacetabular impingement. Clinical Nuclear Medicine. 2008;**33**(11):757

[3] Ganz R, Parvizi J, Beck M, Leunig M, Nötzli H, Siebenrock KA. Femoroacetabular impingement: A cause for osteoarthritis of the hip. Clinical Orthopaedics and Related Research. 2003;**417**:112-120

[4] Beaulé P, Zaragoza E, Motamedi K, Copelan N, Dorey F. Three-dimensional computed tomography of the hip in the assessment of femoroacetabular impingement. Journal of Orthopaedic Research. 2005;**23**(6):1286-1292

[5] Hinzpeter J, Barrientos C, Barahona M, Diaz J, Zamorano A, Salazar A, Catalan J. Fluid extravasation related to hip arthroscopy: A prospective computed tomography-based study. Orthopaedic Journal of Sports Medicine. 2015;**3**(3):2325967115573222

[6] Kassarjian A, Brisson M, Palmer WE. Femoroacetabular impingement. European Journal of Radiology. 2007;**63**(1):29-35

[7] Beall DP, Sweet CF, Martin HD, Lastine CL, Grayson DE, Ly JQ, et al. Imaging findings of femoroacetabular impingement syndrome. Skeletal Radiology. 2005;**34**(11):691-701

[8] Kang AC, Gooding AJ, Coates MH, Goh TD, Armour P, Rietveld J. Computed tomography assessment of hip joints in asymptomatic individuals in relation to femoroacetabular impingement. The American Journal of Sports Medicine. 2010;**38**(6):1160-1165

[9] Tannast M, Siebenrock KA, Anderson SE. Femoroacetabular impingement: Radiographic diagnosis — What the radiologist should know. American Journal of Radiology. 2007;**188**(6): 1540-1552

[10] Barton C, Salineros MJ, Rakhra KS, Beaulé PE. Validity of the alpha angle measurement on plain radiographs in the evaluation of cam-type femoroacetabular impingement. Clinical Orthopaedics and Related Research. 2011;**469**(2):464-469

[11] Notzli HP, Wyss TF, Stoecklin CH, Schmid MR, Treiber K, Hodler J. The contour of the femoral head-neck junction as a predictor for the risk of anterior impingement. The Journal of Bone and Joint Surgery. British Volume. 2002;**84**(4):556-560

[12] Hack K, Di Primio G, Rakhra K, Beaulé PE. Prevalence of cam-type femoroacetabular impingement morphology in asymptomatic volunteers. The Journal of Bone and Joint Surgery. 2010;**92**(14):2436-2444

[13] Allen D, Beaulé PE, Ramadan O, Doucette S. Prevalence of associated deformities and hip pain in patients with cam-type femoroacetabular impingement. The Journal of Bone and Joint Surgery. British Volume. 2009;**91**(5):589-594

[14] Barrientos C, Diaz J, Brañes J, Chaparro F, Barahona M, Salazar A, Hinzpeter J. Hip morphology characterization: Implications in femoroacetabular impingement in a Chilean population. Orthopaedic Journal of Sports Medicine. 2014;**2**(10):2325967114552800

[15] Pollard TC, Villar RN, Norton MR, Fern ED, Williams MR, Simpson DJ, Carr AJ. Femoroacetabular impingement and classification of the cam deformity: The reference interval in normal hips. Acta Orthopaedica. 2010;**81**(1):134-141

[16] Kleinbaum DG, Kupper LL, Muller KE. Applied Regression Analysis and Other Multivariate Analysis Methods. Boston: PWS-Kent Publishing Company; 1988

[17] Hosmer DW Jr, Lemshow S. Applied Logistic Regression. John Wiley & Sons; New York, USA. 2004

[18] Burgueño MJ, García-Bastos JL, González-Buitrago JM. Las curvas ROC en la evaluación de las pruebas diagnósticas. Medicina Clínica (Barcelona). 1995;**104**(17):661-670

[19] Sutter R, Dietrich TJ, Zingg PO, Pfirrmann CWA. How useful is the alpha angle for discriminating between symptomatic patients with cam-type femoroacetabular impingement and asymptomatic volunteers? Radiology. 2012;**264**(2):514-521

[20] Perreira AC, Hunter JC, Laird T, Jamali AA. Multilevel measurement of acetabular version using 3-D CT-generated models: Implications for hip preservation surgery. Clinical Orthopaedics and Related Research. 2010;**469**(2):552-561

[21] Bosse HJP, Lee D, Henderson ER, Sala DA, Feldman DS. Pelvic positioning creates error in CT acetabular measurements. Clinical Orthopaedics and Related Research. 2011;**469**(6):1683-1691

[22] Siebenrock KA, Kalbermatten DF, Ganz R. Effect of pelvic tilt on acetabular retroversion: A study of pelves from cadavers. Clinical Orthopaedics and Related Research. 2003;**407**:241

[23] Nakahara I, Takao M, Sakai T, Nishii T, Yoshikawa H, Sugano N. Gender differences in 3D morphology and bony impingement of human hips. Journal of Orthopaedic Research. 2011;**29**(3):333-339

[24] Dudda M, Kim Y-J, Zhang Y, Nevitt MC, Xu L, Niu J, et al. Morphologic differences between the hips of Chinese women and white women: Could they account for the ethnic difference in the prevalence of hip osteoarthritis? Arthritis & Rheumatism. 2011;**63**(10): 2992-2999

[25] Gosvig KK, Jacobsen S, Sonne-Holm S, Palm H, Troelsen A. Prevalence of malformations of the hip joint and their relationship to sex, groin pain, and risk of osteoarthritis: A population-based survey. The Journal of Bone and Joint Surgery. 2010;**92**(5):1162-1169

[26] Ganz R, Leunig M, Leunig-Ganz K, Harris WH. The etiology of osteoarthritis of the hip. Clinical Orthopaedics and Related Research. 2008;**466**(2):264-272

[27] Ito K, Minka-II MA, Leunig M, Werlen S, Ganz R. Femoroacetabular impingement and the cam-effect: A MRI-based quantitative anatomical study of the femoral head-neck offset. Journal of Bone and Joint Surgery. British Volume. 2001;**83**(2):171

[28] Konishi N, Mieno T. Determination of acetabular coverage of the femoral head with use of a single anteroposterior radiograph. The Journal of Bone and Joint Surgery. American Volume. 1993;**75**:1318-1333

[29] Toogood PA, Skalak A, Cooperman DR. Proximal femoral anatomy in the normal human population. Clinical Orthopaedics and Related Research. 2009;**467**(4):876

[30] Gosvig KK, Jacobsen S, Palm H, Sonne-Holm S, Magnusson E. A new radiological index for assessing asphericity of the femoral head in cam impingement. Journal of Bone and Joint Surgery. British Volume. 2007;**89**(10):1309-1316

6

Non-contrast CT in the Evaluation of Urinary Tract Stone Obstruction and Haematuria

Mohammad Hammad Ather, Wasim Memon,

Wajahat Aziz and Mohammad Nasir Sulaiman

Abstract

Non-contrast computed tomography (CT) abdomen has emerged as a first line investigation in suspected upper urinary tract obstruction. Underlying causes can usually be ascertained on computed tomography of kidneys, ureters and bladder (CT KUB). However, further investigations may be required to delineate/confirm underlying pathology like ureteropelvic junction obstruction (UPJ), differentiation between obstruction and residual dilatation. Actual protocol of CT KUB for evaluation of stone disease and haematuria vary on institutional guidelines. CT KUB is not only extremely sensitive and specific in the diagnosis of stone; it is now used in the pre-operative nomograms in predicting success of various endourological interventions like percutaneous nephrolithotomy (PCNL) and shock wave lithotripsy (SWL). Determination of stone density, stone volume, stone composition, skin to stone distance, presence of ureteral wall oedema, perinephric oedema are highly predictive of stone free rate. CT recognition of various anomalies, presence of retro-renal colon, horse-shoe kidney, malrotation, etc. can help in better planning to avoid complications. One of the major limitations of CT is the radiation dose, besides cost and availability. Modification in technique and technological innovation has resulted in significant dose reduction from 4.5 to about 1 mSv.

Keywords: CT KUB, non-contrast-enhanced CT, low-dose CT, endourology, PCNL, SWL, NCCT

1. Introduction

Computed tomography of kidneys, ureters and bladder (CT KUB) is a quick non-invasive technique for diagnosis of stone disease. It was initially used in the evaluation of radiolucent stones only however, Smith et al. [1] in 1995 showed CT has superiority over intravenous urography (IVU). CT KUB subsequently became the first choice in the diagnostic imaging of urinary tract for obstruction of stones. It has replaced IVU almost completely in the last two decades [2]. It is usually considered the initial imaging modality for suspected acute renal colic and dipstick positive haematuria in an emergency setting and initial diagnostic evaluation of upper tract obstruction. CT KUB has certain clear advantages over other urinary tract imaging for stones. It is not dependent on stone chemical composition; all stones are well seen on CT except for the Indinavir stones [3], it does not require contrast, it can be rapidly performed and can be used in planning endourological treatment.

Actual protocol of CT KUB for evaluation of stone disease and haematuria will vary depending on institutional guidelines. The general parameters are (i) non-contract examination is performed on multi-detector computed tomography scanner; (ii) supine or supine and prone patient positioning (prone has the advantage of assessing stones near the VUJ); (iii) data interpretation with the use of axial, coronal, sagittal and sometimes curved oblique images for proper evaluation; (iv) scan parameters which includes slice thickness(recommended 5 mm or less), field of view: patient size algorithm: standard technique (120 kV/Auto MA .5 rotation); Anatomical start point: 1 cm above the liver Anatomical stop through inferior pubic rami).

2. Technique/protocols

CT KUB is a quick non-invasive technique for diagnosis of stone disease. It is usually considered the initial imaging modality for suspected acute renal colic and dipstick positive haematuria in an emergency setting. Unenhanced CT is also increasingly being used for treatment planning and post-treatment surveillance for stone recurrence.

This is a study without intravenous or oral contrast, relatively low-dose (in CT terms), and has a very high sensitivity for the detection of renal and ureteric stones. CT KUB allows a rapid, contrast-free, anatomically accurate diagnosis of urolithiasis with a sensitivity of 97–98% and a specificity of 96–100%.

The effective dose of a standard CT KUB examination has been estimated to be between 3 and 5 mSv, which is up to three times that for intravenous pyelography. However, radiation dose in CT KUB is gradually decreasing with the introduction of ultra-low radiation dose CT KUB (0.5–0.7 mSv). These doses are almost comparable to plain film KUB and have shown favourable outcomes similar to standard radiation dose CT KUB. Reductions in CT dose inherently create an increase in image noise. Therefore, a balance has to be found between image quality (signal-to-noise ratio) and restraining the radiation dose.

In comparison to conventional CT, spiral CT is significantly faster. It thus allows acquisition of a complete data set in a single breath-hold and prevents the misregistration of slice location that is typical of conventional CT. In addition, multi-slice spiral CT reduces the time needed for image acquisition, allowing for thinner slice collimation and retrospective reconstruction of thin slices to review challenging areas of analysis.

From the top of the kidneys through the base of the bladder (mid-liver [T-12] through symphysis pubis), data acquisition is uninterrupted using a maximum of 5-mm collimation with table speed of 5 mm/s. Slice collimation with multi-slice CT is usually 2.5–3 mm with table speed up to 5 mm/s.

Multislice technique allows slices as thin as 1 mm to be obtained for problem solving. The thinner slices can be viewed retrospectively without rescanning the patient. Thin slices enable identification of extremely small sized calculi that may be overlooked if the slices are thicker.

Turning the patient to a prone position permits differentiation of stones impacted at the ureterovesical junction from stones that have already passed into the bladder.

Actual protocol of CT KUB for evaluation of stone disease and haematuria will vary depending upon institutional guidelines but following are the general parameters:

- Non-contrast examination is performed on multi-detector computed tomography scanner.

- Supine or prone patient positioning. Prone has the advantage of assessing stones near the VUJ. Some institutions may perform a limited pelvic scan in prone if the supine scan shows a calculus near the VUJ.

- Data interpretation with the use of axial, coronal, sagittal and sometimes curved oblique images for proper evaluation.

Scan parameters:

- Slice thickness: 5 mm

- Field of view: patient size

- Algorithm: standard

- Technique: 120 kV/Auto MA .5 rotation

- Anatomical start: 1 cm above the liver

- Anatomical stop: through inferior pubic rami

- Filming/windowing: soft-tissue window with 3 mm coronal and sagittal reconstructions.

Dual-energy CT scanning is a new technique that can more correctly distinguish different stone types. It involves acquiring CT data at two different X-ray energies (80 and 140 peak kilovoltage [kVp]). Post-processing software can make use of the different attenuation properties of calculi of various chemical compositions at low and high X-ray energies.

Decreased exposure is most commonly achieved by modifying tube current and applying new image reconstruction algorithms. Low-dose CT has been shown to maintain diagnostic accuracy compared with standard-dose CT, even in overweight and obese patients when using automated tube current modulation.

2.1. Indication and uses of CT KUB

A clinical decision to order CT KUB has to be made in two different clinical presentations. First is a patient with flank pain presenting in emergency department. The classic clinical presentation of a young man writhing in pain is usually distinctive. However, atypical presentations are not uncommon. CT KUB is still reasonable first-line investigation for all patients presenting in emergency with flank pain as it increases diagnostic accuracy in atypical cases and can detect other pathologies. In a study of 1500 consecutive CT examinations in patients with flank pain, 14% had CT findings other than stone requiring immediate or deferred treatment [4]. Although this diagnostic superiority of CT KUB for flank pain is well established, recent studies have questioned whether it influences management decision in emergency setting. A multicentre, randomised controlled trial of carefully selected patients with suspected nephrolithiasis compared ultrasound with CT KUB and concluded that initial ultrasound decreases cumulative radiation exposure by obviating need of CT in some patients without significant difference in missing high-risk diagnoses, serious adverse events and re-admissions [5].

In a clinical setting, the choice of CT KUB versus ultrasound for initial diagnostic imaging in patients with flank pain should be individualised. Patients who are obese, clearly sick or have associated gross/microscopic haematuria are more likely to benefit from CT scan. On the other hand, children, pregnant women and those assessed to have musculoskeletal pain clinically are more appropriate for ultrasound first approach. Available local resources, for example, expert sonologist should also be taken into account when making this decision.

3. Evaluation of obstruction

Second clinical setting requiring CT KUB is incidental finding of hydronephrosis on ultrasound. The decision to request CT KUB will depend on information available on ultrasound and suspected cause of underlying obstruction. In some cases, ultrasound will provide sufficient information to decide further management. For instance, in classic ureteropelvic junction obstruction (UPJO) in a child, ultrasound alone would provide enough anatomical detail to proceed for radionuclide imaging. Similarly small ureterovesical junction stone seen clearly on ultrasound combined with clinical picture is usually sufficient to proceed for management decision. CT KUB is suitable if renal or ureteric stones are suspected as underlying cause of hydronephrosis or a benign pathology, for example, ureteric stricture/retroperitoneal fibrosis is presumed after history and examination. If an upper tract tumour or extrinsic malignant obstruction is suspected, a contrast-enhanced study is more appropriate.

Upper tract obstruction may lead to derangement in renal function and it is not uncommon to find raised creatinine in such patients especially if obstruction is bilateral. European Society of Urogenital Radiology recommends that an estimated glomerular filtration rate (eGFR) of less than 45 ml/min/1.73 m^2 particularly with other risk factors, for example, diabetic nephropathy and dehydration increases the risk of contrast-induced nephropathy (CIN) [6]. This effectively precludes contrast-enhanced study in such patients. CT KUB is helpful in excluding calculi and may even provide a definitive diagnosis in up to 40% cases of non-calculus obstruction [7]. MR urography will be required for making a definitive diagnosis in remaining cases.

CT KUB is currently considered as the first line imaging in the evaluation of stone and obstruction (**Figure 1**) and is preferred over an IVU [2]. This is in view of high sensitivity and specificity of CT over other imaging modalities. It is particularly useful in the diagnosis of ureteral stones (**Figures 1** and **2**) with sensitivity of 95–98% and specificity of 96–98% [8, 9]. It is of particular value in patients with renal failure, which precludes use of intravenous contrast, and ultrasound has limited value [10]. The sensitivity of ultrasound in the evaluation

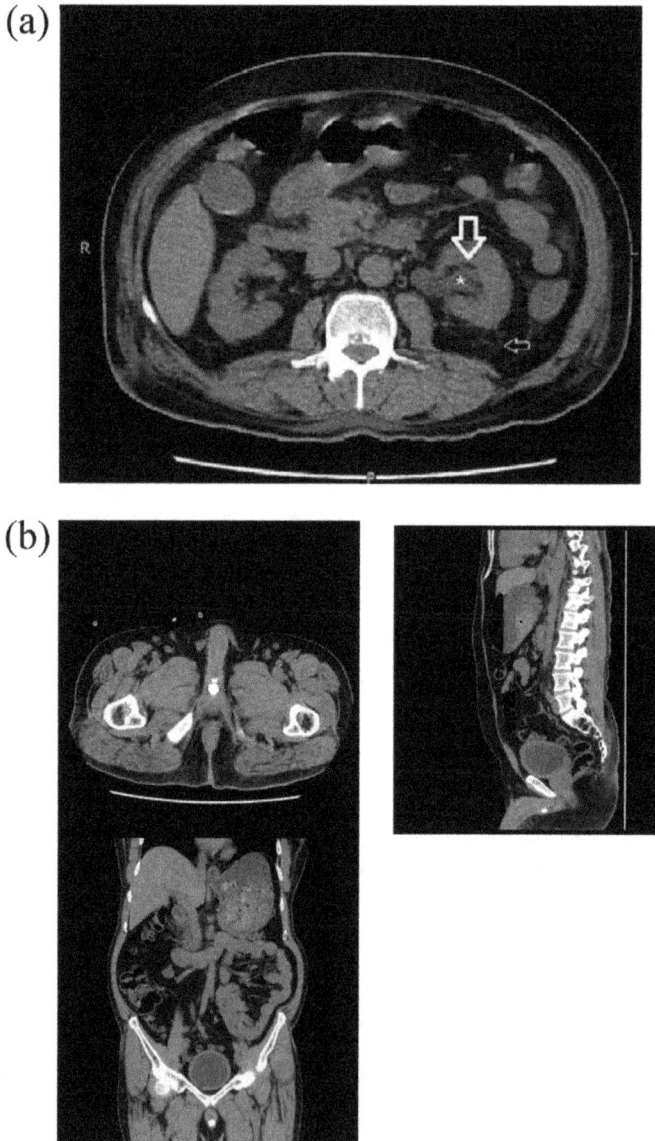

Figure 1. (a) Hydronephrosis (asterik), reduced peripelvic fat (white arrow) and increased perinephric fat stranding (black arrow) as compared to contralateral side and (b). CT KUB axial, sagittal and coronal sections demonstrating multiple calcific densities near the bulbar urethra likely representing urethral diverticulum with stone formation.

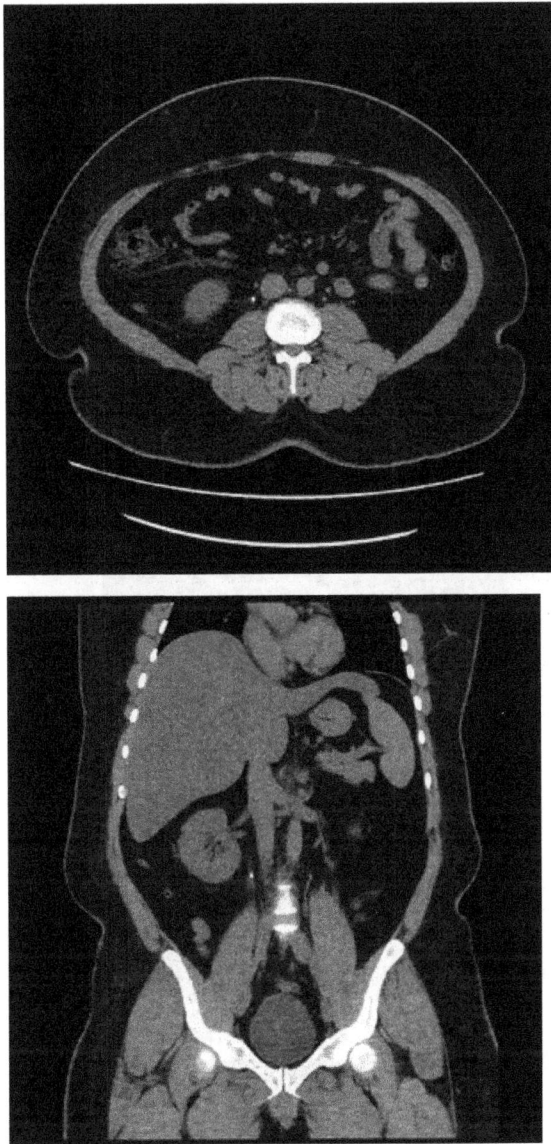

Figure 2. CT KUB axial and coronal sections demonstrating an obstructing right proximal ureteric calculus.

of ureteral stones when compared with CT KUB is only 46% and for hydroureter in half of the cases. CT KUB in the evaluation of ureteral stones is able to identify ureteral dilation in 83%, hydronephrosis in 80% and perinephric oedema in 59%, and ipsilateral nephromegaly in 57.2% of cases [11].

4. Evaluation of haematuria

In addition to diagnosis of stone and obstruction, it is also used in the work up haematuria. Asymptomatic micro-haematuria (AMH) is relatively common and is often not associated with urinary tract malignancies. The current guidelines indicate evaluation of upper urinary tract with contrast-enhanced CT (CECT). This often leads to identification of extra-urinary tract abnormalities. The diagnoses of such conditions often require extensive work for most conditions, which are inconsequential [12]. These are often observed on non-contrast CT imaging as well [13]. In vast majority of cases, ASH is idiopathic followed small renal stones (**Figure 3**) and other benign causes. Ultrasound is often the initial imaging, however, CT KUB can be used in lieu.

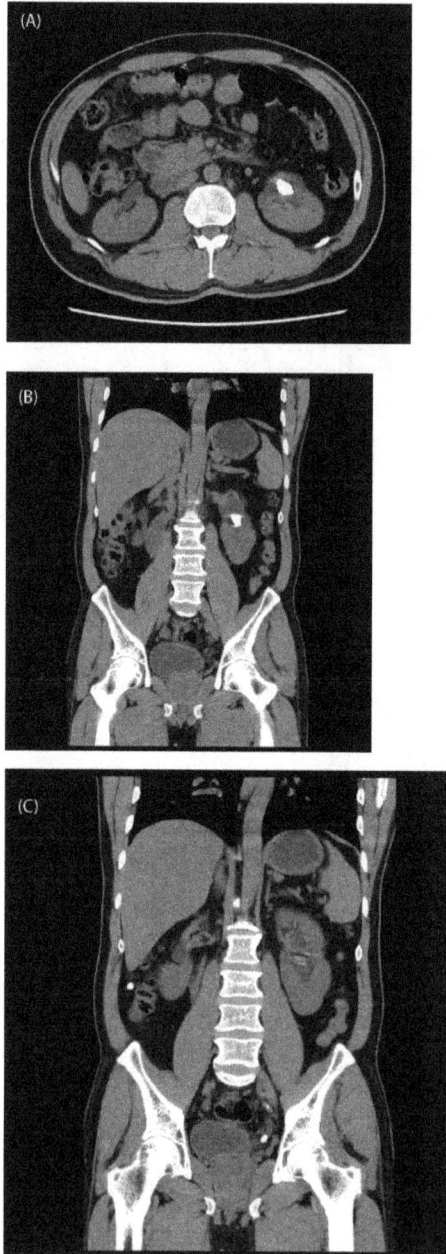

Figure 3. CT KUB axial and coronal sections demonstrating a left renal pelvis calculus (a and b) and left distal ureteric calculus (c).

4.1. In emergency room setting

Acute onset flank pain suggestive of ureteral obstruction is a common presentation in the emergency room (ER) setting. Introduction of CT has decreased the time in decision-making [14] about the possible aetiology of cause of flank pain [15, 16]. Clinical evaluation and ultra-sound often makes it difficult to differentiate ureteral obstruction from other pathologies. However, CT not only quickly identifies urolithiasis but also identifies other causes of flank pain [17]. This includes both genitourinary and extra-genitourinary abnormalities. Stones from ureter-vesical junction sometimes pass into the urethra (**Figure 4**) without significant changes in symptoms, these can be diagnosed by careful inspection of the CT.

Initial clinical evaluation including dipstick test for micro-haematuria also lack sensitivity. Li et al. [18] noted during the period of 4 years that there were 159,083 emergency visits. During this period, 397 had urolithiasis, in these patients absence of haematuria was noted in 9% (95% confidence interval 7–12%). The next step in the management of patients with stone

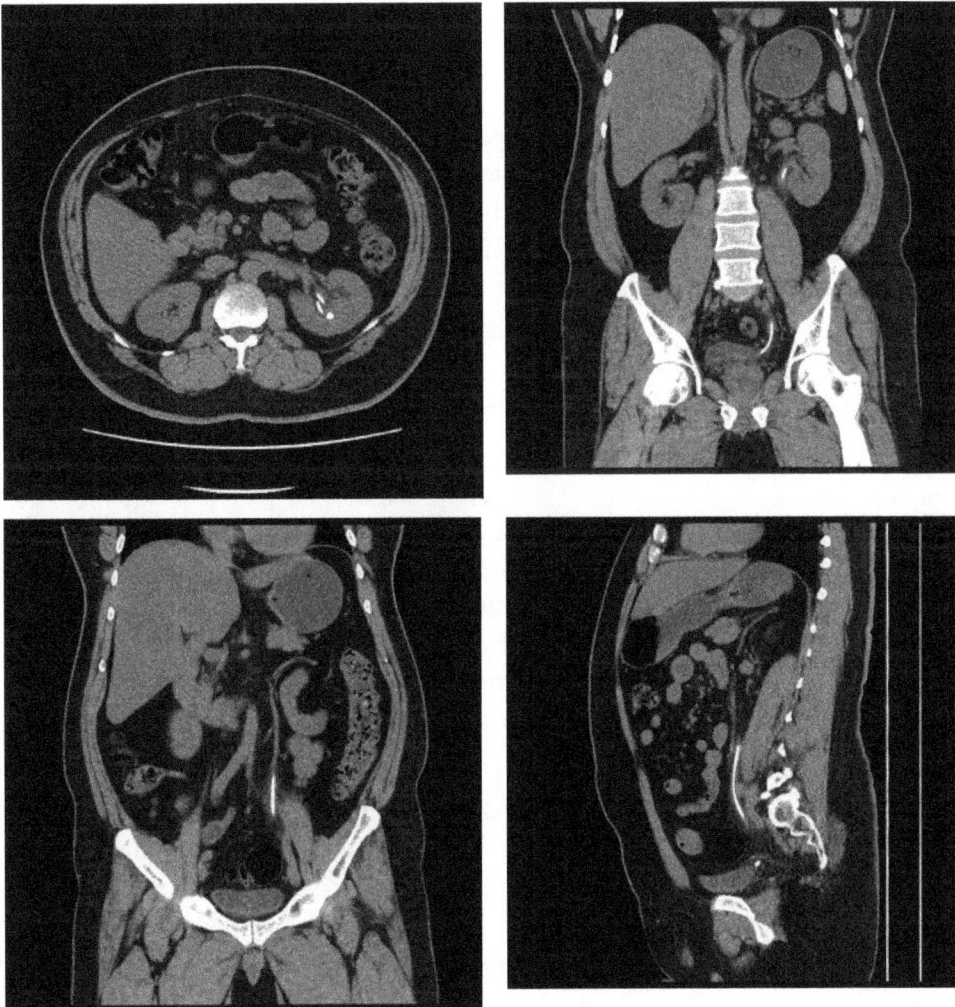

Figure 4. CT KUB axial, coronal and sagittal sections demonstrating a calculus in the prostatic urethra.

is to determine the extent of obstruction and of any complications from obstruction and stone. None of the conventional imaging, that is, IVU, ultrasound and plain X-ray KUB is sensitive enough to answer the question. CT KUB due to its high specificity and sensitivity to diagnose ureteral stones is ideal imaging in such a situation. However, CT without contrast has limitations being a non-contrast study. Secondary signs of obstruction like perinephric, periureteral stranding and unilateral nephromegaly are sometimes helpful. Bird et al. [19] in a study assess the significance of secondary signs of obstruction on CT KUB and noted that they do not correlate with degrees of obstruction on MAG-3. The authors suggested use of CT KUB in combination with radioisotope scans [9]. This is cumbersome particularly in an emergency room setting. As an alternate, Kravchick et al. [20] suggested the use of dynamic renal sonography in combination with CT KUB, particularly in patients with raised white cell count and stone larger than 4 mm. This is particularly useful in triaging patients who need admission in the hospital.

4.2. In elective clinical situation

Modern endourological interventions are becoming increasingly minimally invasive. Percutaneous nephrolithotomy is performed with 24–30 Fr. Amplatz; however, finer nephroscope has led to the introduction of mini (2001), micro (2011) and ultra mini (2013) [21]. Planning for these interventions require precise pre-operative assessment of stone size, location and anatomical abnormalities including caliceal narrowing, presence of caliceal diverticulum, etc. CT can be instrumental in making pre-operative assessment. It has been seen that increasing stone volume can influence post-operative complication rate. It is being observed that >4 cm stones are associated with significantly higher rate of post-operative pyrexia and need for transfusion [13].

4.3. Radiological signs of urinary obstruction

4.3.1. CT beyond the diagnosis of stone

The sensitivity and specificity of CT in the diagnosis of stone is well established. Even small stones, which would otherwise be missed on most other imaging, can be identified on CT. However, CT has utility beyond recognising the presence of stone in the urinary tract. It can be used in planning endourological interventions. Stone size, composition, location, skin to stone distance, etc. are some of the well recognised parameters used in the risk stratification and predicting success of treatment [22].

Shock wave lithotripsy (SWL) is the most minimally invasive treatment in the management of urolithiasis. Prediction of success for renal stones is often done on a CT KUB using estimation of stone volume, density (using Hounsfield Units) and skin to stone distance [23]. In a recent work, Park et al. [24] noted that BMI and perinephric oedema in addition to stone density are independent predictors of success of SWL. Ureteral stones requiring interventional treatment are either treated by SWL or ureteroscopy. Success of ureteral stone is dependent on stone size [25]. The success of treatment is assessed not only by stone free rate but also need for ancillary treatment and number of sessions required to clear the stone [26]. One important factor responsible for failed medical SWL for ureteral stone is stone impaction, defined as stone stuck in one location for over 1 month. Sarica et al. [27] recently noted that of all the evaluated stone- and patient-related factors, only ureteral wall thickness at the impacted stone site independently predicted shock wave lithotripsy success.

Stone size is one of the most important parameter in deciding the management of ureteral stone. In a recent work, Soomro et al. [28] compared the mean stone size, as measured on bone window versus standard soft-tissue window setting using multi-detector computed tomography (MDCT) in patients with a solitary ureteric stone. They noted that the stone size measured using the soft-tissue window setting on a MDCT is significantly different from the measurement on the bone windows. Earlier work also indicated that the transverse stone diameter on axial images of CT KUB underestimates the size of ureteric stone [29]. The authors suggested that coronal re-formatted images be used for size estimation.

Percutaneous nephrolithotomy (PCNL) is a minimally invasive treatment modality used in the management of >20 mm kidney stones, and as such, is considered as the primary modality by EAU and AUA guidelines [30, 31]. Predicting complications and success of percutaneous surgery for urolithiasis can now be reliably done using one of the several nephrolithom-etry scores [22]. Nephrolithometry scoring systems are based on pre-operative stone and patient features and they demonstrate and stratify relationships between kidney's anatomy and stones. Currently there are three scoring systems; Guy's score [32] described in 2011, S.T.O.N.E. nephrolithometry system [33] and CROES nephrolithometry nomogram [34] in 2013. In a recent work by Choi et al. comparing these three scoring systems for tubeless PCNL, noted that Guy's stone score was the only significant predictive factor for stone free and complication rates. However, Tailly et al. [35] earlier noted no difference in the ability to predict stone free rate comparing the three scoring systems after PCNL.

PCNL is safe surgical procedure and is not associated with high grade on Clavien grading. The most frequently reported complication following PCNL is infection and haemorrhage, however one of the most devastating complication is a surrounding organ injury includ-ing bowel injury. According to the Clavien-Dindo classification of surgical complications, colonic injury is regarded as a stage IVa complication. The incidence of colon injury is reported to be 0.3–0.5%, however in a large recently reported series, AslZare et al. [36] noted 11 cases in 5260 cases of PCNL. Colonic injuries are seen in patients with retro-renal colon, the prevalence of retro-renal colon in males to be 13.6% on the right and 11.9% on the left, whilst in females it was 13.4% on the right and 26.2% on the left [37]. CT KUB is instrumental in recognising retro-renal colon prior to PCNL. Most of the colonic injuries are now managed conservatively with drainage of colon via percutaneous drain, insertion of JJ stent to drain kidney, intravenous antibiotics and bowel rest by giving intravenous nutrition.

4.4. Features of upper tract obstruction

Once a CT KUB abdomen is ordered for suspected upper tract obstruction, it should be reviewed for secondary radiological signs of obstruction, site of obstruction and underly-ing pathology. Moreover, associated findings, for example, dilated appendix, ovarian cysts, spinal pathologies should be considered and systematically reviewed.

Classic secondary radiological signs on CT KUB suggesting upper tract obstruction include: dilatation of renal pelvis, dilated ureter and perinephric stranding (**Figure 1a** and **b**). Renal pelvis is identifiable as area of low attenuation compared to adjacent renal parenchyma. Dilatation of renal pelvis (hydronephrosis) usually appears as anterior and medial bulging of this low attenuation structure. In some cases, dilated renal pelvis may be difficult to differentiate from a prominent extra renal pelvis. However, dilated calices that obliterate the renal sinus fat help in making this differentiation. CT is also valuable in differentiating between stone and stent (**Figure 5**), particularly with the use of bone windows.

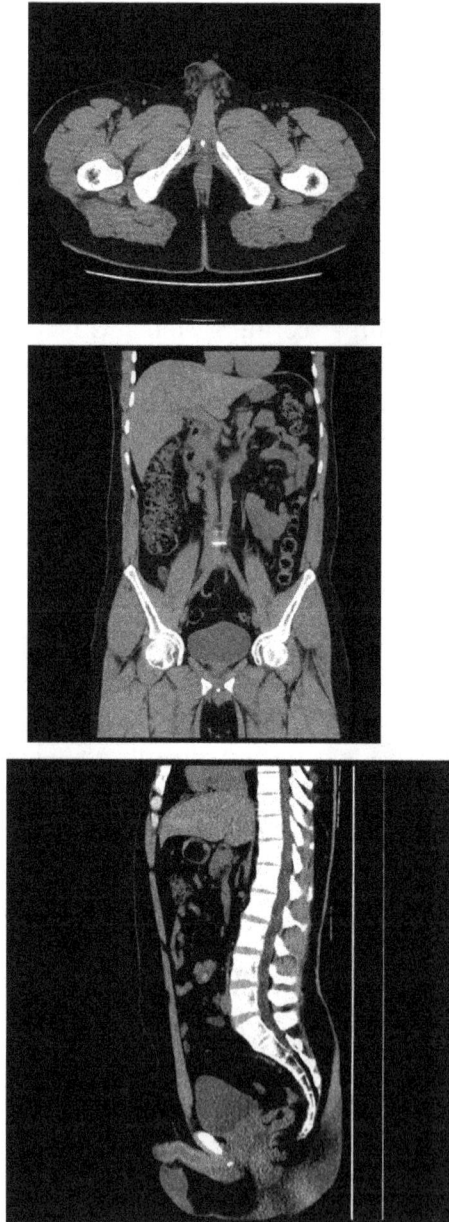

Figure 5. CT KUB axial, coronal and sagittal sections demonstrating a left-sided double J stent in place.

An assessment of degree of obstruction can also be made on CT KUB (**Table 1**). The Society of Foetal Ultrasound first described the grading system for hydronephrosis [38]. Similar description has also been applied to other imaging modalities like intravenous urography and CT [39].

Dilatation of ureter when present should be traced down to the site of obstruction, to differentiate between phlobolith and stone (**Figure 6**). The dilated ureter is usually traceable from

Grade	Degree	Description
Grade 0		No dilation caliceal walls opposed to each other
Grade 1	Mild	Dilation of renal pelvis without dilation of the calyces
Grade 2	Mild	Dilation of renal pelvis and calyces, no cortical thinning
Grade 3	Moderate	Dilation of the renal pelvis and calices with blunting of papillary impression with or without cortical thinning
Grade 4	Severe	Gross dilation of the renal pelvis and calices with associated cortical thinning

Table 1. Degree and grade of hydronephrosis and its description.

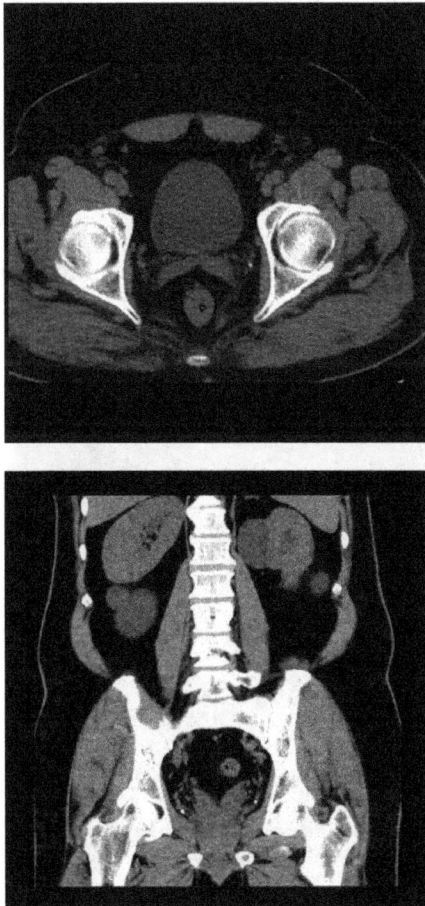

Figure 6. CT KUB axial and coronal sections demonstrating s in the pelvis.

ureteropelvic junction when viewing coronal sections at a workstation. However, combining information from both axial and coronal images may be needed, especially for the lower ureter obscured by bowel loops or iliac vessels (**Figure 6**). Curved planar re-formatted images have been utilised to provide images mimicking a contrast-enhanced study and improve diagnostic yield for ureteric lesions [40]. UVJ stones could be differentiated from vesical stones by prone CT of the bladder area (**Figure 7**).

Once tracing the dilatation of ureter identifies site of obstruction, it should be reviewed for intraluminal, luminal or extra luminal obstructing lesions. Intraluminal pathologies include stones, blood clot and papilla. Fortunately the most common obstructing lesion, that is, stone is almost always CT dense and easily identifiable. In the absence of obstructing stone and positive radiological signs of obstruction, one should consider differential diagnosis of passed

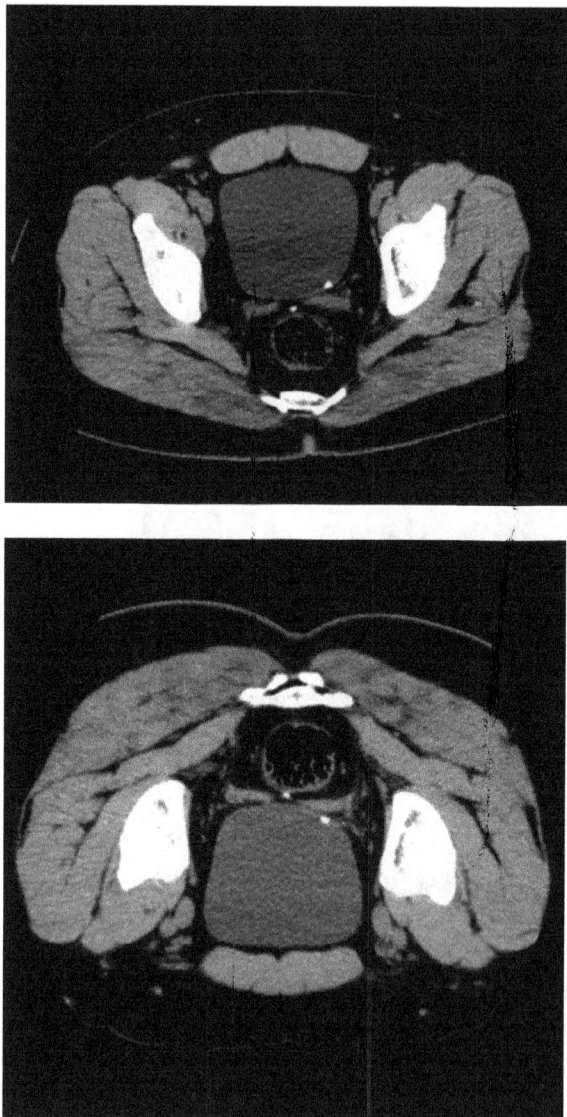

Figure 7. CT KUB axial supine and prone positions demonstrating a left-sided VUJ calculus.

stone, pyelonephritis or obstruction caused by lesion not visible on CT KUB. Such lesions include blood clot, papilla and Indinavir stone. Reviewing clinical picture can narrow these differentials. For instance, Indinavir stone occurs only in patients treated with this protease inhibitor for HIV and papillary necrosis is more common in diabetic patients with analgesic nephropathy.

Presence of ureteric thickening or narrowing at the site of obstruction is suggestive of ureteric stricture. Differentiating benign from malignant strictures would require a contrast-enhanced study or endoscopy. Extramural lesions causing obstruction include pelvic tumour, retroperitoneal mass and retroperitoneal fibrosis. Retroperitoneal fibrosis is classically seen as irregular, well-defined iso-dense mass surrounding aortic bifurcation. It usually follows the common iliac arteries and expands laterally to trap ureters. Differentiation from retroperitoneal malignancies may be difficult even after contrast-enhanced study. Enhancement after contrast administration is variable and depends on degree of metabolic activity and on-going fibrosis. Presence of bone destruction and displacement of major vessels will be suggestive of malignant process [41].

4.5. Limitations of CT KUB in diagnosis

Limitations of CT KUB include the fact that CT has limited spatial resolution. Therefore, its negative predictive value in completely excluding sub-millimetre calculi and small stone fragments is significantly less than its negative predictive value in excluding larger calculi (>4 mm). In addition, repeated use of CT in patients with recurrent urolithiasis can result in a substantial cumulative dose.

Details of pelvicalyceal anatomy may not be apparent on non-contrast-enhanced study. Intravenous urography or CT urography may be required if specific anatomical details are needed for making a management decision, for example, bifid system, stone in a calyceal diverticulum or narrow lower pole infundibulum.

CT KUB is a static study and the abnormalities related to urinary dynamics, that is, UPJ obstruction, obstructive versus residual dilatation of the collecting system, etc. cannot be appreciated. Complementing CT KUB with either MAG3 scan or dynamic Doppler ultrasound are some of the modifications recommended.

The other major limitation of the CT KUB is the risk of radiation exposure. Dose reduction by various technical modifications has been recommended [42]. In a systematic review, Xiang et al. [43] noted that lowering the dose of radiation of CT does not negatively impact the sensitivity and specificity in the diagnosis of stone and obstruction. They noted that low dose CT KUB has a cumulative sensitivity of 93% and specificity of about 97% [19].

In a meta-analysis reported by Niemann and colleagues [44] some 9 yeas back, they noted that dose reduction attempts resulted in mean dose of less than 3 mSv without jeopardizing the pooled sensitivity (97%) and specificity (95%). However in the last decade, there has been significant interval improvement with iterative reconstruction techniques, detector series and arrangements. These modifications have allowed a further reduction in dose to <1 mSv [45]. This is quite comparable to plain X-ray KUB at 0.7 mSv [46].

5. Conclusions

Non-contrast CT abdomen has emerged as first line investigation in suspected upper tract obstruction. Underlying cause can usually be ascertained on CT KUB. However, further investigations may be required to delineate/confirm underlying pathology like UPJ obstruction, differentiation between obstruction and residual dilatation, etc. CT KUB is not only extremely sensitive and specific in the diagnosis of stone; it is now used in the pre-operative nomograms in predicting success of various endourological interventions like PCNL an SWL. Determination of stone density, stone volume, stone composition, skin to stone distance, presence of ureteral wall oedema, perinephric oedema are highly predictive of stone free rate. CT recognition of various anomalies, presence of retro-renal colon, horse-shoe kidney, malrotation, etc. can help in better planning to avoid complication. One of the major limitations of CT is the radiation dose. Modification in technique and technological innovation has resulted in significant dose reduction from 4.5 mSV to about 1 mSv.

Author details

Mohammad Hammad Ather*, Wasim Memon, Wajahat Aziz and Mohammad Nasir Sulaiman

*Address all correspondence to: hammad.ather@aku.edu

Aga Khan University, Karachi, Pakistan

References

[1] Smith RC, Rosenfield AT, Choe KA, Essenmacher KR, Verga M, Glickman MG, Lange RC. Acute flank pain: Comparison of non-contrast-enhanced CT and intravenous urography. Radiology. 1995;**194**(3):789-794

[2] Ahmed F, Zafar AM, Khan N, Haider Z, Ather MH. A paradigm shift in imaging for renal colic—Is it time to say good-bye to an old trusted friend? International Journal of Surgery. 2010;**8**(3):252-256

[3] Sundaram CP, Saltzman B. Urolithiasis associated with protease inhibitors. Journal of Endourology. 1999;**13**(4):309-312

[4] Hoppe H, Studer R, Kessler TM, Vock P, Studer UE, Thoeny HC. Alternate or additional findings to stone disease on unenhanced computerized tomography for acute flank pain can impact management. The Journal of Urology. 2006;**175**(5):1725-1730

[5] Smith-Bindman R, Aubin C, Bailitz J, Bengiamin RN, Camargo Jr CA, Corbo J, Dean AJ, Goldstein RB, Griffey RT, Jay GD, Kang TL. Ultrasonography versus computed tomography for suspected nephrolithiasis. New England Journal of Medicine. 2014;**371**(12):1100-1110

[6] Thomsen HS, Morcos SK. Contrast media and the kidney: European Society of Urogenital Radiology (ESUR) guidelines. British Journal of Radiology. 2003;**76**(908):513-518

[7] Shokeir AA, El-Diasty T, Eassa W, Mosbah A, El-Ghar MA, Mansour O, Dawaba M, El-Kappany H. Diagnosis of ureteral obstruction in patients with compromised renal function: The role of noninvasive imaging modalities. Journal of Urology. 2004;**171**(6):2303-2306

[8] Smith RC, Verga M, McCarthy S, et al. Diagnosis ofacute flank pain: Value of unenhanced helical CT. AJR. American Journal of Roentgenology. 1996;**166**(1):97-101

[9] Dalrymple NC, Verga M, Anderson KR, et al. The value of unenhanced helical computerized tomography in the management of acute flank pain. Journal of Urology. 1998;**159**(3):735-740

[10] Ather MH, Jafri AH, Sulaiman MN. Diagnostic accuracy of ultrasonography compared to unenhanced CT for stone and obstruction in patients with renal failure. BMC Medical Imaging. 2004;**4**(1):2

[11] Ege G, Akman H, Kuzucu K, et al. Acute ureterolithiasis: Incidence of secondary signs on unenhanced helical CT and influence on patient management. Clinical Radiology. 2003;**58**(12):990-994

[12] Ziemba J, Guzzo TJ, Ramchandani P. Evaluation of the patient with asymptomatic microscopic hematuria. Academic Radiology. 2015;**22**(8):1034-1037

[13] Khan N, Ather MH, Ahmed F, Zafar AM, Khan A. Has the significance of incidental findings on unenhanced computed tomography for urolithiasis been overestimated? A retrospective review of over 800 patients. Arab Journal of Urology. 2012;**10**(2):149-154

[14] Millet I, Sebbane M, Molinari N, Pages-Bouic E, Curros-Doyon F, Riou B, Taourel P. Systematic unenhanced CT for acute abdominal symptoms in the elderly patients improves both emergency department diagnosis and prompt clinical management. European Radiology. 2017;**27**(2):868-877

[15] Ahmad NA, Ather MH, Rees J. Incidental diagnosis of diseases on un-enhanced helical computed tomography performed for ureteric colic. BMC Urology. 2003;**3**:2

[16] Ather MH, Faizullah K, Achakzai I, Siwani R, Irani F. Alternate and incidental diagnoses on noncontrast-enhanced spiral computed tomography for acute flank pain. Urology Journal. 2009;**6**(1):14-18

[17] Ather MH, Memon W, Rees J. Clinical impact of incidental diagnosis of disease on non-contrast-enhanced helical CT for acute ureteral colic. Seminars in Ultrasound, CT and MRI. 2005;**26**(1):20-23

[18] Li J, Kennedy D, Levine M, Kumar A, Mullen J. Absent hematuria and expensive computerized tomography: Case characteristics of emergency urolithiasis. Journal of Urology. 2001;**165**(3):782-784

[19] Bird VG, Gomez-Marin O, Leveillee R, Sfakianakis G, Rivas LA, Amendola MA. A comparison of unenhanced helical computerized tomography findings and renal obstruction determined by furosemide 99m-technetium mercaptoacetyltriglycine diuretic scintirenography for patients with acute renal colic. Journal of Urology. 2002;**167**(4):1597-1603

[20] Kravchick S, Stepnov E, Lebedev V, Linov L, Leibovici O, Ben-Horin CL, Trejo L, Peled R, Cytron S. Non-contrast computerized tomography (CT KUB) and dynamic renal scintigraphy (DRS) in the patients with refractory renal colic. European Journal of Radiology. 2006;**58**(2):301-306

[21] Ghani KR, Andonian S, Bultitude M, Desai M, Giusti G, Okhunov Z, Preminger GM, de la Rosette J. Percutaneous nephrolithotomy: Update, trends, and future directions. Europen Journal of Urology. 2016;**70**(2):382-396

[22] Farhan M, Nazim SM, Salam B, Ather MH. Prospective evaluation of outcome of percutaneous nephrolithotomy using the 'STONE' nephrolithometry score: A single-centre experience. Arab Journal of Urology. 2015;**13**(4):264-269

[23] Gökce MI, Esen B, Gülpınar B, Süer E, Gülpınar Ö. External validation of triple D score in an elderly (≥65 Years) population for prediction of success following shockwave lithotripsy. Journal of Endourology. 2016;**30**(9):1009-1016

[24] Park HS, Gong MK, Yoon CY, Moon du G, Cheon J, Choi YD. Computed tomography-based novel prediction model for the outcome of shockwave lithotripsy in proximal ureteral stones. Journal of Endourology. 2016;**30**(7):810-816

[25] Akhtar S, Ather MH. Appropriate cutoff for treatment of distal ureteral stones by single session in situ extracorporeal shock wave lithotripsy. Urology. 2005;**66**(6):1165-1168

[26] Ather MH, Memon A. Therapeutic efficacy of Dornier MPL 9000 for prevesical calculi as judged by efficiency quotient. Journal of Endourology. 2000;**14**(7):551-553

[27] Sarica K, Kafkasli A, Yazici Ö, Çetinel AC, Demirkol MK, Tuncer M, Şahin C, Eryildirim B. Ureteral wall thickness at the impacted ureteral stone site: A critical predictor for success rates after SWL. Urolithiasis. 2015;**43**(1):83-88

[28] Soomro HU, Hammad Ather M, Salam B. Comparison of ureteric stone size, on bone window versus standard soft-tissue window settings, on multi-detector non-contrast computed tomography. Arab Journal of Urology. 2016;**14**(3):198-202

[29] Nazim SM, Ather MH, Khan N. Measurement of ureteric stone diameter in different planes on multidetector computed tomography—Impact on the clinical decision making. Urology. 2014;**83**(2):288-292

[30] Preminger GM, Assimos DG, Lingeman JE, Nakada SY, Pearle MS, Wolf Jr JS, AUA Nephrolithiasis Guideline Panel). Journal of Urology. 2005;**173**(6):1991-2000

[31] Zanetti SP, Boeri L, Catellani M, Gallioli A, Trinchieri A, Sarica K, Montanari E. Retrograde intrarenal surgery (RIRS), regular and small sized percutaneous nephrolithot-

omy (PCNL) in daily practice: European Association of Urology Section of Urolithiasis (EULIS) Survey. Archivio Italiano di Urologia, Andrologia. 2016 Oct 5;88(3):212-216

[32] Thomas K, Smith NC, Hegarty N, Glass JM. The Guy's stone score—Grading the complexity of percutaneous nephrolithotomy procedures. Urology. 2011;**78**:277-281

[33] Okhunov Z, Friedlander JI, George AK, Duty BD, Moreira DM, Srinivasan AK, Hillelsohn J, Smith AD, Okeke Z. S.T.O.N.E. nephrolithometry: Novel surgical classification system for kidney calculi. Urology. 2013;**81**:1154-1159

[34] Smith A, Averch TD, Shahrour K, Opondo D, Daels FP, Labate G, Turna B, de la Rosette JJ. A nephrolithometric nomogram to predict treatment success of percutaneous nephrolithotomy. Journal of Urology. 2013;**190**:149-156

[35] Tailly TO, Okhunov Z, Nadeau BR, Huynh MJ, Labadie K, Akhavein A, Violette PD, Olvera-Posada D, Alenezi H, Amann J, Bird VG, Landman J, Smith AD, Denstedt JD, Razvi H. Multicenter external validation and comparison of stone scoring systems in predicting outcomes after percutaneous nephrolithotomy. Journal of Endourology. 2016;**30**(5):594-601

[36] AslZare M, Darabi MR, Shakiba B, Gholami-Mahtaj L. Colonic perforation during percutaneous nephrolithotomy: An 18-year experience. Canadian Urological Association journal. 2014;**8**(5-6):E323–E326

[37] Chalasani V1, Bissoon D, Bhuvanagir AK, Mizzi A, Dunn IB. Should PCNL patients have a CT in the prone position preoperatively? Canadian Journal of Urology. 2010;**17**(2):5082-5086

[38] Fernbach SK, Maizels M, Conway JJ. Ultrasound grading of hydronephrosis: Introduction to the system used by the Society for Fetal Urology. Pediatric Radiology. 1993;**23**(6):478-480

[39] Ito Y, Kikuchi E, Tanaka N, Miyajima A, Mikami S, Jinzaki M, Oya M. Preoperative hydronephrosis grade independently predicts worse pathological outcomes in patients undergoing nephroureterectomy for upper tract urothelial carcinoma. The Journal of Urology. 2011;**185**(5):1621-1626

[40] Atta H, Abdel-Gawad EA, ElAzab A, Saleh M, Abbas WA, Soliman R, Imam H. Whole ureteric course delineation assessment using noncontrast curved sagittal oblique reformatted CT. The Egyptian Journal of Radiology and Nuclear Medicine. 2016;**47**(3):1103-1110

[41] Cronin CG, Lohan DG, Blake MA, Roche C, McCarthy P, Murphy JM. Retroperitoneal fibrosis: A review of clinical features and imaging findings. American Journal of Roentgenology. 2008;**191**(2):423-431

[42] Ather MH, Memon WA. Stones: Impact of dose reduction on CT detection of urolithiasis. Nature Review Urology. 2009;**6**(10):526-527

[43] Xiang H, Chan M, Brown V, Huo YR, Chan L, Ridley L. Systematic review and meta-analysis of the diagnostic accuracy of low-dose computed tomography of the kidneys, ureters and bladder for urolithiasis. Journal of Medical Imaging and Radiation Oncology. 2017

[44] Niemann T, Kollmann T, Bongartz G. Diagnostic performance of low-dose CT for the detection of urolithiasis: A meta-analysis. AJR American Journal of Roentgenology. 2008;**191**:396-401. Jan 31. doi: 10.1111/1754-9485.12587

[45] Wall BF, Hart D. Revised radiation doses for typical X-ray examinations. Report on a recent review of doses to patients from medical X-ray examinations in the UK by NRPB. National Radiological Protection Board. British Journal of Radiology. 1997;**70**:437-439

[46] Mettler FA, Huda W, Yoshizumi TT, Mahesh M. Effective doses in radiology and diagnostic nuclear medicine. Radiology. 2008;**248**:254-263

7

Advances in Cardiac Computed Tomography

Karthik Ananthasubramaniam, Nishtha Sareen and
Gjeka Rudin

Abstract

Coronary cardiac computed tomography (CCTA) has seen rapid improvements in technology including hardware and postprocessing techniques that have contributed to its rapid growth and enabled it to remain in the forefront on diagnostic imaging. Important technological advances include wider detectors for greater coverage with less gantry rotation times, dual-source computed tomography (CT) with improved temporal resolution, dual-energy CT where simultaneous imaging at different energies to increase the contrast difference between different tissues enhances diagnostic accuracy, and emergence of spectral CT to enhance atherosclerotic imaging through nanoparticle technology. Software advances include iterative reconstruction methodologies to reduce noise and radiation doses, plaque imaging and quantification tools to assess plaque morphology and stenosis severity. Processing advances using computational fluid dynamics now enables the determination of fractional flow reserve (FFR). Another important advancement in CCTA physiologic imaging is CCTA perfusion imaging to detect ischemia and compares favorably with myocardial perfusion imaging and coronary angiographic stenosis. Finally, large registry studies and single-center studies have now been published assessing the incremental value of coronary calcium score, CT plaque severity of disease and have demonstrated that the CCTA carries strong prognostic value over and above traditional risk assessment in predicting adverse outcomes.

Keywords: coronary computed tomography angiography, CT advances, CT perfusion imaging, CT fractional flow reserve, prognosis

1. Introduction

Cardiac computed tomography (CT), specifically coronary CT angiography (CCTA), has made major progress and currently is one of the leading noninvasive modalities for diagnosis of coronary artery disease (CAD) during the past years. The progress can be attributed to many reasons but chief among them are progressive establishment of CCTA as a front-line imaging modality for diagnosis and prognosis of coronary artery disease. This was shown by randomized trials and multicenter registry-based evidence totaling tens of thousands of patients. The second important factor contributing to the rapid rise of CT is advancements in CT technology in hardware and new software solutions, such as refined image reconstruction methods. Due to such advances, CCTA has enjoyed progressive enhancements in image quality and achieved better temporal and spatial resolution. Most importantly, CCTA is now possible with much lower radiation doses than a traditional SPECT scan. Furthermore, with some advanced scanners and scanning methodologies current doses approach the 1-milliseivert range which is a mind-boggling advance since the inception of the technique not too long ago in early 2000.

2. Historical perspective

The first CCTA was performed using electron-beam CT in the 1990s [1]. X-ray beams were produced by an electron beam, and were directed toward stationary targets around the patient. This image was produced at a temporal resolution of 100 ms but was insufficient to image coronaries given a slice thickness of 1.5–3 mm. However, this laid the groundwork for manufacturers to move the field forward with the multislice CST (MSCT), and the first four-slice CT in 2000 for coronary visualization had a gantry rotation time of 500 ms and a temporal resolution of 250 ms [2]. Subsequently, this evolved into 16-, 40-, and then 64-slice CT. There was slight improvement in slice thickness but now with an ability to image the heart in 4–8 heart beats. This led to reduction in less breath hold times, lesser artifacts, higher speed of contrast use, and thus lesser contrast volume. Multiple studies have now established the diagnostic accuracy of 64-slice CCTA using retrospective helical acquisition techniques [3, 4].

3. Equipment advances in CCTA

Although 64-slice CCTA remains the workhorse of coronary imaging, manufacturers have worked continuously to move technology forward. While some have just increased the number of slices in detectors which then translates to greater scan coverage and thus acquisition of the image needed in shorter number of heart beats, others have used dual-scanner technology (dual-source CT at 90° angle) to enable increasing temporal resolution by a factor of 2.

1. **Wide detector CT:** By increasing the number of CT scanner detector width (number of slices), a great amount of coverage of the heart in a single gantry rotation can be achieved. Each detector row has a width (collimation) of 0.5–0.6 mm. So, a 64-slice detector can cover 64 × 0.5 = about 38 mm of scan coverage. Thus, a wider detector array such as 320-detector CT would provide a single gantry rotation coverage of 320 × 0.5 = 160 mm. Since the approximate coverage to scan the entire heart is about 120 mm, a 65-slice scanner would need about 4 gantry rotations, and a 320-slice scanner could cover the entire heart in one rotation. The disadvantage of wide detector CT is that due to extra rotation at the beginning and end of scan to avoid cone beam reconstruction artifact (over ranging), there is extra radiation burden to patient and also additionally areas not in the field of interest also being exposed

to radiation. **Table 1** provides a comparison of CT scan characteristics and acquisition parameters over a wide range of detector widths, and **Figure 1** provides a comparative illustration of detector coverage depending on the number of detector rows in MSCT.

2. **Dual-source CT:** The principle behind dual-source CT scanners is two sources of radiation with the corresponding detectors set at 90° to each other. Thus, image acquisitions are much faster cutting short time by 50% which is a key factor in improving image quality by decreasing artifacts related to breath hold [5]. Furthermore, temporal resolution is also improved (83 ms). Whereas a 64-slice single-detector MSCT requires half of gantry rotation (180°) for image reconstruction, the same information can be obtained with a DSCT for one-fourth of the gantry rotation (90°). The heart rate factor also is of less importance with DSCT although HR has to be steady and significant tachycardia is not optimal [6]. Another important factor is that radiation doses are also decreased even though two radiation sources are used because the radiation source is on for less than half of the time narrowing electrocardiogram (ECG)-pulsing window for image acquisition given the DSCT technology. Investigators have now pushed the limits of this scanner further with recent high-pitched prospective gated acquisition which enables whole heart acquisition in250 ms in a single heart beat [7]. This if combined with excellent heart rate controls (<60 bpm) can achieve extremely low radiation doses reaching 1 milliseivert [8]. **Figure 2** shows the CT image quality with 320-slice and with high-pitch prospective CT-scanning technology.

3. **Dual-energy CT:** Apart from using dual source, using different energies could have the advantage of assessing iodine from other tissues by varying the voltage (kilovolts). This has the impact of demonstrating the nonlinear variation of different tissues at varying voltages. This could help improve contrast between structures. The dual-energy concept can either be with two sources alternating the voltages or by using detectors with elements capable of detecting varying energies. Although the full role of this technique is not clear, it could help in separating calcium from contrast-enhanced lumen and in detecting perfusion defects in CT perfusion imaging [9]. One other intriguing advantage of dual energy is in radiation reduction. By using virtual-unenhanced image reconstruction (VUE) techniques employing iodine subtraction algorithms, early studies have shown that it is possible to obtain calcium score and contrast-enhanced corona angiographic information from a single image which can translate to dose reduction ranging from 20 to 50% by avoiding non-contrast calcium score scans [10, 11]. **Table 2** outlines some of the applications of dual-energy CT technology

4. **Spectral CT:** Along the same lines as dual-source CT, spectral CT also adopts the principle of varying photo energies to characterize different tissues and can be used in conjunction with nanoparticles to further characterize atherosclerosis. In contrast to two levels of energy in dual source which poses limits to detecting different energy spectra, a photon-sensitive spectral CT detector can sample a bin the incident photon based on the current pulse generated at a specific energy level. This allows multiple photon energies to be sampled. This technology is in its earliest stages but studies are being done and detector technology is being evaluated [12, 13]. **Table 2** outlines some of the applications of spectral energy CT technology.

5. **Flat panel CT:** Flat panel CT as the name implies employ a flat panel of digital detectors achieving isotropic resolution (0.2 mm) and represent a totally different technology from the current generation of CT scanners in every aspect. These provide volumetric coverage

Number of detector slices	4	16	64	256	320
Detector collimation (mm)	4 × 1 4 × 1.25	16 × 0.5 16 × 0.625 16 × 0.75	64 × 0.5 64 × 0.65 2 × 32 × 0.6*	2 × 128 × 0.625*	320 × 0.5
Slice width (mm)	1.3	0.8–1.0	0.5–0.8	0.6	0.5
Spatial resolution (mm)	1	0.6	0.4–0.6	0.4	0.35
Rotation time (s)	0.5	0.375–0.420	0.33–0.40	0.27	0.35
Temporal resolution (ms)	250	188–210	165–200‡	135	175§
z-axis coverage (mm)	4–5	8–12	32–40	80	160
Scan time to cover the entire heart volume (s)	40	15–20	6–12	1–2	>1

* Double z-sampling. ‡Temporal resolution can be improved to 83 ms with dual source acquisitions in single-energy applications. §Temporal resolution can be improved to 58 ms with multisegment acquisition and multisegment reconstruction

Abbreviation: MDCT, multidetector CT

Schuleri K.H. *et al. Nat. Rev. Cardiol.*

Table 1. Technical and acquisition parameters for cardiac examinations with MDCT.

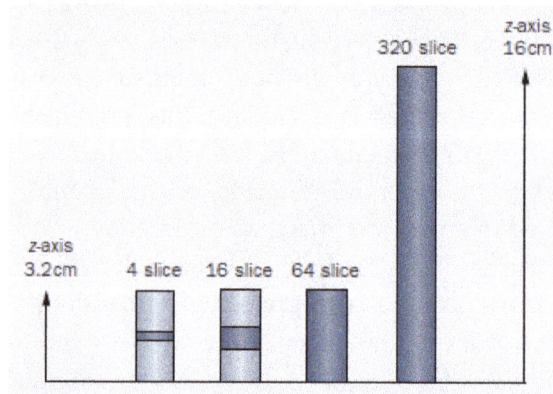

Figure 1. Technical progression of scanner technology. Improvement in coverage of the z-axis with 4-, 16-, and 64-slice detector rows, relative to wide-range 320-slice detector rows. With the wide-range technology, the entire heart is covered in one gantry rotation. Schuleri, K. H. *et al. Nat. Rev. Cardiol.* **6**, 699–710 (2009); doi:10.1038/nrcardio.2009.172.

of the entire heart and deliver extremely high spatial resolution capable of imaging distal small coronary arteries, much better stented lumen delineation, and less artifacts from calcium. The major limitations currently are poor temporal resolution (2 s) and poor contrast resolution (5–10 Hounsfield units compared to 1 Hounsfield unit for MSCT) [14]. Currently as most evidence is limited to preclinical and animal studies, further research and studies are needed in this field.

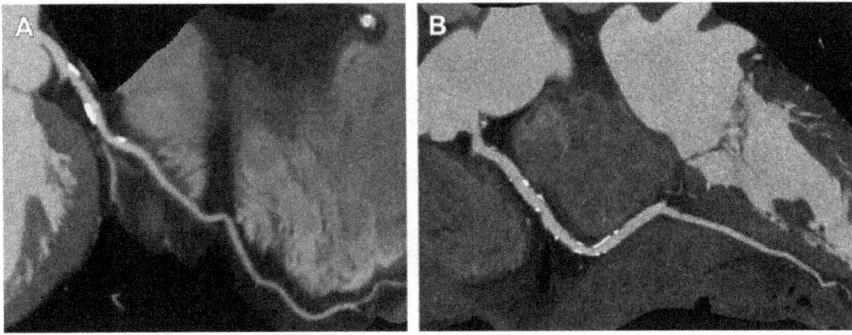

Figure 2. (A) Coronary CT with 320-slice CT. (B) Coronary CT with high-pitch prospective scanning. Achenbach S et al. Cardiol Clin 30 (2012) 1–8.

Parameter	Dual source	kVp switching	Double-layer detector
Method	Two X-ray tubes with 90° offset each tube can operate at a two different kVp energy levels	One X-ray tube voltage switches between low- and high-energy setting (e.g., 80 and 140 kVp) continuously during spiral 360° acquisitions	One X-ray tube exposes a detector system consisting of two layers. The first (top) layer encountered by photons absorbs most of the low energy (soft spectrum), whereas the bottom detector layer absorbs the remaining higher energy (hard spectrum)
Advantages	No significant lag time between low-energy and high-energy scans	No image mis-registration Monochromatic image acquisitions possible	No time lag for kVP switching; suitable for rapid imaging in cardiac motion Photon counting possible to sort spectral subranges in order to form images based on their attenuation profile; enables high-sensitivity acquisitions for targeted contrast agents
Disadvantages	Image mis-registration possible Reduced temporal resolution Currently only polychromatic image acquisitions	Dual-energy time lag between low and high energy depends on switching time Limited temporal resolution Currently only polychromatic image acquisitions	X-rays are generated as polychromatic beam Limited temporal resolution

Schuleri, K. H. *et al. Nat. Rev. Cardiol.*

Table 2. Current applications of dual-energy and spectral CT techniques.

4. Advances in temporal and spatial resolution

Continuing advances are being made in the development of faster scanners and in the pipeline is GE.

Revolution CT TM (GE Healthcare, Milwaukee, WI) with a wider z-axis coverage and a gantry rotation time of 0.2 s providing wider z-axis coverage and single beat image acquisition (Revolution CT 2014; available at www.gehealthcare) and the Seimens Somatom Force TM

(Seimens AG, Erlangen, Germany) providing very high temporal resolution of 66 ms and spatial resolution of 0.24 s and able to image the heart in a single beat with Turbo Flash mode with the need for breath hold. These superb technological advances need formal clinical validation (Somatom Force TM available at www.seimens.com).

Typical MSCT detectors have solid-state ceramic detectors which help to convert X-rays to visible light followed by conversion to analog electrical signal which then gets converted to a digital signal for image formation. The detectors all have septate electric boards which are all then linked to each other.

However, with breakthrough in technology one vendor has introduced a new detector system called Stellar Detector (Stellar Detector TM, Siemens AG, Erlangen, Germany) which combines all detectors into single electric board and claims superior spatial resolution and decrease in image noise.

GE has introduced Gemstone Detector which is a garnet-based substance which has much shorter decay and after-glow times enabling much rapid processing of signal improving spatial resolution and decreasing image noise. This concept has proven useful in reading CTAs in stent, determining intrastent diameter and area due to decrease in image noise [15]. It appears to be compatible with dual-energy scanners too.

5. Software advances in CCTA

a. **Iterative reconstruction (IR):** Although filtered back-projection remains a common method of reconstruction, IR techniques are more commonly being used where image information is used to simulate expected image based on CT measurements and then these simulated data are modified in subsequent image reconstruction. This technique has been shown to reduce image noise and reduction in radiation doses [16, 17]. **Figure 3** shows an example of noise reduction with IR.

b. **Motion correction:** Motion artifact is one of the most important limitations in CCTA affecting overall accuracy. Techniques such as heart rate control and faster scanning with wide detector and dual source technologies are ways to limit motion artifact. Recently, GE Healthcare has introduced Snapshot FreezeTM where the software evaluates multiple adjacent cardiac phases within the same cardiac cycle to evaluate and plot coronary artery motion and eliminate residual coronary motion artifact. This promises to further minimize motion artifact improving the image quality and interpretability [18].

c. **Arrhythmia detection:** Occurrence of arrhythmias causes significant issues with missing data and artifacts in CCTA. Advances in arrhythmia detection include using of complex arrhythmia detection algorithms to enable stopping the scan when arrhythmia occurs and restarting scans after arrhythmia subsides to enable capturing data in the right cardiac cycles (Seimens Healthcare, Forcheim, Germany). Other advances include image reconstruction using identical filling concepts isovolumetric phases (which contain best image data) are used in image reconstruction [19].

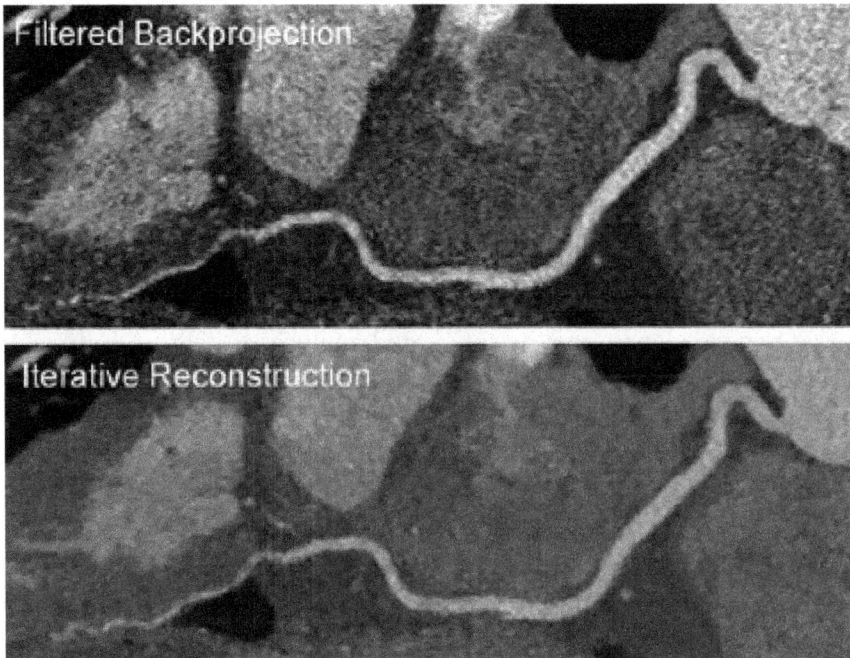

Figure 3. Image noise reduction with iterative reconstruction technology. Achenbach S et al. Cardiol Clin 30 (2012) 1–8.

d. **Radiation reduction:** Apart from prospective gating, traditional ECG tube current modulation, wide detector coverage, and dual source high-pitch-scanning techniques all of which dramatically reduce radiation; further advances are being done to do real-time modulation of attenuation-based adjustments in tube potential, thus driving radiation doses down even further (Care Dose4D TM; Seimens Healthcare, Forcheim, Germany).

6. Advances in CCTA beyond traditional noninvasive coronary angiography

CCTA has been recognized as a cost-effective noninvasive diagnostic modality [20]. Evolving literature has established that revascularization has clinical benefit when performed in stenosis with hemodynamic significance [21, 22]. An intermediate stenosis on CT scan is not a good predictor of physiological significance [23–25]; this calls for additional tools which can provide complementary physiological data to available anatomy. Noninvasive fractional flow reserve (FFR) evaluation on CT, myocardial CT perfusion, and transluminal attenuation gradient (TAG) are the three techniques with clinical evidence. We will talk briefly about these in this section of the chapter.

6.1. Noninvasive fractional flow reserve evaluation on CCTA: physiology

FFR is defined as the ratio of the mean coronary pressure distal to a coronary stenosis to the mean aortic pressure during maximal coronary blood flow. An FFR value of 0.80 or less suggests lesion-specific hemodynamic significance [26]. Incorporation of FFR in CT does not call for any modification of CCTA protocols, additional image acquisition, or administration of medications. The calculation is performed by segmentation of coronary tree and left ventricular mass and application of computational fluid dynamics (see **Figure 4**). While no adenosine administration is performed, the conditions to simulate the same can be established.

6.1.1. Clinical evidence

FFR incorporation into routine CT has been compared to visual estimation alone in multiple studies. We now have evidence from an integrated analysis of data from three prospective, international, and multicenter trials, which assessed the diagnostic performance of FFR CT using invasive FFR as a reference standard [27]. The key trials outlining the value of CT FFR were the DISCOVER-FLOW, DeFACTO, and the NXT trials. These studies with cumulative over 600 patients concluded that with intermediate coronary stenosis, FFR CT remained both highly sensitive and specific with respect to the diagnosis of ischemia. Specifically, CT FFR had higher sensitivity than CT (81 vs. 53%) Additionally, when compared to invasive FFR evaluation, FFR CT had higher diagnostic accuracy (86 vs. 71%) in the identification of hemodynamically significant lesions.

More exciting data have suggested an economic benefit associated with a 12% reduction in adverse cardiovascular events at 1 year with the use of CT FFR when compared to angiography with stenosis-based PCI [28]. In their study, Hlatky et al. applied a decision analysis comparing five clinical strategies constructed as follows: (1) angiography with stenosis-based PCI; (2) angiography with FFR-guided PCI; (3) coronary CTA followed by angiography and

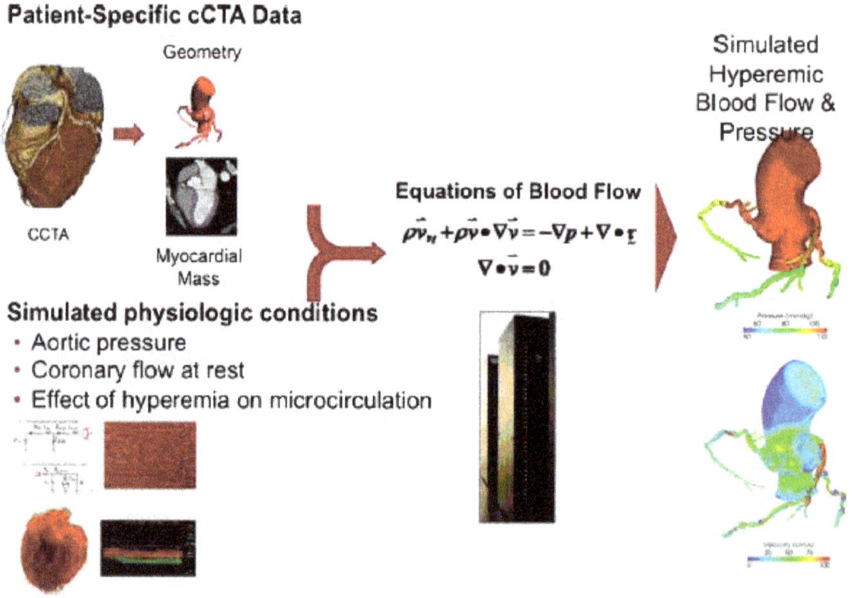

Figure 4. Simplified scheme of computational fluid dynamic techniques for simulating hyperemic flow and pressure applied to CTA data. Min JK. JCCT 2011;5(5);301-9.

stenosis-based PCI; (4) coronary CTA followed by angiography and FFR-guided PCI and (5) coronary CTA–FFR CT followed by FFR CT-guided PCI. The projected initial management costs were highest for angiography with stenosis-based PCI and lowest for the coronary CTA–FFR CT followed by FFR CT-guided PCI. Inspired from this concept, we now have a prospective, controlled utility trial evaluating patients with an intermediate likelihood of CAD PLATFORM (Prospective Longitudinal Trial of FFR CT: Outcome and Resource IMpacts) [29]. Patients referred for noninvasive evaluation formed the first cohort and those referred for invasive coronary angiogram comprised the second cohort. These were evaluated by using standard care approach (first phase) and coronary CTA with physiologic FFR evaluation (second stage). The primary result was that among those with intended ICA (FFRCT-guided = 193; usual care = 187), no-obstructive CAD was found at ICA in 24 (12%) in the CTA/FFRCT arm and 137 (73%) in the usual care arm ($P < 0.0001$), with similar mean cumulative radiation exposure (9.9 vs. 9.4 mSv, $P = 0.20$). Invasive coronary angiography was cancelled in 61% after receiving CTA/FFRCT results. Clinical event rates within 90 days were low in both the arms. This is just another example of how CT FFR is a feasible and safe alternative to invasive angiography and was associated with a significantly lower rate of invasive angiography showing no-obstructive CAD (**Figure 5a** and **b**).

We await the results of the multicentric registry ADVANCE (assessing diagnostic value of noninvasive FFRCT in coronary care) which will evaluate the clinical and economic impacts of FFR CT (NCT02499679).

6.1.2. Clinical applications

Enhanced specificity and accuracy in the available data has established FFR incorporation to CT as a promising new dimension in noninvasive modalities. It may serve as a "gate-keeper" to escalation to invasive coronary angiography in suitable patient population. We await many more exciting studies to define the niche for its role in daily clinical practice.

6.1.3. Limitations

1. Presence of heavy calcification, mis-registration, and motion artifacts may affect FFR calculation with CT since the calculation relies on accurate anatomic models.

2. Computational simulation of adenosine-induced hyperemia is performed without the actual use of adenosine which may incorporate errors, especially in the presence of microvascular dysfunction.

3. Presence of viable or scarred myocardium also affects the FFR value.

6.2. Myocardial CT perfusion (myocardial CTP)

Myocardial CTP protocol is composed of a stress phase acquisition and a rest phase acquisition, as with nuclear myocardial perfusion imaging [30]. Iodinated contrast is administered in both the stress and rest acquisition (60–75 ml for each acquisition), for a total contrast dose of

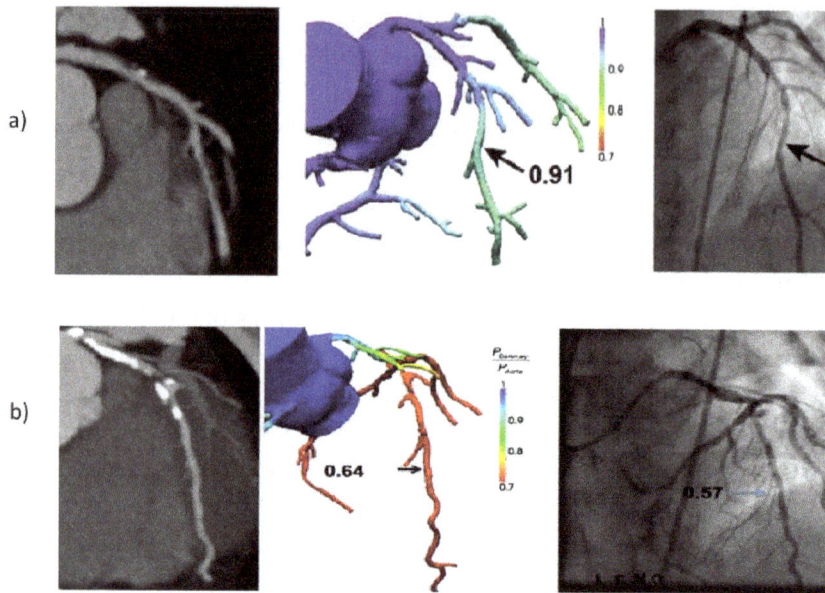

Figure 5. (a) Examples of a no-obstructive CAD on CTA and corresponding normal CT FFR and correlative coronary angiographic FFR of patient from the DeFACTO study. (b) Example of patient with obstructive coronary disease in left anterior descending coronary artery on CTA and corresponding abnormal CT FFR and correlative coronary angiographic FFR from the DeFACTO study.

approximately 130–150 ml. The pharmacological stress agents include adenosine, dipyridamole or regadenosin. Although it has been shown in many studies that pharmacological and exercise stress testing have comparable diagnostic characteristics, exercise is the preferred method of stress in myocardial perfusion imaging when possible [31].

There are two ways in which to set up a stress and rest myocardial CTP protocol based on the order of scan acquisition, namely stress phase first followed by rest phase, or vice versa (as illustrated in **Figure 6**).

As expected, the main consideration is that the first scan will be a "clean" acquisition, and that the contrast used in the first acquisition can cross-contaminate the second acquisition if the interval between the scans is less than approximately 30 min. On the other hand, when doing a stress phase acquisition first, the detection of myocardial ischemia is optimized by not having contamination of contrast; however, the second scan can underestimate the presence of infarct in the myocardium if a short scan interval is used. This is so because the contrast from the stress scan would accumulate in an area of myocardial infarct due to the slow wash-out phenomenon, leading to persistent perfusion defect during rest imaging. Thus, possible underestimation of myocardial infarction specifically if the second scan is done within 10 min of the first one. A coronary CTA acquisition can be acquired simultaneously with the rest acquisition, and beta-blockers and sublingual nitroglycerin can be given to optimize the second scan (**Table 3**)

6.2.1. Clinical evidence

The smaller initial studies have been conducted at various institutions with differences in protocols and reference standards. The unifying conclusion is that perfusion defects on myocardial

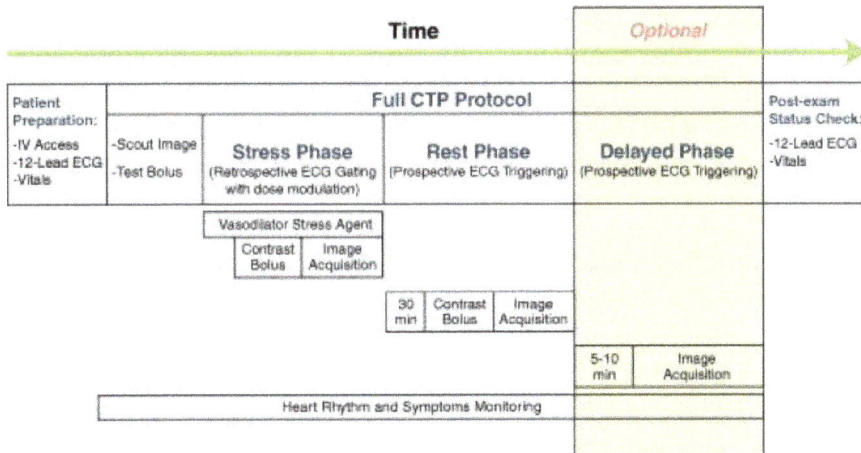

Figure 6. Full CTP Protocol: The protocol includes patient preparation and post-examination checkup (including an optional delayed phase acquisition (shaded box). All steps are as listed in sequence. Heart rhythm and symptoms are monitored throughout the entire examination. (Adopted with permission from Ref [31]).

Sequence	Advantages	Disadvantages
Stress → Rest	Better sensitivity of stress scan (ability to detect ischemia). Coronary CTA can be optimized with second acquisition by giving medications without interfering with perfusion assessment	Contrast contamination, leading to appearance of late-contrast enhancement during rest acquisition (decreased sensitivity for infarct)
Rest → Stress	Ability to stop protocol after rest phase (if no or minimal disease is evident). Better sensitivity of rest scan (ability to detect infarct)	Contrast contamination, leading to appearance of late-contrast enhancement during stress acquisition (decreased sensitivity for ischemia). Beta-blocker given during first acquisition can underestimate myocardial ischemia

Table 3. Advantages and disadvantages of different CTP protocol sequences (adopted with permission [30]).

CTP correlate well with those on SPECT and also in some studies with stenosis on quantitative coronary angiography. We briefly present some of these studies.

George et al. [32] used a 64-detector MDCT or a 256-detector MDCT for image acquisition with adenosine as the stress agent. The combined analysis of all patients (including both scanner types) in this study showed a per-vessel territory sensitivity, specificity, positive-predictive value (PPV), and negative-predictive value (NPV) of 75, 87, 60, and 93%, respectively, when compared with QCA and SPECT. Using the same stress agent, Blankstein et al. [33] acquired myocardial CTP images using a dual-source CT scanner, which has higher temporal resolution. They confirmed that myocardial CTP is equivalent to SPECT in detecting coronary artery stenosis by QCA, with comparative sensitivity and specificity to prior study. One interesting derivation from this study was similar radiation exposure with full myocardial CTP when compared to SPECT MPI. Rocha-Filho et al. [34] demonstrated that adding perfusion information obtained from stress myocardial CTP to coronary CTA improves all diagnostic characteristics of CTA alone, with most significant impact on specificity and PPV. The size and severity evaluation of perfusion defect at rest and stress have been shown to be concordant between myocardial CTP and SPECT [35]. This concordance has been further validated in the form of excellent validation by a five-point scale and a total perfusion deficit score [36]. Myocardial CTP has proven equivalent to SPECT in the detection of stenosis found on QCA (sensitivity and specificity: 88 and 79% for myocardial CTP and 69 and 71% for SPECT, p = NS) with dipyridamole on a 64-detector MDCT scanner [37].

An additional concept is the utilization of dynamic myocardial perfusion. Ho et al. [38] demonstrated that stress and rest dynamic perfusion imaging can detect myocardial perfusion defect with good diagnostic accuracy when compared with SPECT MPI (per-segment sensitivity, specificity, PPV, and NPV of 83, 78, 79, and 82%, respectively) and with QCA (per-segment sensitivity, specificity, PPV, and NPV of 95, 65, 78, and 79%, respectively) and allows for defining time-attenuation curves with the potential for quantification of myocardial blood flow. This comes at the price of a much higher radiation dose when compared to static imaging.

6.2.2. Limitations

1. CT-related artifacts should be recognized in an attempt to minimize them. One major culprit is beam hardening, which is a phenomenon that occurs when X-ray beams pass through objects of high density, leading to a selective attenuation of lower-energy beams and increased mean energy of the remaining beams. The resulting appearance is a hypoenhanced region that may mimic areas of true perfusion defect. Such hypoenhanced region is usually triangular and appears to originate from the region of high attenuation next to it, and does not conform to vascular territories [39]. A particularly common location includes the basal inferolateral wall, due to proximity to the descending aorta with iodinated contrast and dense vertebral bodies. Attempts to develop an algorithm to minimize beam-hardening artifacts are ongoing, with the use of iterative reconstruction.

2. Myocardial CTP is also prone to motion artifacts similar to coronary CTA, particularly during the stress phase acquisition, due to the increased heart rate. Cardiac motion during the acquisition leads to hypoenhanced areas that can mimic true perfusion defects. Enhanced temporal resolution of CT has led to marked decrease in this artifact.

It cannot be emphasized enough that a careful review of multiple phases of the cardiac cycle is a robust method to differentiate a true perfusion defect from an artifact.

In summary,

- Myocardial CTP has the potential to become a robust clinical tool for the evaluation of chest pain patients.

- The available literature is in a very preliminary stage with only single-center preliminary experiences. These are flawed by referral bias and absence of any standardized protocol.

- More research is needed in order to further define, optimize, and validate the modality.

7. Transluminal attenuation gradient

TAG is a modality that is based upon the kinetics of iodinated contrast media within coronary arteries. It is the linear regression coefficient between the lumen attenuation and axial distance along the vessel from the ostium. This method is based upon the contrast attenuation difference across a stenosis which may predict functional significance [40].

7.1. Clinical evidence

Changes in coronary opacification across a stenosis were found to predict abnormal resting coronary blood flow in a study by Chow et al. [41]. The comparison of coronary opacification after normalization to aorta was performed to severity of stenosis and thrombolysis in myocardial infarction flow in the coronary arteries at invasive coronary angiography. TAG significantly improves both sensitivity and specificity over CCTA stenosis degree alone [40].

7.2. Clinical applications

The addition of TAG to CCTA may supplement detection of hemodynamic significance of coronary stenosis especially in severely calcified lesions. An advantage of TAG over FFR supplementation of CT is that there is no complex computation required [42].

7.3. Limitations

The evidence on the role of TAG in CCTA is limited. Further validation of both diagnostic and prognostic role of this approach is required in larger studies.

8. Take home points

The single most attractive characteristic of the summarized techniques is that they provide both anatomical and functional assessments of CAD. The current studies have demonstrated that these methods are feasible for noninvasive assessment of CAD and have the potential to provide incremental value in detecting functionally significant coronary stenosis over CCTA alone. The available data are preliminary, but definitely promising. This calls for dedicated research to identify the prognostic value and clinical outcomes of decision making based on these techniques.

9. CCTA and prognosis

In an era where coronary artery disease (CAD) is the leading cause of death worldwide, noninvasive cardiac imaging is essential for the diagnosis and prognosis of patient with suspected or known coronary artery disease. While nuclear positron emission tomography (PET), SPECT, cardiac magnetic resonance imaging, and stress echocardiography are well-established modality with excellent diagnostic accuracy, coronary computed tomographic angiography (CCTA) has emerged in the past couple of decades and is rapidly growing as noninvasive testing modality for the detection of coronary artery disease (CAD). CCTA provides excellent anatomic information that is comparable with invasive coronary angiography and in addition can provide significantly more information about subclinical atherosclerosis [43–46].

This has attracted particular interest to explore prognostic implication of the CCTA in cardiology field. Several single- and multiple-center studies, including meta-analysis of large registry, have been done to evaluate its prognostic value and compare it to the traditional risk factors [47].

9.1. Clinical evidence

Prognostic value of the CCTA was studied in a variety of patient population including symptomatic and asymptomatic subset of patients. Hadamitzky et al. analyzed large patient population of 17,793 from the international CONFIRM registry in patient with suspected coronary artery disease. Combining the CCTA data and the clinical risk scores, a modeled score was developed with end-point assessment being all-cause mortality at 2-year follow-up. The optimized score developed improved risk stratification and overall risk prediction beyond the clinical risk scores. Incremental prognostic value was noted particularly with plaque burden and vessel stenosis, with a proportional correlation for proximal segment involvement [48]. Similar outcome was replicated at longer 5-year follow-up studies [49].

Other studies evaluated the prognostic value of the CCTA based on the plaque location and whether the atherosclerotic plaque is obstructive or not and the number of vessels involved. Cheruvu et al. analyzed the CCTA prognosis in asymptomatic patients without modifiable cardiovascular risk factors [50]. A total number of 1884 patients from 12 different centers were enrolled and followed up for approximately 5 years. Both obstructive and non-obstructive CADs were found to predict MACE with increased HR associated with higher degree of stenosis. MACE ranged from 5.6% in patients with no CAD to 36.28% in patients with obstructive CAD. **Figure 7** shows the obstructive severity on CTA and clinical implications. **Table 4** provides a summary of some of prognostic studies in CCTA.

The additive information of the CCTA on atherosclerotic plaque features offers the promise to provide a more comprehensive view on total plaque burden. In emergent data, atherosclerotic plaque characteristics have been associated with plaque vulnerability; hence, several observational and prospective studies are done to correlate their ability to predict future cardiovascular events [51–54]. Feuchtner et al. characterized CTA features associated with worse clinical outcomes. The evaluation of the CTA findings was based on lesion severity, plaque types (the spectrum from different degrees of calcified to non-calcified), and high-risk plaque criteria (low attenuation by HU, napkin-ring, spotty calcification, and remodeling index). The study concluded that the low attenuation plaque of <60 HU and napkin-ring sign were the most powerful predictors for MACE. Prognosis was established as excellent long term if CTA is negative but worsens with increasing non-calcifying plaque component [55]. Similar

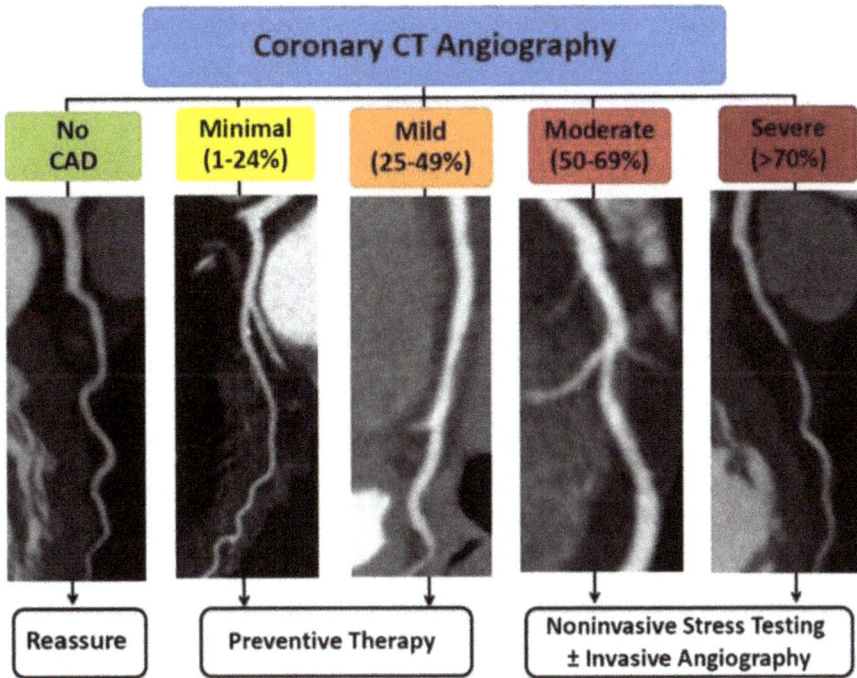

Figure 7. Coronary artery disease (CAD) severity identified by coronary CT angiography and recommended management. Patients with a normal coronary CT angiography can be safely reassured. Follow-up for preventive therapy is recommended for non-obstructive (<50%) CAD. For obstructive CAD (≥50% stenosis), further testing is recommended to guide management [55].

concept was entertained by Nadjiri et al., who performed a semi-quantitative analysis of all non-calcified plaques or partially calcified plaques to quantify the low attenuation plaque volume (LAPV), total non-calcified plaque volume, and remodeling index. All these plaque characteristics were associated with increased MACE independently from the clinical risk presentation. The strongest prognosis was associated with LAPV, which carried additional information beyond the calcium score and the conventional coronary CTA [56]. High-risk plaque and plaque progression were also found to be independent risk factors for predicting ACS [57, 58]. **Figures 8–10** demonstrate images of different histologic plaque types, their quantitative measurements, and plaque-specific-associated risk.

Considering the well-known correlation of the diabetes mellitus and CAD, particular attention was directed of the CCTA implication in diagnosing diabetic patients with subclinical CAD and assessing the prognostic value in this subset of patients. On prospective evaluation of 525 asymptomatic diabetic patients, Van den Hoogen et al. found a proportional increase in event rates in patients with increased CAC category and coronary stenosis severity. What was even more importantly noted was that patients with normal CTA had an excellent prognosis [59]. Whether or not asymptomatic diabetic patients would benefit from screening for CAD remains controversial. Muhlestein et al. demonstrated in a prospective study of 900 patients that CTA screening showed no survival benefit compared to optimized medical therapy in asymptomatic patients with type 1 and type 2 diabetes mellitus [60].

Study	Study aim	Patients (N)	Population characteristics	Major findings
Puchner S. et al. [58] (ROMICATII TRIAL)	Plaque characteristics predicting ACS.	472	Acute chest pain, low risk for ACS.	Presence of high-risk plaques was an independent *predictor of ACS*
Hadamitzky M et al. [48, 49]	Predict cardiac events at 5 years follow-up.	1584	Suspected CAD, not previously diagnosed	Severity of CAD and total plaque score predicted cardiac events over standard clinical events
Feuchtner G et al. [55]	Prospective assessment of the CCTA and MACE.	1469	Low to intermediate risk patients for CAD	Strongest predictors for MACE were LAP and napkin-ring sign with HR of 4.96 and 3.85, respectively.
Nadjiri J et al. [56]	Plaque characteristics and associated prognosis	1168	Patient with suspected CAD	Napkin-ring sign lesions and LAVP found to be predictors for MACE with LAVP carrying the strongest prognostic value HR 1.12, p < 0.0001
Cheruvu C et al. [50]	Predict MACE in long-term follow-up.	1884	Symptomatic patient with angina-equivalent	MACE were 5.6% in patients with non-obstructive CAD and 36.28% in patients with obstructive CAD
Van den Hoogen IJ et al. [59]	Prognostic assessment of the CCTA in patient with diabetes mellitus	525	Asymptomatic diabetic patients with no known history of CAD	Excellent prognosis in patient with CCTA negative. Prognosis was worse and directly proportional to the *number and severity of stenosis*
Linde et al. [61] (CATCH TRIAL)	CCTA-guided management and clinical outcomes.	600	Symptomatic patient with chest pain but negative troponin and ECG	CCTA-guided strategy appears to improve clinical outcomes in these patient population with HR: 0.36; $p = 0.04$

CCTA, coronary computed tomographic angiography; *CAD*, coronary artery disease; *HR*, hazard ratio; *LAVP*, low attenuation volume plaque; *LAP*, low attenuation plaque; *MACE*, major adverse cardiac events.

Table 4. Major studies assessing prognostic value of CCTA.

Symptomatic patients are another subgroup of patients where the role of CTA and its clinical implication was assessed. ROMICATT II and CCATCH trials [61, 62] addressed the clinical impact of CTA-guided therapy in patients with acute chest pain and negative ECG and cardiac biomarkers were evaluated in 600 randomized patients. Almost half underwent CTA guided and other half standard care (exercise MPI/EKG). MACE (cardiac death, myocardial infarction, hospitalization for unstable angina, symptom-driven revascularization, and readmission for chest pain) was significantly better in CTA group.

In conclusion, the above review has summarized the advances in CCTA and emerging data reflecting the very promising role CCTA carries in diagnosis and prognosis over the traditional risk assessment. Its unique ability to provide complete assessment of anatomy, plaque characteristics, and prognosis makes the CCTA's future very promising and crucial in enhancing patient care.

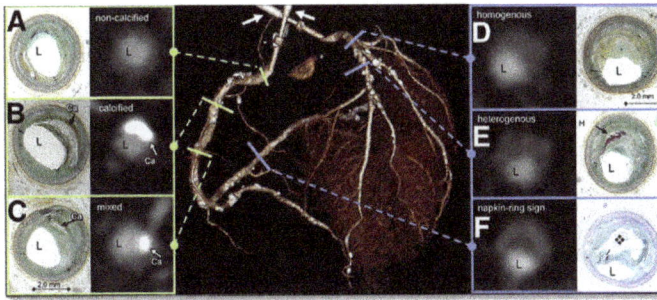

Figure 8. CCTA image of the coronaries with traditional plaque classification and the corresponding histology slides. There are non-calcified (A), calcified (B), and mixed plaque (C) noted. Based on plaque attenuation, there is homogeneous (D), heterogeneous (E), and napkin-ring sign (F) plaques [56].

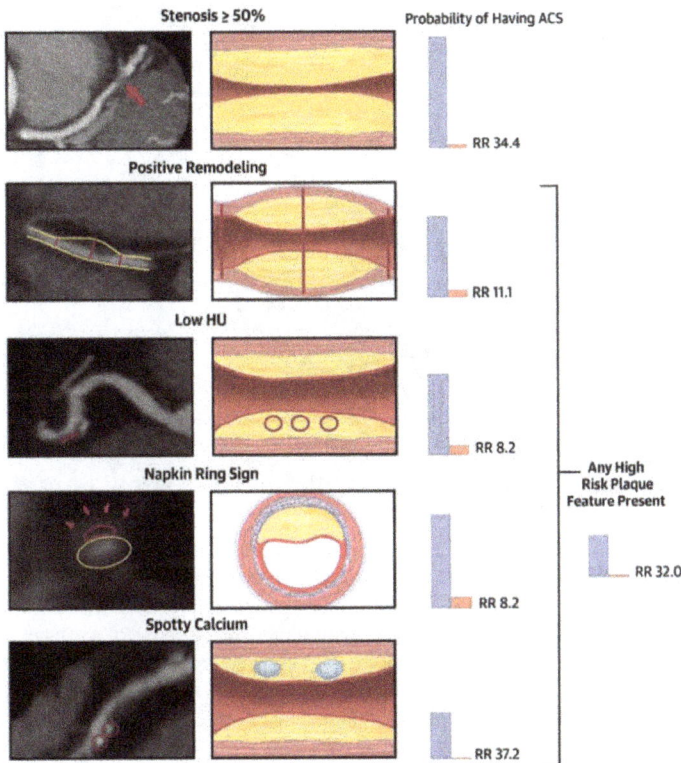

Figure 9. Probability of having acute coronary syndrome during the index hospitalization according to coronary computed tomography characteristics. Central Illustration: Significant stenosis and high-risk coronary plaque features and their association with the probability of having acute coronary syndrome during the index hospitalization. Stenosis of ≥50%—Severe stenosis of the mid-left anterior descending coronary artery (Bold arrow). Non-calcified plaque with positive remodeling in the distal right coronary artery (arrowhead). Positive remodeling—The two dotted red lines (image insert) demonstrate the vessel diameters at the proximal and distal reference (both 1.8 mm) and the full red line demonstrates the maximal vessel diameter in the mid portion of the plaque (2.7 mm)—the remodeling index is 1.5 Low HU plaque—Partially calcified plaque in the mid-right coronary artery with low <30 HU plaque. The red circles demonstrate the three regions of interest with the mean CT number of 22, 19, and 20 HU Napkin-ring sign—Napkin-ring sign plaque in the mid-left anterior descending coronary artery. Schematic cross-sectional view of the napkin-ring sign. The red line demonstrates the central low HU area of the plaque adjacent to the lumen (ellipse) surrounded by a peripheral rim of the higher CT attenuation (arrows). Spotty calcium—Partially calcified plaque in the mid-right coronary artery with spotty calcification (diameter of <3 mm in all directions; circles) [58].

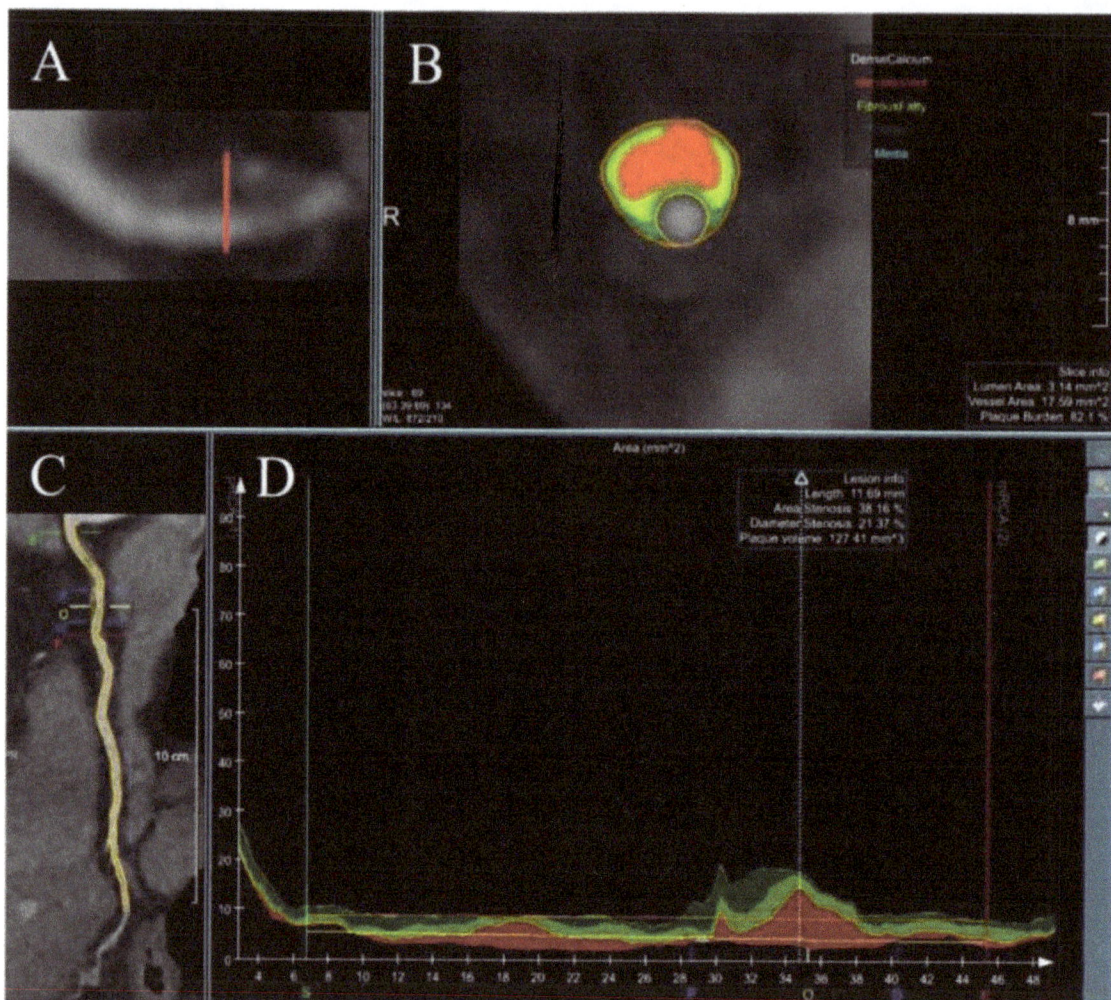

Figure 10. An example of the quantitative plaque measurements. **Panel A** – The large coronary plaque in the proximal right coronary artery (RCA) showed in long-axis view in the multiplanar reformatted image. **Panel B** – The cross-sectional view of the proximal RCA demonstrates a large plaque. The software detects plaque components with low CT attenuation <30HU, 31 to 60HU and 61 to 130HU. **Panel C** – The curved multiplanar reformatted image of the RCA. The proximal and distal normal cross sections are selected manually by the reader to mark the beginning and end of the plaque. The software automatically selects the minimal luminal area (stenosis). **Panel D** – The software provides quantitative measurements of the selected coronary plaque including total plaque volume (127 mm³), remodeling index (2.04), stenosis degree (21%) and plaque length (11.7 mm). The volumes of plaque subcomponents are also reported [62].

Author details

Karthik Ananthasubramaniam*, Nishtha Sareen and Gjeka Rudin

*Address all correspondence to: kananth1@hfhs.org

1 Department of Medicine, Heart and Vascular Institute, Henry Ford Hospital, Detroit, Michigan, USA

2 Division of Cardiology, St. Joseph Mercy Hospital Oakland, Michigan, USA

References

[1] Schmermund A, Rensing BJ, Sheedy PF, et al. Intravenous electron-beam computed tomographic coronary angiography for segmental analysis of coronary artery stenoses. Journal of American College of Cardiology. 1998 Jun;**31**(7):1547-1554

[2] Achenbach S, Giesler T, Ropers D, Baum U, et al. Detection of coronary artery stenoses by contrast-enhanced, retrospectively electrocardiographically-gated, multislice spiral computed tomography. Circulation. 2001 May 29;**103**(21):2535-2538

[3] Budoff MJ, Dowe D, Jollis JG, et al. Diagnostic performance of 64-multidetector row coronary computed tomographic angiography for evaluation of coronary artery stenosis in individuals without known coronary artery disease: Results from the prospective multicenter ACCURACY (Assessment by Coronary Computed Tomographic Angiography of Individuals Undergoing Invasive Coronary Angiography) trial. Journal of American College of Cardiology. 2008 Nov 18;**52**(21):1724-1732

[4] Miller JM, Rochitte CE, Dewey M, et al. Diagnostic performance of coronary angiography by 64-row CT. New England Journal of Medicine. 2008 Nov 27;**359**(22):2324-2336

[5] Flohr TG, McCollough CH, Bruder H, et al. First performance evaluation of a dual-source CT (DSCT) system. European Radiology. 2006 Feb;**16**(2):256-268. Epub 2005 Dec 10

[6] Ropers U, Ropers D, Pflederer T, et al. Influence of heart rate on the diagnostic accuracy of dual-source computed tomography coronary angiography. Journal of American College of Cardiology. 2007 Dec 18;**50**(25):2393-2398

[7] Conigliaro J, Whittle J, Good CB, Hanusa BH, et al. Understanding racial variation in the use of coronary revascularization procedures: The role of clinical factors. Archives of the International Medicine. 2000 May 8;**160**(9):1329-1335

[8] Sohns D, Kruse S, Vollmann D, et al. Accuracy of 64-multidetector computed tomography coronary angiography in patients with symptomatic atrial fibrillation prior to pulmonary vein isolation. European Heart Journal – Cardiovascular Imaging. 2012;**13**:263-270

[9] Schwarz F, Ruzsics B, et al. Dual-energy CT of the heart--principles and protocols. European Journal of Radiology. 2008 Dec;**68**(3):423-433

[10] Yamada Y, Jinzaki M, Okamura T, et al. Feasibility of coronary artery calcium scoring on virtual unenhanced images derived from single-source fast kVp-switching dual-energy coronary CT angiography. Journal of Cardiovascular & Computed Tomography. 2014 Sep–Oct;**8**(5):391-400

[11] Fuchs TA, Stehli J, et al. Coronary artery calcium quantification from contrast enhanced CT using gemstone spectral imaging and material decomposition. International Journal of Cardiovascular Imaging. 2014 Oct;**30**(7):1399-1405

[12] Schlomka JP, Roessl E, et al. Experimental feasibility of multi-energy photon-counting K-edge imaging in pre-clinical computed tomography. Physics in Medicine and Biology. 2008 Aug 7;**53**(15):4031-4047

[13] Ronaldson JP, Zainon R, et al. Toward quantifying the composition of soft tissues by spectral CT with Medipix3. Medical Physics. 2012 Nov;**39**(11):6847-6857. doi: 10.1118/1.4760773

[14] Hassan A, Nazir SA, Alkadhi H. Technical challenges of coronary CT angiography: Today and tomorrow. European Journal of Radiology. 2011 Aug;**79**(2):161-171

[15] Min JK, et al. High-definition multidetector computed tomography for evaluation of coronary artery stents: Comparison to standard-definition 64-detector row computed tomography. Journal of Cardiovascular & Computed Tomography. 2009 Jul–Aug;**3**(4): 246-251

[16] Bittencourt MS, Schmidt B, Seltmann M, Muschiol G, Ropers D, Daniel WG, et al. Iterative reconstruction in image space (IRIS) in cardiac computed tomography: initial experience. International Journal of Cardiovascular Imaging. 2011 Oct;**27**(7):1081-1087

[17] Leipsic J, Labounty TM, Heilbron B, Min JK, et al. Adaptive statistical iterative reconstruction: Assessment of image noise and image quality in coronary CT angiography. American Journal of Roentgenology. 2010 Sep;**195**(3):649-654

[18] Leipsic J, Labounty TM, Hague CJ, et al. Effect of a novel vendor-specific motion-correction algorithm on image quality and diagnostic accuracy in persons undergoing coronary CT angiography without rate-control medications. Journal of Cardiovascular & Computed Tomography. 2012 May–Jun;**6**(3):164-171

[19] Reinartz SD, Diefenbach BS, Allmendinger T, et al. Reconstructions with identical filling (RIF) of the heart: A physiological approach to image reconstruction in coronary CT angiography. European Radiology. 2012 Dec;**22**(12):2670-2678

[20] Shaw LJ, Hausleiter J, Achenbach S, et al. Coronary computed tomographic angiography as a gatekeeper to invasive diagnostic and surgical procedures: Results from the multicenter confirm (coronary ct angiography evaluation for clinical outcomes: an international multicenter) registry. Journal of the American College of Cardiology. 2012;**60**(20):2103-2114

[21] Pijls NHJ, De Bruyne B, Peels K, et al. Measurement of fractional flow reserve to assess the functional severity of coronary-artery stenoses. The New England Journal of Medicine. 1996;**334**(26):1703-1708

[22] Tonino PAL, Fearon WF, de Bruyne B, et al. Angiographic versus functional severity of coronary artery stenoses in the FAME study fractional flow reserve versus angiography in multivessel evaluation. Journal of the American College of Cardiology. 2010;**55**(25):2816-2821

[23] Rispler S, Keidar Z, Ghersin E, et al. Integrated single-photon emission computed tomography and computed tomography coronary angiography for the assessment of hemodynamically significant coronary artery lesions. Journal of the American College of Cardiology. 2007;**49**(10):1059-1067

[24] Schuijf JD, Wijns W, Jukema JW, et al. Relationship between noninvasive coronary angiography with multi-slice computed tomography and myocardial perfusion imaging. Journal of the American College of Cardiology. 2006;**48**(12):2508-2514

[25] Di Carli MF, Dorbala S, Curillova Z, et al. Relationship between CT coronary angiography and stress perfusion imaging in patients with suspected ischemic heart disease assessed by integrated PET-CT imaging. Journal of Nuclear Cardiology. 2007;**14**(6):799-809

[26] Pijls NHJ, De Bruyne B. Coronary pressure measurement and fractional flow reserve. Heart. 1998;**80**(6):539-542

[27] Xu R, Li C, Qian J, Ge J. Computed tomography-derived fractional flow reserve in the detection of lesion-specific ischemia: An integrated analysis of 3 pivotal trials. Medicine (Baltimore). 2015 Nov;**94**(46):e1963

[28] Hlatky MA, Saxena A, Koo BK, Erglis A, Zarins CK, Min JK. Projected costs and consequences of computed tomography-determined fractional flow reserve. Clinical Cardiology. 2013;**36**:743-748

[29] Douglas PS, Pontone G, Hlatky MA, et al., for the PLATFORM Investigators. Clinical outcomes of fractional flow reserve by computed tomographic angiography-guided diagnostic strategies vs. usual care in patients with suspected coronary artery disease: The prospective longitudinal trial of FFRct: Outcome and resource impacts study. European Heart Journal. 2015 Sep 1 [E-pub ahead of print]

[30] Techasith T, Cury RC. Stress myocardial CT perfusion: An update and future perspective. Journal of American College of Cardiology: Cardiovascular Imaging. 2011;**4**(8):905-916

[31] Santos-Ocampo CD, Herman SD, Travin MI, et al. Comparison of exercise, dipyridamole, and adenosine by use of technetium 99m sestamibi tomographic imaging. Journal of Nuclear Cardiology. 1994;**1**:57-64

[32] George RT, et al. Adenosine stress 64-and 256-row detector computed tomography angiography and perfusion imaging: A pilot study evaluation the transmural extent of perfusion abnormalities to predict atherosclerosis causing myocardial ischemia. Circulation: Cardiovascular Imaging. 2009;**2**:174-182

[33] Blankstein R, et al. Adenosine-induced stress myocardial perfusion imaging using dual-source cardiac computed tomography. Journal of American College of Cardiology. 2009;**54**:1072-1084

[34] Rocha-Filho JA, Blankstein R, Shturman LD, et al. Incremental value of adenosine-induced stress myocardial perfusion imaging with dual-source CT at cardiac CT angiography. Radiology. 2010;**254**:410-419

[35] Okada DR, Ghoshhajra BB, Blankstein R, et al. Direct comparison of rest and adenosine stress myocardial perfusion CT with rest and stress SPECT. Journal of Nuclear Cardiology. 2010;**17**:27-37

[36] Tamarappoo BK, Dey D, Nakazato R, et al. Comparison of the extent and severity of myocardial perfusion defects measured by CT coronary angiography and SPECT myocardial perfusion imaging. Journal of American College of Cardiology Imaging. 2010;**3**:1010-1019

[37] Cury RC, Magalhaes TA, Borges AC, et al. Dipyridamole stress and rest myocardial perfusion by 64-detector row computed tomography in patients with suspected coronary artery disease. American Journal of Cardiology. 2010;**106**:310-315

[38] Ho KT, Chua KC, Klotz E, Panknin C. Stress and rest dynamic myocardial perfusion imaging by evaluation of complete time-attenuation curves with dual-source CT. Journal of American College of Cardiology Imaging. 2010;**3**:811-820

[39] George RT, Silva C, Cordeiro MA, et al. Multidetector computed tomography myocardial perfusion imaging during adenosine stress. Journal of American College of Cardiology. 2006;**48**:153-160

[40] Wong DTL, Ko BS, Cameron JD, et al. Transluminal attenuation gradient in coronary computed tomography angiography is a novel noninvasive approach to the identification of functionally significant coronary artery stenosis: A comparison with fractional flow reserve. Journal of the American College of Cardiology. 2013;**61**(12):1271-1279

[41] Chow BJW, Kass M, Gagn O, et al. Can differences in corrected coronary opacification measured with computed tomography predict resting coronary artery flow? Journal of the American College of Cardiology. 2011;**57**(11):1280-1288

[42] Xu L, Sun Z, Fan Z. Noninvasive physiologic assessment of coronary stenoses using cardiac CT. BioMed Research International. 2015;**4**:435737

[43] Thomas MD, Branch KR, Cury RC. PROMISE of coronary CT angiography: Precise and accurate diagnosis and prognosis in coronary artery disease. South Medical Journal. 2016 Apr;**109**(4):242-247

[44] Doris M, Newby DE. Coronary CT angiography as a diagnostic and prognostic tool: Perspectives from the SCOT-HEART Trial. Current Cardiology Reports. 2016 Feb;**18**(2):18

[45] Eckert J, Schmidt M, Magedanz A, et al. Coronary CT angiography in managing atherosclerosis. International Journal of Molecular Science. 2015 Feb 9;**16**(2):3740-3756

[46] Aljizeeri A, Cocker MS, Chow BJ. CT vs SPECT: CT is the first-line test for the diagnosis and prognosis of stable coronary artery disease. Journal of Nuclear Cardiology. 2013 Jun;**20**(3):465-472

[47] Otaki Y, Berman DS, Min JK. Prognostic utility of coronary computed tomographic angiography. Indian Heart Journal. 2013 May–Jun;**65**(3):300-310

[48] Hadamitzky M, Achenbach S, Al-Mallah M, et al. CONFIRM Investigators. Optimized prognostic score for coronary computed tomographic angiography: Results from the CONFIRM registry (COronary CT Angiography EvaluatioN For Clinical Outcomes: An

InteRnational Multicenter Registry). Journal of American College of Cardiology. 2013 Jul 30;**62**(5):468-476

[49] Hadamitzky M, Täubert S, Deseive S, et al. Prognostic value of coronary computed tomography angiography during 5 years of follow-up in patients with suspected coronary artery disease. European Heart Journal. 2013 Nov;**34**(42):3277-3285

[50] Cheruvu C, Precious B, Naoum C, et al. Long term prognostic utility of coronary CT angiography in patients with no modifiable coronary artery disease risk factors: Results from the 5-year follow-up of the CONFIRM International Multicenter Registry. Journal of Cardiovascular & Computed Tomography. 2016 Jan–Feb;**10**(1):22-27

[51] Hou ZH, Lu B, Gao Y, et al. Prognostic value of coronary CT angiography and calcium score for major adverse cardiac events in outpatients. Journal of American College of Cardiology: Cardiovascular Imaging. 2012 Oct;**5**(10):990-999

[52] Tesche C, et al. Prognostic implications of coronary CT angiography-derived quantitative markers for the prediction of major adverse cardiac events. Journal of Cardiovascular & Computed Tomography. 2016 Nov–Dec;**10**(6):458-465

[53] Divakaran S, Cheezum MK, Hulten EA, et al. Use of cardiac CT and calcium scoring for detecting coronary plaque: Implications on prognosis and patient management. British Journal of Radiology. February 2015;**88**(1046):20140594

[54] Maurovich-Horvat P, Schlett C, Alkadhi H, et al. The napkin-ring sign indicates advanced atherosclerotic lesions in coronary CT angiography. JCMG. 2012 Dec 12;.03.019

[55] Feuchtner G, et al. The high-risk criteria low-attenuation plaque <60 HU and the napkin-ring sign are the most powerful predictors of MACE: A long-term follow-up study. European Heart Journal: Cardiovascular Imaging. 2016 Aug 07. DOI: 10.1093/ehjci/jew167

[56] Nadjiri J, et al. Incremental prognostic value of quantitative plaque assessment in coronary CT angiography during 5 years of follow up. Journal of Cardiovascular Computed Tomography. 2016 Mar-Apr;**10**(2):97-104. doi: 10.1016/j.jcct.2016.01.007

[57] Motoyama S, et al. Plaque characterization by coronary computed tomography angiography and the likelihood of acute coronary events in mid-term follow-up. Journal of American College of Cardiology. 2015 Jul 28;**66**(4):337-346

[58] Puchner SB, Liu T, Mayrhofer T, et al. High-risk plaque detected on coronary computed tomography angiography predicts acute coronary syndrome independent of significant stenosis in patients with acute chest pain results from ROMICAT II Trial. Journal of American College of Cardiology. 2014 August 19;**64**(7):684-692

[59] Van den Hoogen IJ, et al. Prognostic value of coronary computed tomography angiography in diabetic patients without chest pain syndrome. Journal of Nuclear Cardiology. 2016 Feb;**23**(1):24-36

[60] Muhlestein JB, Lappé DL, Lima JA, et al. Effect of screening for coronary artery disease using CT angiography on mortality and cardiac events in high-risk patients with
diabetes: The FACTOR-64 randomized clinical trial. Journal of the American Medical
Association. 2014 Dec 3;**312**(21):2234-2243

[61] Linde JJ, Hove JD, Sørgaard M, et al. Long-term clinical impact of coronary CT angi-
ography in patients with recent acute-onset chest pain: The randomized controlled
CATCH trial. Journal of American College of Cardiology: Cardiovascular Imaging. 2015
Dec;**8**(12):1404-1413

[62] Ferencik M, Mayrhofer T, Puchner SB, Lu MT, et al. Computed tomography-based
high-risk coronary plaque score to predict acute coronary syndrome among patients
with acute chest pain--Results from the ROMICAT II trial. Journal of Cardiovascular &
Computed Tomography. 2015 Nov–Dec;**9**(6):538-545

8

Cone-Beam Computed Tomography for Oral and Maxillofacial Imaging

Ufuk Tatli and Burcu Evlice

Abstract

The invention of computed tomography (CT) technique revolutionized diagnostic imaging. Compared to conventional X-ray imaging procedures, CT involves higher radiation doses. Recently, cone-beam CT (CBCT) specifically designed for maxillofacial imaging was introduced. CBCT technique is based on a cone-shaped X-ray beam centered on a two-dimensional (2D) detector. The detector system performs one rotation around the patient, producing a series of 2D images which are then reconstructed in a 3D data set. The contemporary knowledge regarding CBCT and its proper application guides the practitioner for improvement in diagnostic purposes and treatment planning. The aim of this chapter is to focus on the details, advantages, drawbacks, and clinical applications of CBCT as a headmost CT imaging technique in the oral and maxillofacial (OMF) region. The main clinical applications of CBCT in the OMF region are dentistry including dentoalveolar and maxillofacial surgery, orthodontics, endodontics, and periodontics; and otolaryngology. The aforementioned clinical use of CBCT was described in detail with illustrated sample cases. In most of the cases in OMF region, CBCT takes the place of multi-slice CT. Thus, clinicians should know the clinical applications and capabilities of CBCT technique with its drawbacks.

Keywords: cone-beam computed tomography, dentistry, maxillofacial imaging, maxillofacial surgery, otolaryngology

1. Introduction

Accurate diagnostic imaging is a key factor for diagnosis and treatment planning. The invention of computed tomography (CT) technique revolutionized diagnostic imaging. Since the inception of CT in the 1970s, it has become one of the commonly used imaging methods [1]. Three-dimensional (3D) imaging provided by CT technology gives the opportunity to the clinician to examine the oral and maxillofacial (OMF) region without superimposition and distortion of the image. Compared to conventional 2D imaging procedures, CT involves higher radiation doses. Recently, cone-beam computed tomography (CBCT) specifically designed for maxillofacial imaging was introduced to offset some of the limitations of conventional CT scanning devices [2].

The contemporary knowledge regarding CBCT and its proper application guides the practitioner for improvement in diagnostic purposes and treatment planning. The aim of this chapter is to focus on the technical features, advantages, drawbacks, limits, and clinical applications of CBCT as a headmost CT imaging technique in the OMF region.

2. Cone-beam technique

The CBCT scanners for maxillofacial region were introduced in the 1990s independently in Japan [3] and in Italy [4]. Although it has been given several names including dental volumetric tomography (DVT), cone-beam volumetric tomography (CBVT), dental computed tomography (DCT), and cone-beam imaging (CBI), the most preferred name is cone-beam computed tomography (CBCT) [5].

CBCT imaging is performed by using a rotating gantry to which an X-ray source and detector are fixed. Cone-beam machines radiate an X-ray beam shaped liked a cone or pyramid, rather than a fan, as in conventional CT machines. The X-ray source and detector rotate around a rotation abutment fixed within the center of the region of interest. The beam exiting the patient is captured on a 2D planar detector, usually an amorphous silicon flat panel or sometimes an image intensifier/charge coupled device (CCD) detector. During the rotation, multiple consecutive planar projection images of the field of view (FOV) are acquired in a complete, or sometimes partial, arc. This procedure varies from a traditional medical CT, which uses a fan-shaped X-ray beam in a helical progression to obtain individual image slices of the FOV and then heaps the slices to get a 3D representation. Each slice requires a separate scan and separate 2D reconstruction. Because CBCT exposure combines the whole FOV, only one rotational turn of the gantry is necessary to acquire enough data for image reconstruction [6, 7]. A cone-beam reconstruction process creates a 3D matrix that can be viewed as a series of 2D cross-sectional images—axial, sagittal, and coronal views. From this data set, the operator can also extract thick or thin, planar or curved reconstructions in any orientation. Axial planes are a series of slices from top to bottom in the volume. Sagittal planes are a series of 2D slices from left to right, and coronal planes are a series of 2D slices from anterior to posterior. In a multi-planar reformation (MPR) window, these three orthogonal planar views are related through intersection lines or crosshairs, allowing for straightforward orientation and navigation (**Figure 1**).

The dose associated with each scan is affected by a number of scan parameters selected by the practitioner, either manually or through preset exposure protocols. For most CBCT systems, the kVp is fixed, and the tube current (mA) and exposure time (s) can be varied depending on the desired image quality and patient size. After reconstruction, CBCT images can be manipulated in different ways to optimize the visualization of anatomical structures and lesions and to isolate certain parts of the image. Basic filtering can also be applied, both during and after reconstruction, in order to smooth or sharpen the image [8]. CBCT has some advantages and disadvantages over conventional CT. These items are summarized below [9–14].

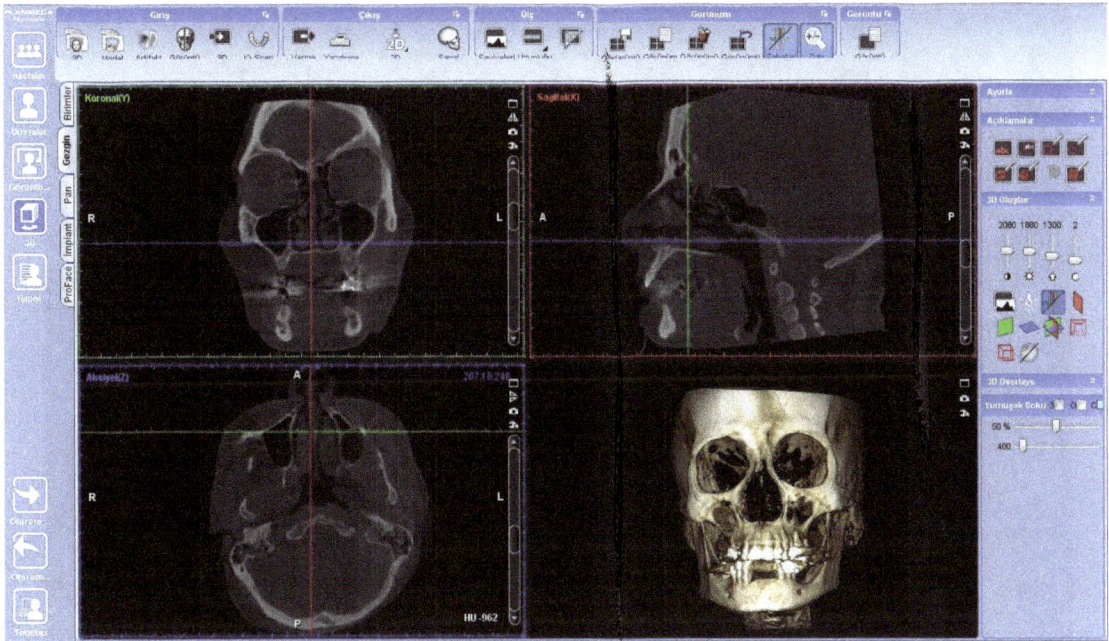

Figure 1. The example of multi-planar CBCT images including coronal, sagittal, axial, and 3D views.

2.1. Advantages of CBCT over conventional CT

- CBCT is less expensive and involves a smaller system, thus providing in-office imaging.

- The X-ray beam is limited, and lower radiation dose is used.

- CBCT provides multi-planar image reconstruction.

- CBCT has higher spatial resolution, providing better visualization of mineralized structures.

- Accurate images are obtained.

- The scan time is more rapid.

- The display modes are exclusive for oral and maxillofacial imaging.

- The imaging artifacts are fewer.

- CBCT has potential for vertical scanning in a natural seated position.

2.2. Disadvantages of CBCT over conventional CT

- Scattered radiation.

- Limited dynamic range of the X-ray detectors.

- Owing to the small detector size, the FOV, and scanned volume are limited.

- Limited contrast resolution.

- Limited soft tissue contrast.

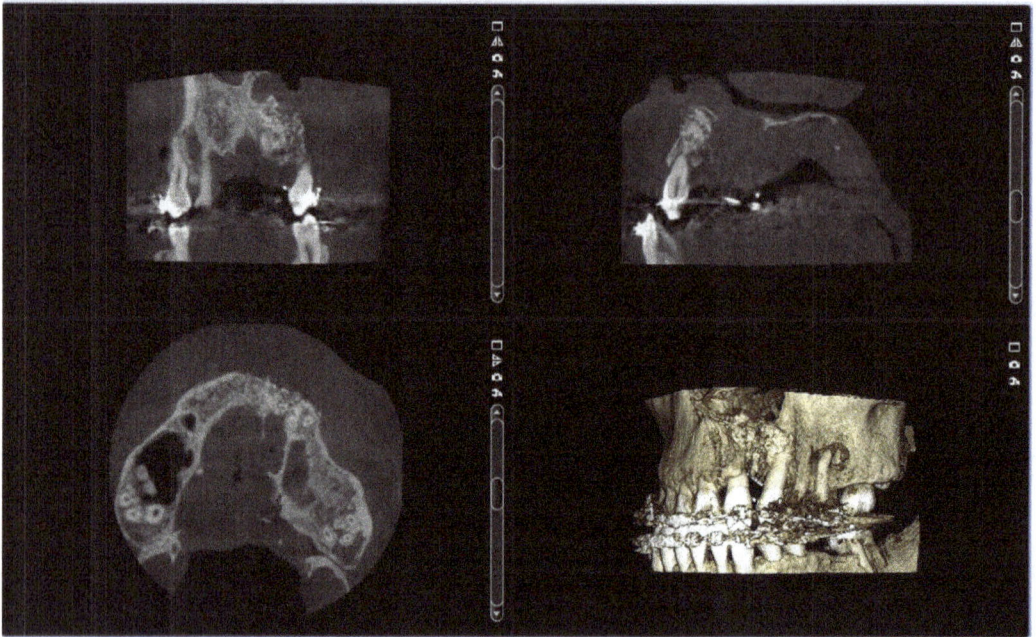

Figure 2. The example of CBCT imaging of an alveolar cleft case showing only the region of interest in order to reduce radiation exposure.

- Bone density values without a linear correlation between different devices.

- Reduced image quality in regions close to high-density neighboring structures such as dental restorations and implants.

According to literature, the subjective image quality was lower on older CBCT units compared to multi-slice CT [15]. However, recent CBCT units with higher resolution showed opposite results [16]. Although new CBCT scanners with flat panel detectors seem to be less prone to metal artifacts, an important problem including susceptibility to movement artifacts still remains [9]. The effective radiation doses for various CBCT devices range from 52 to 1025 micro-sieverts [5]. It was reported that 3D volumetric images obtained with CBCT technology involved up to four times less radiation than conventional CT [17]. Although CBCT requires lower radiation doses compared to CT imaging, the aforementioned radiation doses are still higher than 2D imaging. In order to protect patients and staff during acquisition of images, the selection criteria of CBCT examination should weigh potential benefits against the risks associated with radiation dose. For this purpose, appropriate clinical usage, protective shielding, and the smallest FOV for diagnostic purposes should be obtained (**Figure 2**).

3. Applications of CBCT in oral and maxillofacial region

CBCT is used in all medical and dental disciplines practicing in OMF region, whereas early CBCT devices were dedicated to implantology and dental imaging; nowadays, applications include the whole face and skull. Image analysis function obtains quantifiable accurate data from the image for diagnostic and scientific purposes. Linear, curved, and angular measurements, area and volume calculation, and densitometric analysis can be performed [13, 18–20]. The main clinical applications of CBCT in the OMF region are: dentoalveolar and maxillofacial surgery, maxillofacial pathology, orthodontics, implantology, endodontics, periodontics, and otolaryngology. The CBCT technology can also be used in forensic medicine. The clinical use of CBCT will be reviewed below with illustrated sample cases:

3.1. Oral and maxillofacial surgery

The OMF surgery is the main discipline which uses the CBCT technology. In a literature review, it was reported that 41% of the scientific papers related to the clinical applications of CBCT dealt with the use for maxillofacial surgery [9]. The main topics may be summarized as dental implantology, impacted and supernumerary tooth, OMF pathology, maxillofacial trauma, temporomandibular joint (TMJ) disorders, dentofacial discrepancies, and cleft palate.

3.1.1. Dental implantology

During the preoperative planning of dental implant treatment, radiographic methods for assessment of bone quality and quantity are frequently used. For 2D assessment, orthopantomography (OPG) is frequently used. The American Association of Oral and Maxillofacial Radiology recommends cross-sectional views for evaluation of a potential implant site [14]. CBCT provides the 3D visualization of the alveolar bone height, width, and thickness, and spatial proximity of inferior alveolar and incisive canals, maxillary sinus, and nasal cavity (**Figure 3**). It is the contemporary method used for planning dental implant surgery and bone augmentation

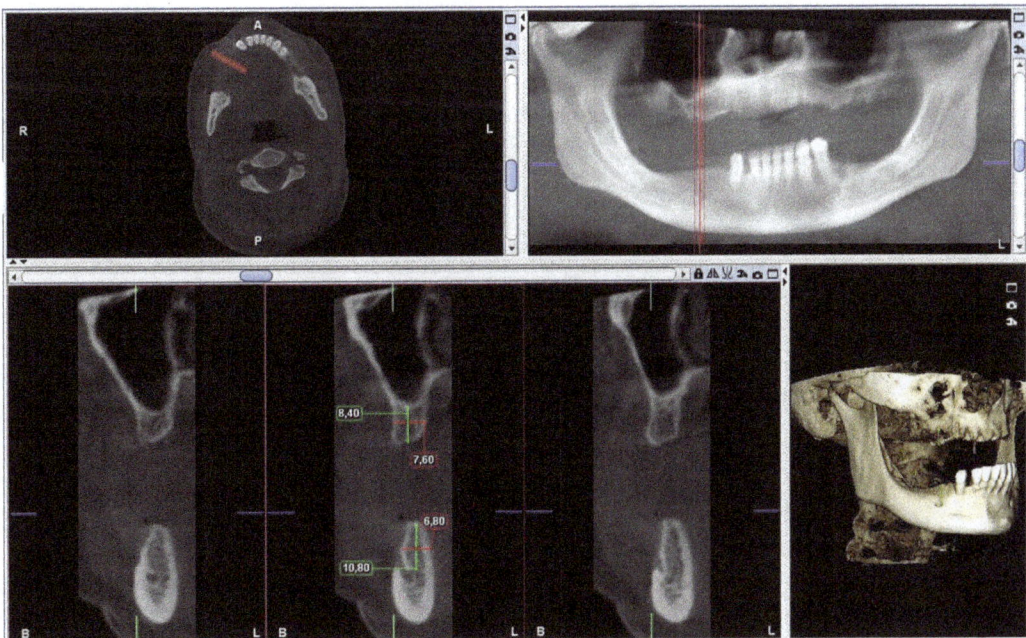

Figure 3. The example of CBCT imaging including cross-sectional view showing the alveolar bone height and width, and localization of maxillary sinus and mental nerve.

procedures (**Figure 4**). As shown in our previous clinical study, accurate measurements can be performed on CBCT images for diagnosis, treatment planning, and evaluation of treatment results of bone augmentation and dental implants [21]. The CBCT images are free from distortion; however, errors in patient positioning may lead to inaccurate measurements which may

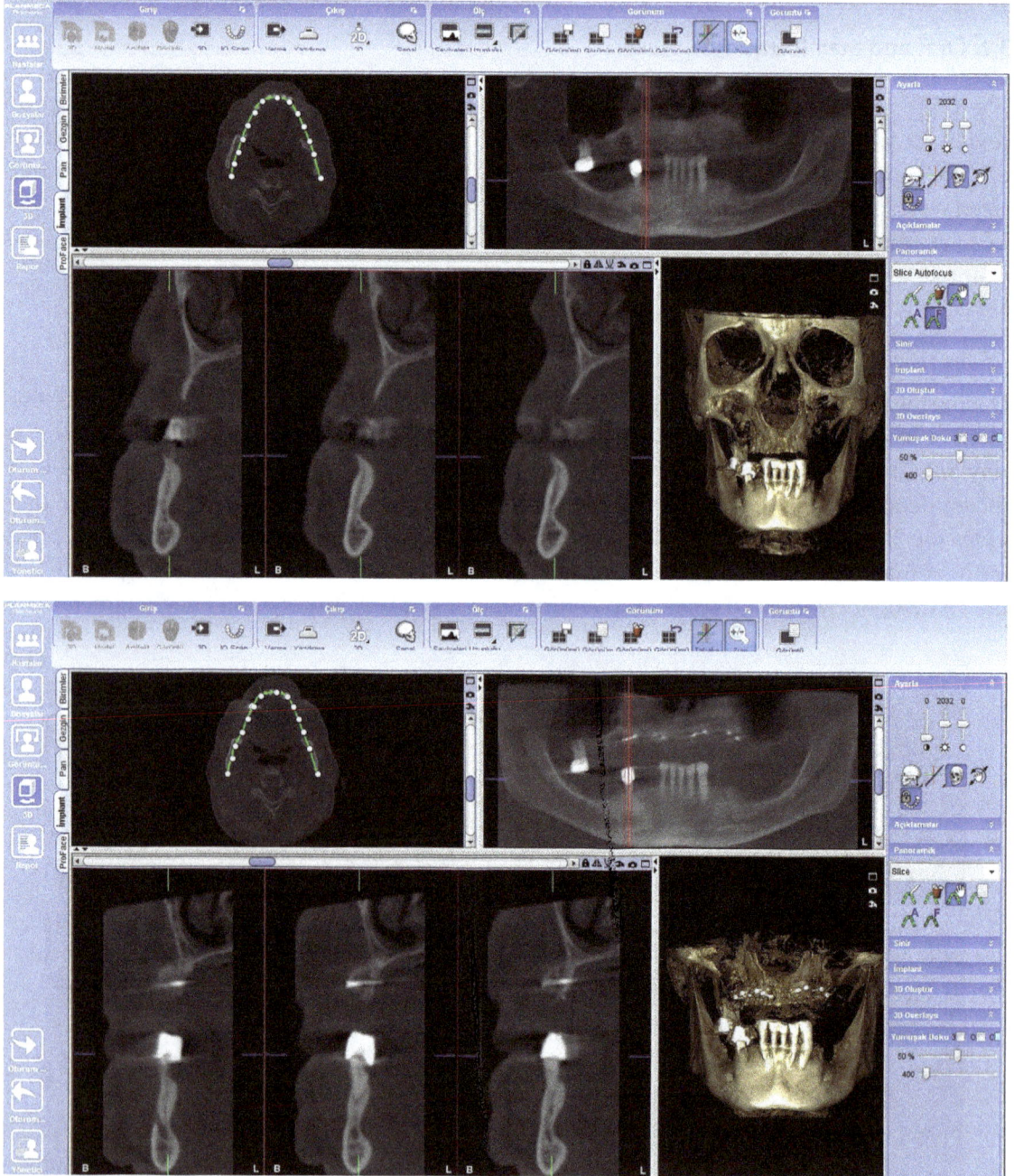

Figure 4. The CBCT imaging of a patient with atrophic maxilla who needs bone augmentation and dental implant treatment. **a.** Before bone augmentation. **b.** After bone augmentation (from iliac crest).

cause damage to anatomical structures. The success of dental implant treatment is influenced by both the quality and quantity of available bone for implant placement. During the past few years, the concept of using CT-derived Hounsfield unit (HU) values had increasing popularity for quantitative assessment of bone density [22, 23]. However, patients are exposed to high radiation during CT scanning. Besides quantitative assessment of bone, CBCT can also be used for evaluation of bone quality (**Figure 5**). In recent studies, significant correlations between the density values of CBCT and HU values of CT were reported [24, 25]. In contrast, controversial results concerning the assessment of bone density using CBCT were also reported in literature [13, 26]. In our previous clinical studies, we observed significant correlation between CBCT-derived bone density and dental implant stability parameters including insertion torque value and resonance frequency analysis [27, 28]. Thus, it seems to be possible to predict bone density, initial implant stability, and possibility of immediate or early loading using CBCT scan prior to implant surgery.

Moreover, it is also possible to perform navigation-guided implant surgery by using specific software and CBCT imaging. The 3D specific navigation system provides surgeons an additional planning tool during implant surgery, offering instant and continuous visualization of drill tip and angle and their relations with neighboring vital structures that have to be respected in the three spatial planes in CBCT images. With the guidance of the dynamic navigation system, surgeon can monitor the 360° view of the relationship among implant drill, inferior alveolar nerve, maxillary sinus, nasal cavity, and buccal and lingual alveolar bone plates during surgery (**Figure 6**).

3.1.2. Impacted and supernumerary tooth

The CBCT is also used for presurgical evaluation of impacted teeth, supernumerary teeth, and their relations with neighboring anatomic structures (adjacent teeth, inferior alveolar nerve,

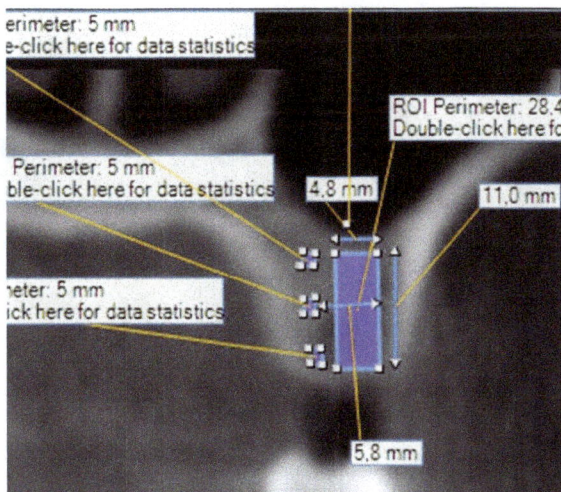

Figure 5. The example of cross-sectional CBCT imaging used to calculate bone density of the designated implant region.

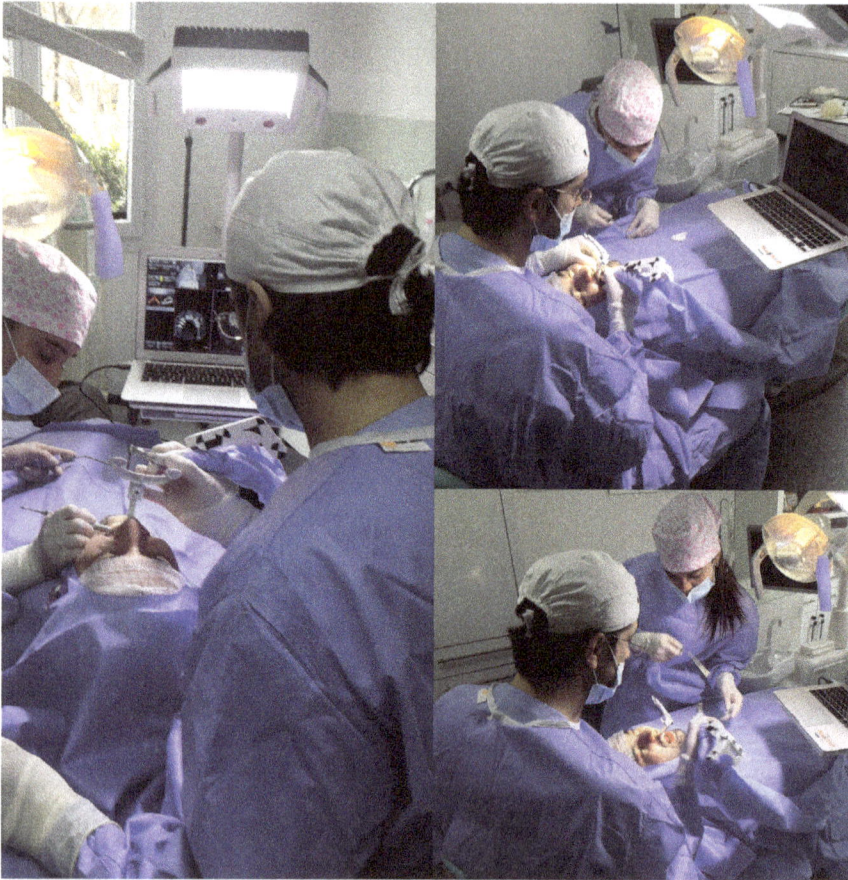

a.

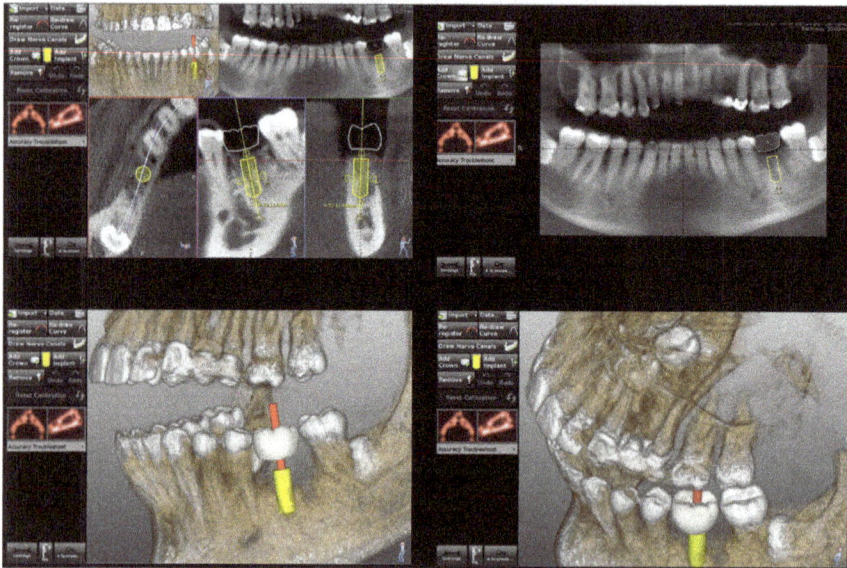

b.

Figure 6. CBCT-based navigation-guided dental implant surgery. **a.** Clinical view. **b.** Software view (by the courtesy of Dr Yakup Üstün).

mental nerve, and maxillary sinus). Thus, clinician is able to plan the surgery and inform the patients about possible risks (**Figure 7**). In a recent clinical study, Jawad et al. reported that CBCT provided improved detection rates (63% versus 45% for plain radiographs) of root resorption associated with impacted canines. The authors also introduced a new root resorption scale for CBCT imaging [29].

3.1.3. Oral and maxillofacial pathology

All kinds of pathologic lesions which affect bone tissue in the OMF region including infection, cysts, tumors, and osteonecrosis can be monitored by CBCT imaging. The CBCT assessment provides maxillofacial surgeon to visualize the accurate localization of pathologic entity and its relation with adjacent vital structures in multi-planar view (**Figure 8**). For medication-related osteonecrosis of the jaws (MRONJ) lesions, the innovative use of routine tumor-surveillance imaging in combination with CBCT imaging was described to provide a high-resolution 3D analysis [30]. The authors interpreted functional imaging information by fusing positron emission tomography/computed tomography (PET/CT) and single-photon emission computed tomography/computed tomography (SPECT/CT) data with CBCT data. Hence, the authors stated that this new composite image analysis, if validated, will facilitate surgical planning by demarcating MRONJ area. The 3D model preparation and adaptation of the reconstruction plates to the jawbone before surgery can also be possible with CBCT imaging for maxillofacial reconstruction patients (**Figure 9**).

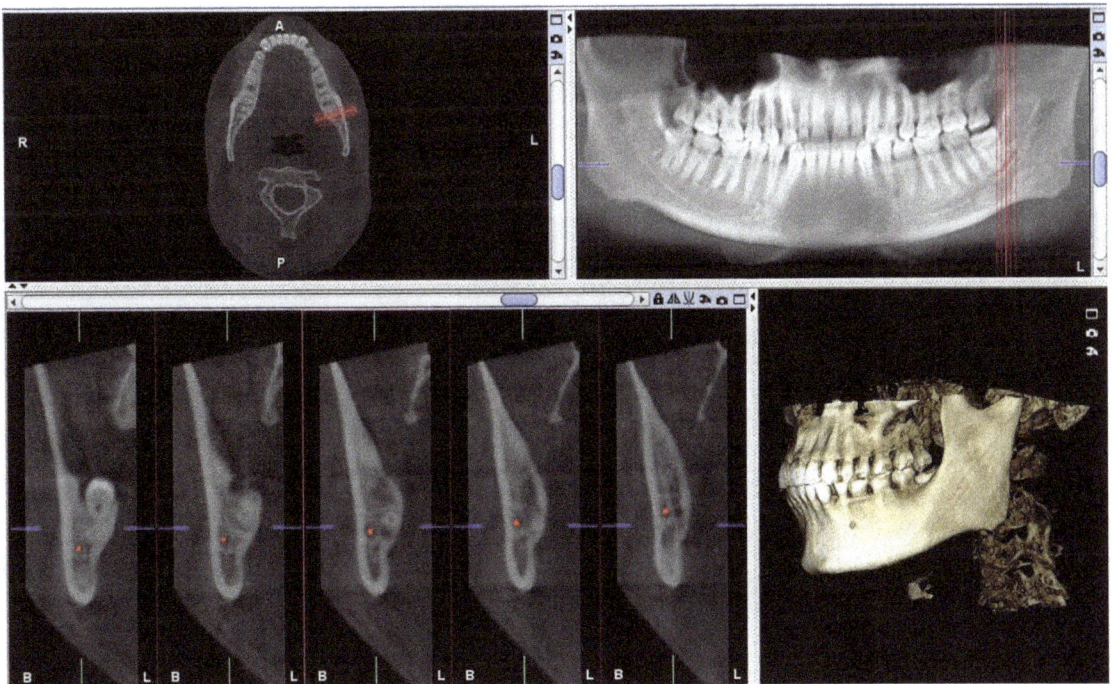

Figure 7. The example of CBC imaging showing the inferior alveolar nerve and its relation with mandibular impacted third molar tooth.

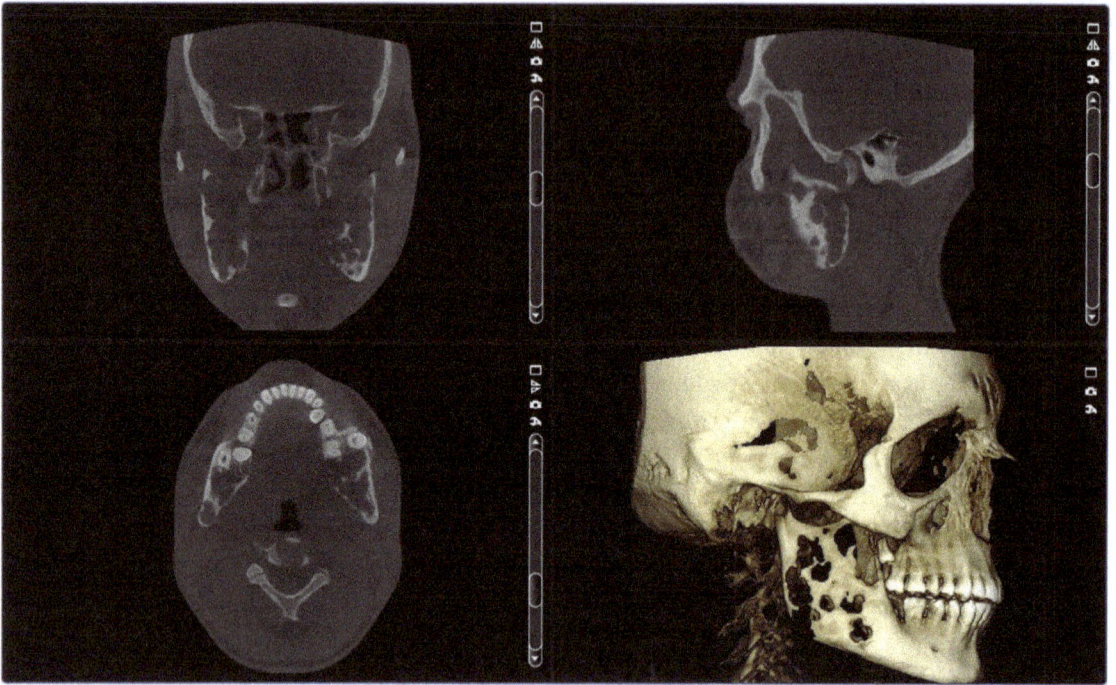

Figure 8. The example of CBCT imaging of a pathologic lesion located in the mandible (reparative giant cell granuloma).

3.1.4. Maxillofacial traumatology

Maxillofacial trauma patients can be assessed with CBCT to plan appropriate treatment method (**Figure 10**). The diagnostic performance of CBCT in detecting orbital floor fractures was reported to be better than ultrasonography. Moreover, it was also reported that CBCT could be used in detecting fractures as a reliable surrogate to CT [31]. The CBCT technology

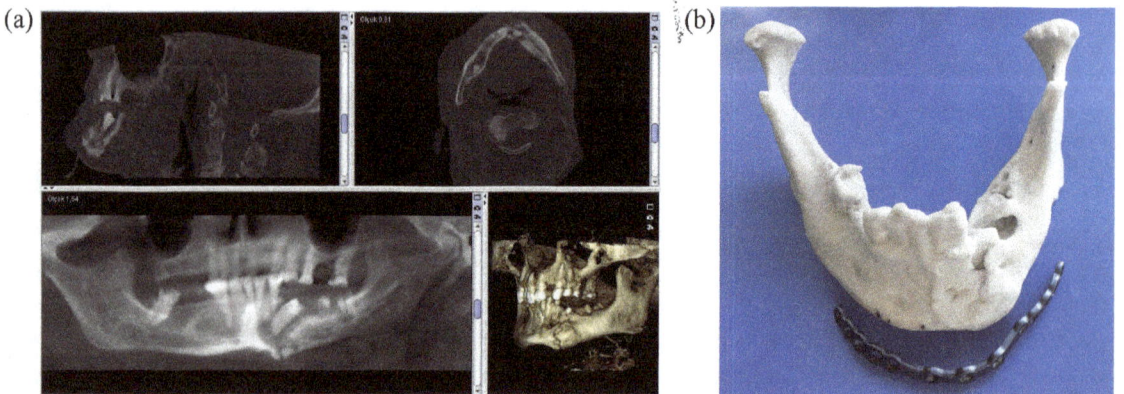

Figure 9. (a) The CBCT imaging of a patient with pathologic mandible fracture due to MRONJ. (b) The CBCT-based 3D model of the patient. Note that bending and adaptation of the titanium plate to the model before surgery can facilitate reconstructive procedures.

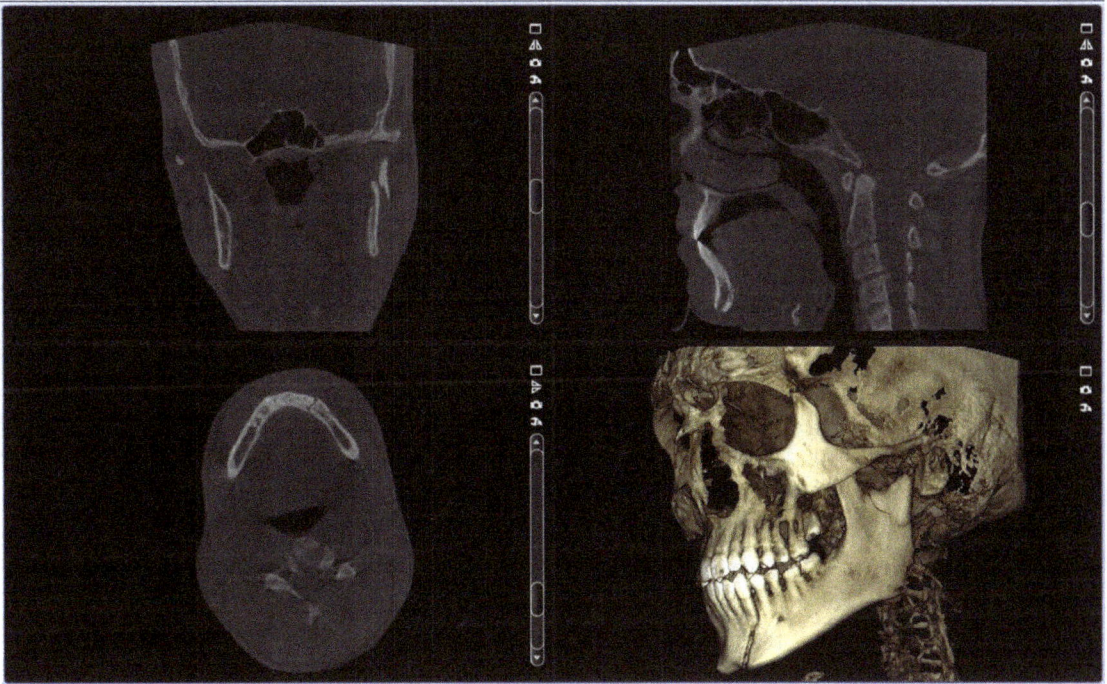

Figure 10. The example of CBCT imaging of a patient with mandibular left parasymphysis and condyle fracture.

can also be used in combination with specific computer software for preoperative virtual planning and fabrication of patient-specific reconstruction plate for mandibular fractures [32]. When CBCT and multi-detector CT were compared in diagnostic imaging of midface, it was concluded that CBCT provided better image quality at lower doses, comparable image quality at higher doses, and superior spatial resolution in standard- and reduced-dose settings [33]. However, in another recent study, it was concluded that CBCT was not optimal for postoperative facial imaging compared to multi-slice CT in terms of visualization of maxillofacial bony structures in the vicinity of osteosynthesis materials [34].

3.1.5. Temporomandibular joint disorders

Temporomandibular disorders associated with degenerative pathologies or abnormalities in the bony structures of condyle, glenoid fossa, and articular eminence such as cortical erosion, articular surface flattening, osteophytes, condiylar hyper-, hypo-, or aplasia, ankylosis, and coronoid process hyperplasia can be visualized with CBCT [9–11]. A CBCT imaging for TMJ complex requires less time and lower radiation doses, it provides the multi-planar views for both TMJs from a single 360° rotation scan, and it simplifies positioning of patient [11]. The linear, angular, and volumetric measurements can also be performed with CBCT imaging software for research purposes. The image-guided puncture technique for TMJ using CBCT can also be used to determine the optimum angle and distance in order to prevent middle cranial fossa damage [35]. These measurements can be used to produce stereographic models and custom-made TMJ prosthesis. The CBCT imaging can only be used to assess the bony structures of TMJ. In general, it is not the imaging of choice for TMJ disorders including myofacial pain dysfunction or internal derangements. The examples of CBCT images acquired for TMJ disorders are shown in **Figures 11–13**.

3.1.6. Dentomaxillofacial discrepancies and cleft palate

The growth abnormalities of maxillofacial bones can be assessed by CBCT imaging (**Figure 14**). The treatment planning and success of the surgical treatments of alveolar cleft patients can be assessed with CBCT imaging (**Figure 15**). As reported in our previous study, it is possible to compare the bone density values of the cleft and non-cleft sites to evaluate the success of alveolar cleft repair using CBCT technology [36]. Moreover, 3D measurement of cleft area including volume of bone defect and outcomes after alveolar grafting in cleft lip and palate patients can also be assessed by CBCT imaging. The dentofacial discrepancies can be visualized, and virtual planning of orthognathic surgeries can be performed with CBCT imaging and special software. Recently, a novel technique for splintless orthognathic surgery, using CBCT imaging with computer-aided design/computer-aided manufacturing (CAD/CAM) technology and virtual planning software, was introduced [37].

The growth abnormalities of head and neck bones can also be scanned using CBCT technology (**Figure 16**). As reported in our previous study, visualization of the styloid process elongation in detail including linear and angular measurements can also be performed with CBCT imaging [18].

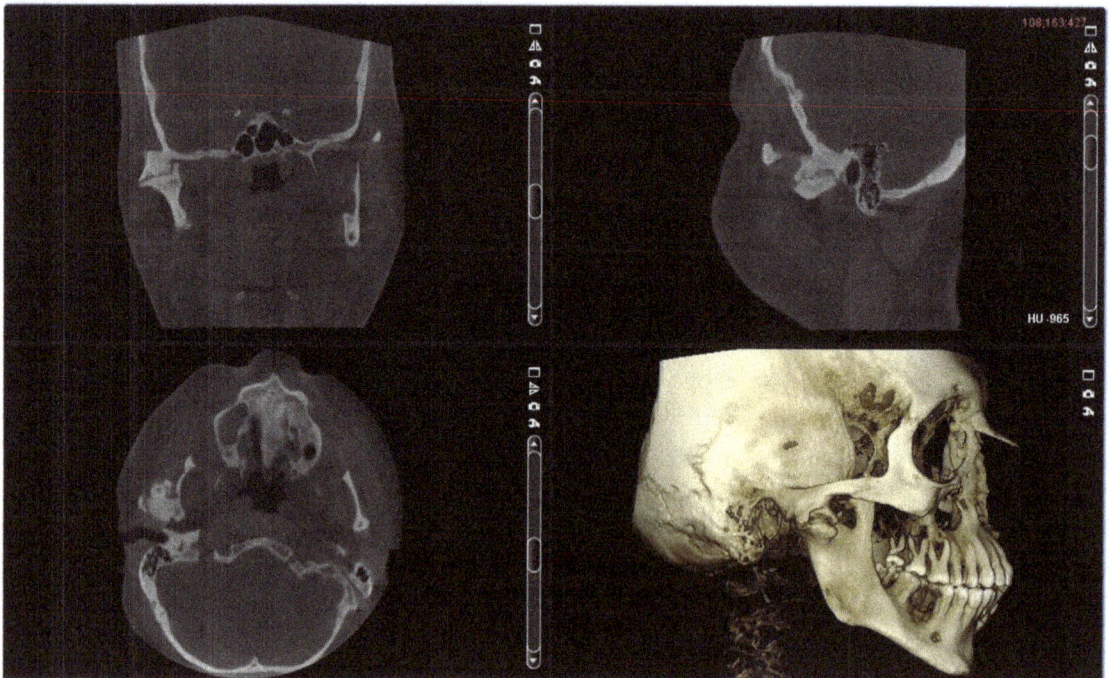

Figure 11. The multi-planar CBCT imaging of a patient with right TMJ ankylosis.

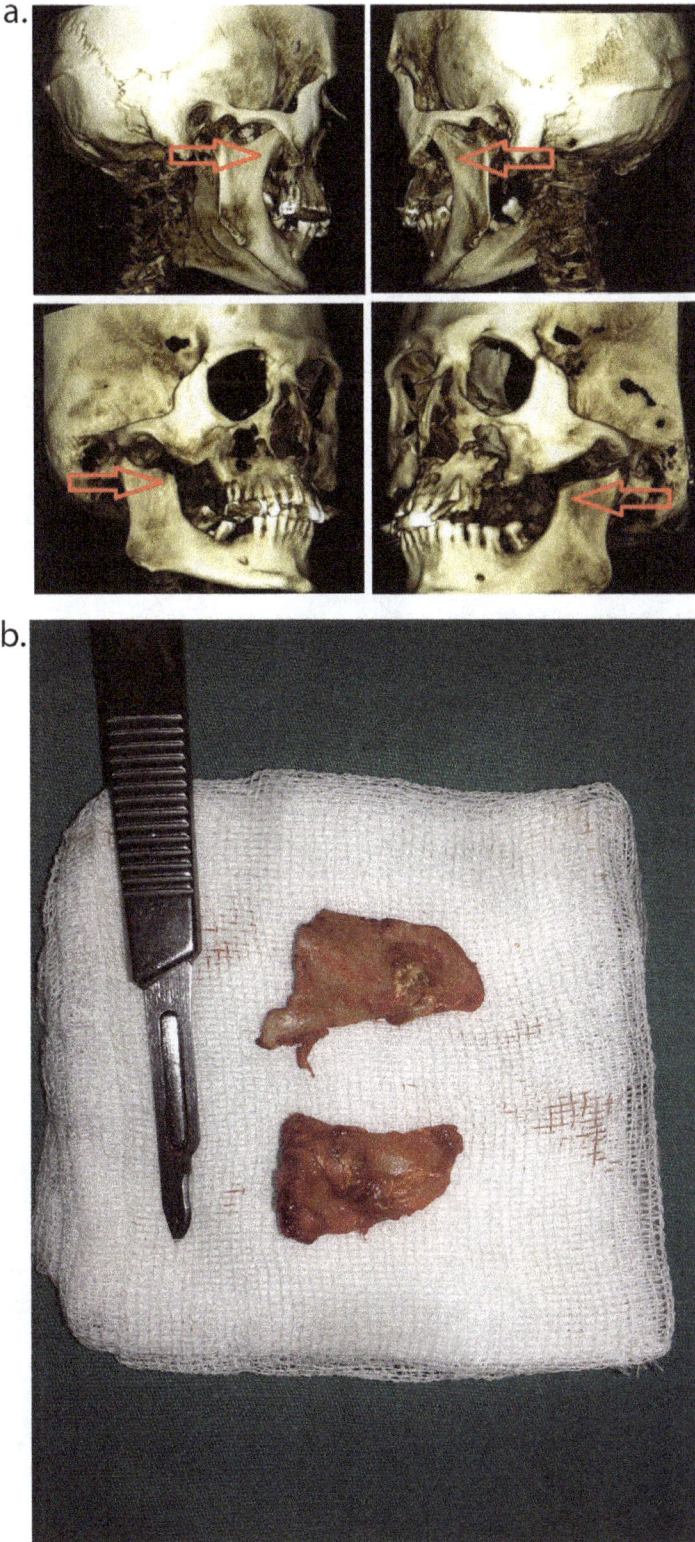

Figure 12. (a) The 3D CBCT views of a patient with bilateral coronoid process hyperplasia before and after coronoidectomy surgery (arrows). (b) The resected bone pieces of coronoid process.

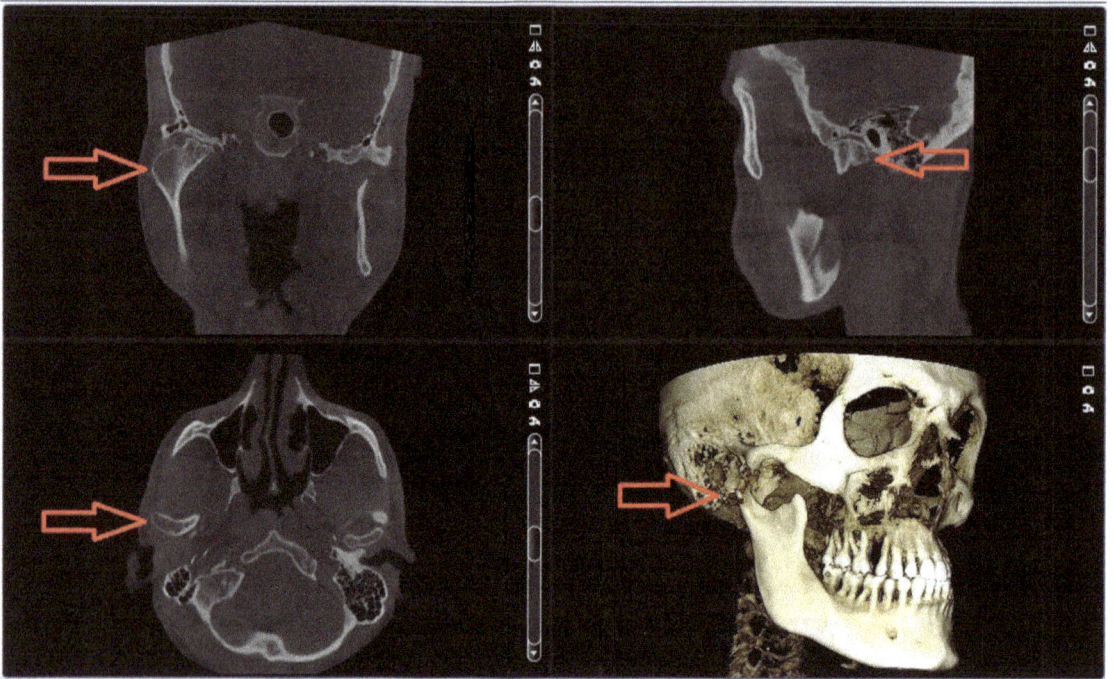

Figure 13. The CBCT imaging of a patient with right mandibular condylar hyperplasia (red arrows).

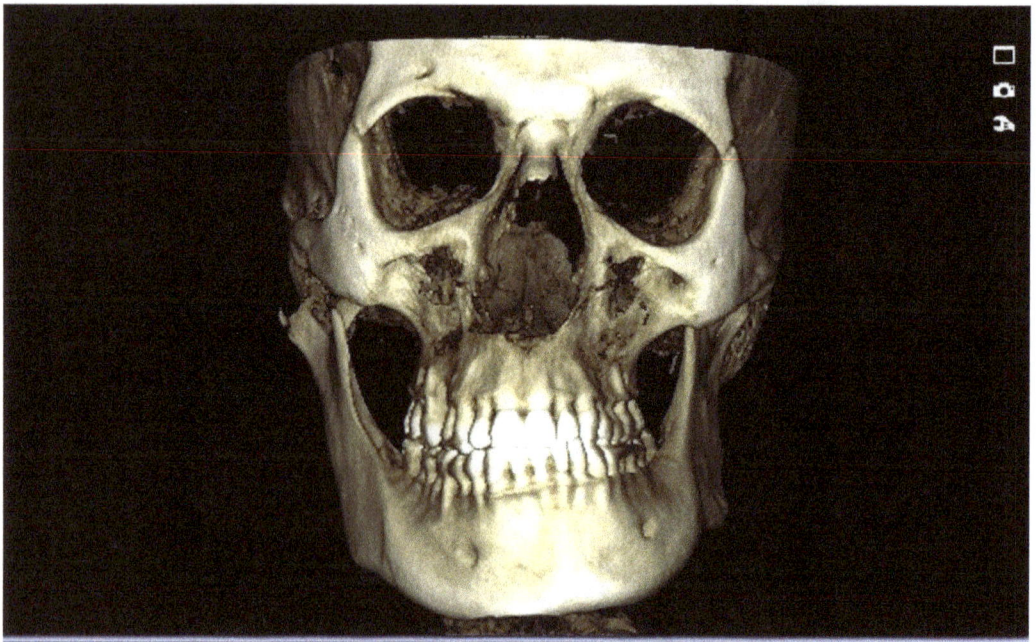

Figure 14. The 3D CBCT imaging of a patient with mandibular asymmetry who needs orthognathic surgery.

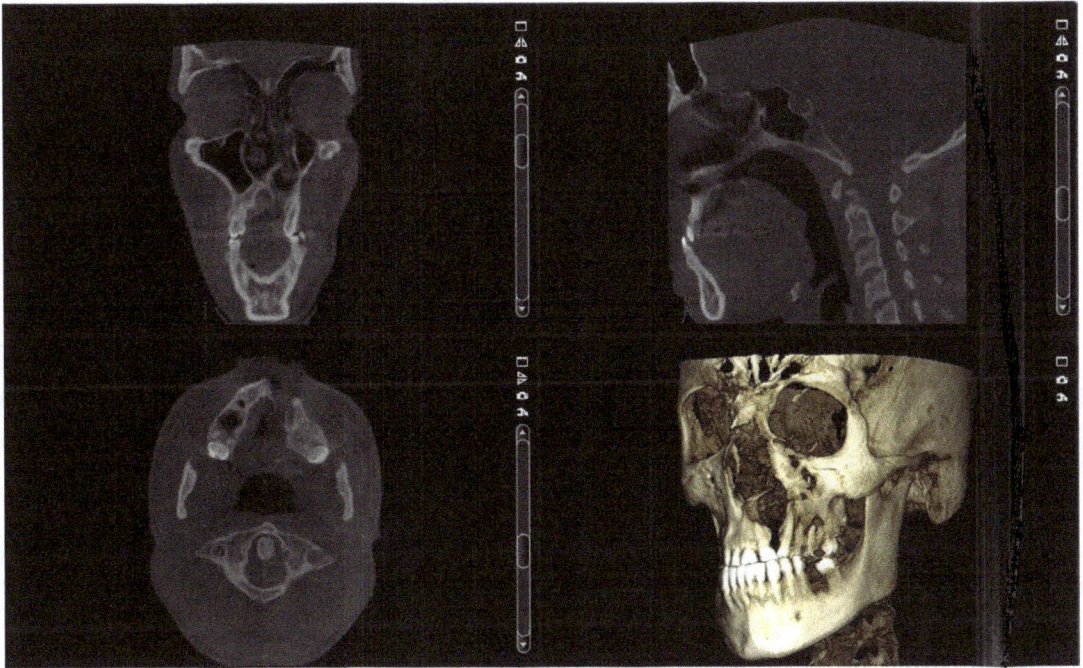

a.

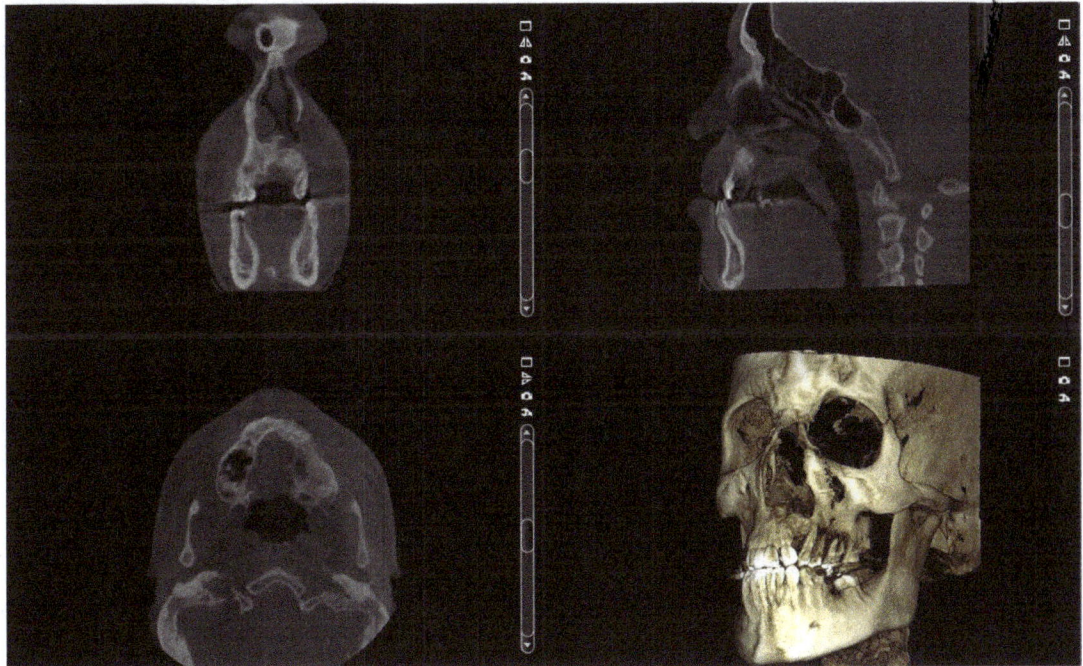

b.

Figure 15. The multi-planar CBCT imaging of a patient with cleft palate on the left site. **a.** Before cleft repair surgery. **b.** After bone augmentation surgery.

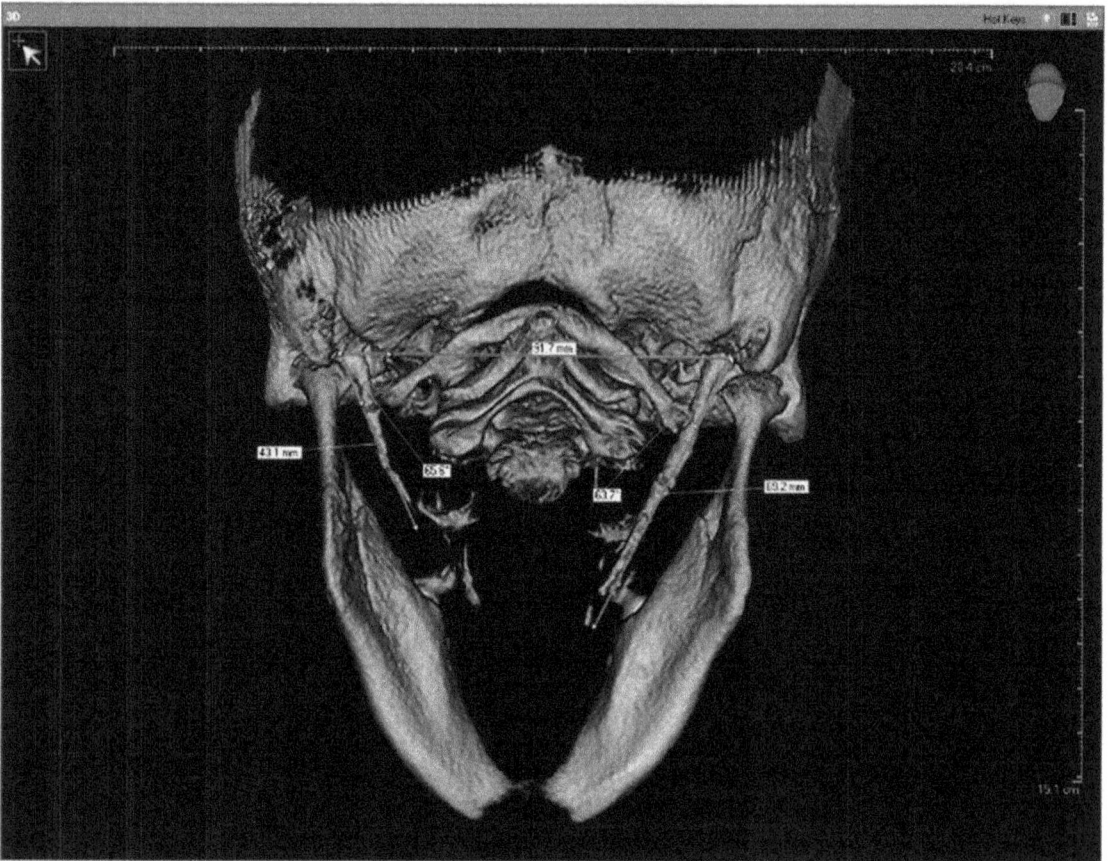

Figure 16. The 3D CBCT imaging of a patient with bilateral elongated styloid process (Eagle syndrome). Note that the length and medial angulations of the styloid process can be measured by using CBCT software.

3.2. Orthodontics

Radiographic analysis is an important aspect for diagnosis and treatment planning in orthodontics. CBCT imaging allows the radiographic assessments in detail with lower radiation doses and without any distortion and superimposition of the other structures. The airway analysis before and after orthognathic surgeries, growth assessment, accurate measurements of cleft area in cleft lip and palate patients, assessment of skeletal and dental structures, assessment of TMJ complex, treatment planning for orthognathic surgery, accurate estimation of space requirement for unerupted or impacted teeth, assessment of orthodontics-induced root resorption, determination of possible regions for mini screw placement, and linear and angular measurements for severe skeletal discrepancies can be performed with CBCT imaging.

The CBCT imaging can be used to assess the amount of interradicular bone, root proximity, the localization of maxillary sinus and inferior alveolar nerve, and density of the available bone, all of which are important in determining the stability and success of orthodontic mini screws. Due to the considerable variation of available bone thickness between individuals, a CBCT imaging is recommended in order to determine the maximum screw length [38]. A CBCT imaging study indicated that vertical facial pattern of the patients should be taken into consideration when adjusting the insertion angle of mini screws at the maxillary buccal site [39].

CBCT can also be used in association with CAD/CAM technology for production of custom-made orthodontic appliances [40].

In terms of evaluation of impacted teeth, small volume of CBCT can be used as a supplement to panoramic imaging in the following cases: when canine inclination in the panoramic X-ray exceeds 30°, when root resorption is suspected at adjacent teeth, and when the canine apex is not clearly seen in the panoramic X-ray [41].

The CBCT scans can be used to evaluate the outcomes of orthodontic treatments and orthognathic surgery. The 3D overlays of superimposed models and 3D color-coded displacement maps provided assessments of treatment changes, displacements of soft and hard tissue during postsurgical follow-up, and amount of relapse [42, 43].

The landmark identification is greatly enhanced in CBCT images. It was reported that reproducibility of cephalometric measurements obtained from CBCT scans was better than that obtained from conventional cephalograms [44]. One of the application areas of CBCT for orthodontics is the growth assessment of patients. The cervical vertebra maturity assessment with CBCT provides reliable assessment of pubertal growth; thus, CBCT can be used to evaluate skeletal maturity for orthodontic treatment [45]. For airway analysis, lateral cephalograms have been routinely used. Axial cuts of 3D CBCT scans provide soft tissue points which are more clearly visible in CBCT sections compared with conventional radiography, thereby enhancing airway assessment [46]. The CBCT-assisted airway analysis also facilitates the diagnosis and treatment planning of obstructive sleep apnea (OSA) [47]. A recent CBCT imaging study concluded that 3D image reconstruction accurately confirmed morphological changes in the upper airway during oral appliance therapy of patients with OSA [48]. In terms of airway analysis with CBCT technology, there are controversial conclusions in literature. A recent systematic review shows that upper pharyngeal airway analysis using CBCT is a reliable method; however, there are some significant limitations including lack of manual orientation of images and selection of threshold sensitivity. Thus, further researches are necessary to adequately establish the reliability of airway analysis with CBCT imaging [49]. A CBCT image used for airway analysis is shown in **Figure 17**.

3.3. Periodontology

The role of CBCT in the diagnosis of periodontal diseases was studied in literature. CBCT displays 2D and 3D images that are necessary for the diagnosis and treatment planning of intrabony defects, furcation involvements, and buccal/lingual bone destructions [50]. In a recent experimental animal study, the diagnostic value of CBCT and digital intraoral radiography for detection of periodontal defects including furcation involvements, one-, two-, three-wall and trough-like intrabony defects, fenestration, and dehiscence were compared. It was concluded that CBCT was superior to digital radiography for detection of grade 1 furcation involvements, three-wall defects, fenestrations, and dehiscences [51]. It is also clinically reported that CBCT imaging provides detailed information about furcation involvement and reliable basis for decision of periodontal treatment [52]. In literature, most of the studies

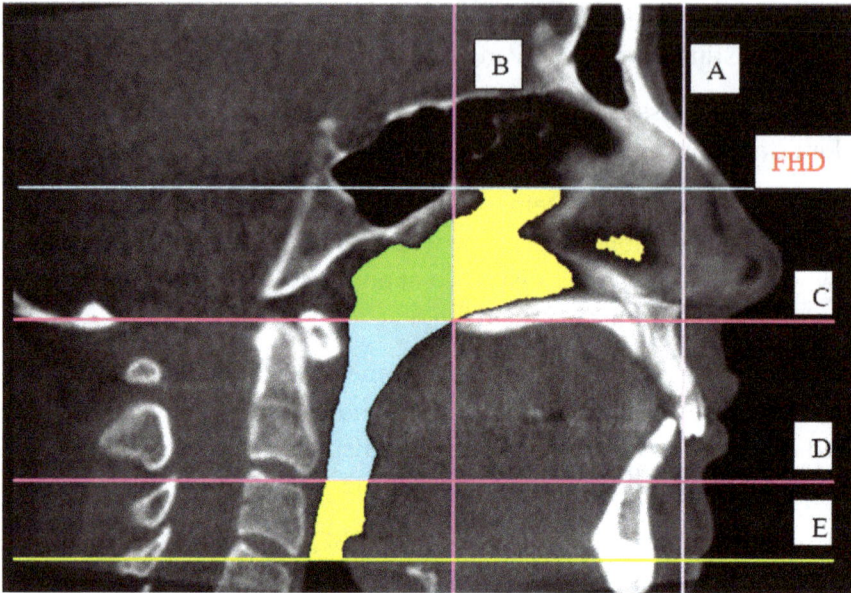

Figure 17. The right lateral view of pharyngeal airway on CBCT image (A: anterior nasal plane, B: posterior nasal plane, C: upper pharyngeal plane, D: middle pharyngeal plane, E: lower pharyngeal plane, FHD: Frankfurt horizontal plane).

concerning the accuracy of CBCT in periodontal diagnosis assessed the efficiency of CBCT in bone defects. However, in our recent study, we concluded that gingival soft tissue thickness and acellular dermal grafts can be consistently evaluated with CBCT technique [53]. The detailed diagnostic imaging of periodontal diseases as well as peri-implantitis may be performed with CBCT technology (**Figures 18** and **19**). Literature shows that optimal detection of peri-implant bone loss is achieved using the smallest FOV, the highest number of acquisition frames, and the smallest voxel [54]. When the CBCT-derived features of peri-implantitis defects compared to the corresponding histomorphometric findings, it is concluded that CBCT represents an accurate diagnostic tool to estimate the histological extent of peri-implantitis [55]. When the performances of different radiographic techniques (intraoral radiography, OPG, CBCT, and CT) in detecting peri-implant bone defects were compared, the highest sensitivity was found with intraoral radiography and CBCT, and the highest specificity was found with intraoral radiography, while CT demonstrated the lowest performance [56].

3.4. Endodontics

The CBCT imaging for endodontic purposes provides the clinicians' wide view in the visualization of periapical lesions, internal or external root resorption, vertical root fractures, and accessory root canals. It was found that CBCT assessment of changes in periapical lesion and mucosal thickening dimensions may reveal useful information regarding endodontic treatment success [57]. The CBCT imaging also guides the clinicians for planning endodontic surgery and in elucidation of causes of fail after endodontic treatment [10, 58]. However, there are two major disadvantages concerning the utilization of CBCT in endodontics: The increased radiation doses, compared to 2D imaging methods, limit its routine usage. Thus, benefits

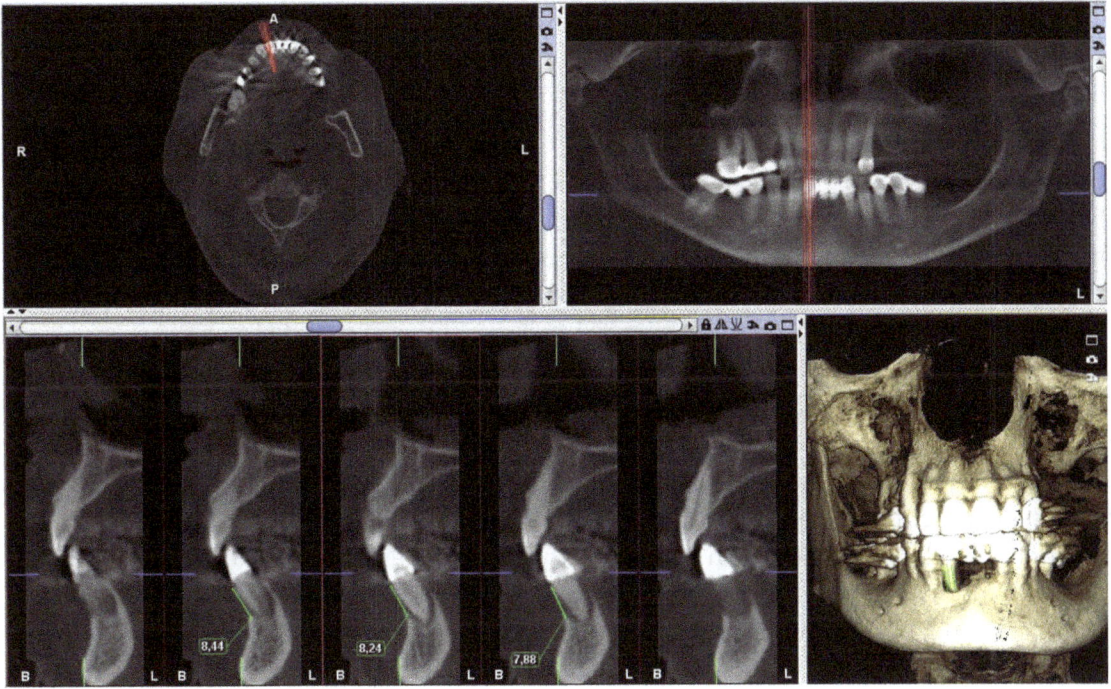

Figure 18. The CBCT imaging of a periodontitis case. Note that the amount of bone resorption around mandibular incisor tooth can be measured in detail using CBCT software.

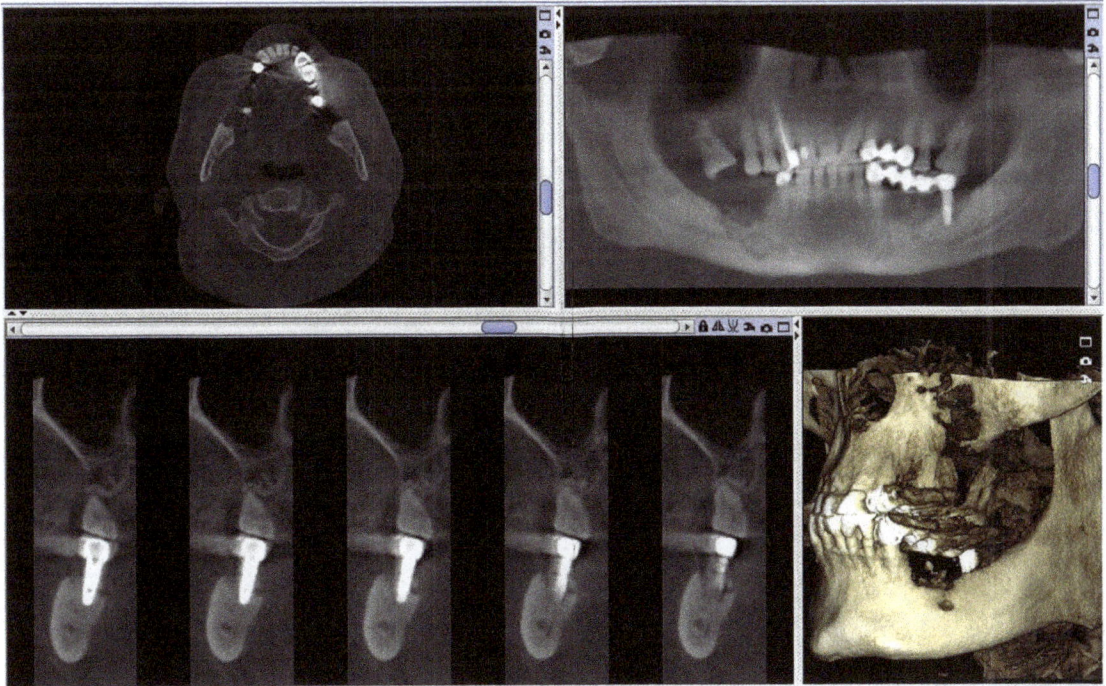

Figure 19. The CBCT imaging of a peri-implantitis case showing bone resorption around dental implant.

getting with CBCT imaging should be carefully evaluated on an individual basis to protect the patients. The other disadvantage is that the radiopaque filling materials and posts crate artifacts which may compromise the diagnosis.

In a recent clinical study, it was reported that CBCT scans had 93% sensitivity, 78% specificity, and 88% accuracy for detection of vertical root fractures in endodontically treated teeth [59]. When CBCT and digital periapical radiography were compared in detecting mandibular molar root perforations, in the non-obturated root canals, the sensitivity and specificity of CBCT scans in perforation detection were better than those of three-angled periapical radiographs. However, in obturated root canals, periapical radiography was reported to be more trustworthy than CBCT for perforation detection [60]. In a recent study, periapical radiographs and CBCT were compared in detecting fractured instruments in root canals with and without filling. The results showed that in the absence of filling, accuracy values were similar in all imaging techniques. In the presence of filling, CBCT had low accuracy [61]. In our recent clinical study, we observed that preoperative CBCT examination demonstrated positive contributions to the endodontic surgery of maxillary first molar teeth [62]. Maxillary posterior teeth have close relationship with maxillary sinus. This may cause the peri-radicular infection to destroy cortical border of the maxillary sinus and spread into the sinus. Such cases may make the clinician to do false or missing diagnosis. In such cases, CBCT imaging allows the practitioner to do appropriate diagnosis of the peri-radicular lesion and its relationship with the adjacent anatomic structures [63]. A CBCT image acquired for planning of endodontic surgery is shown in **Figure 20**.

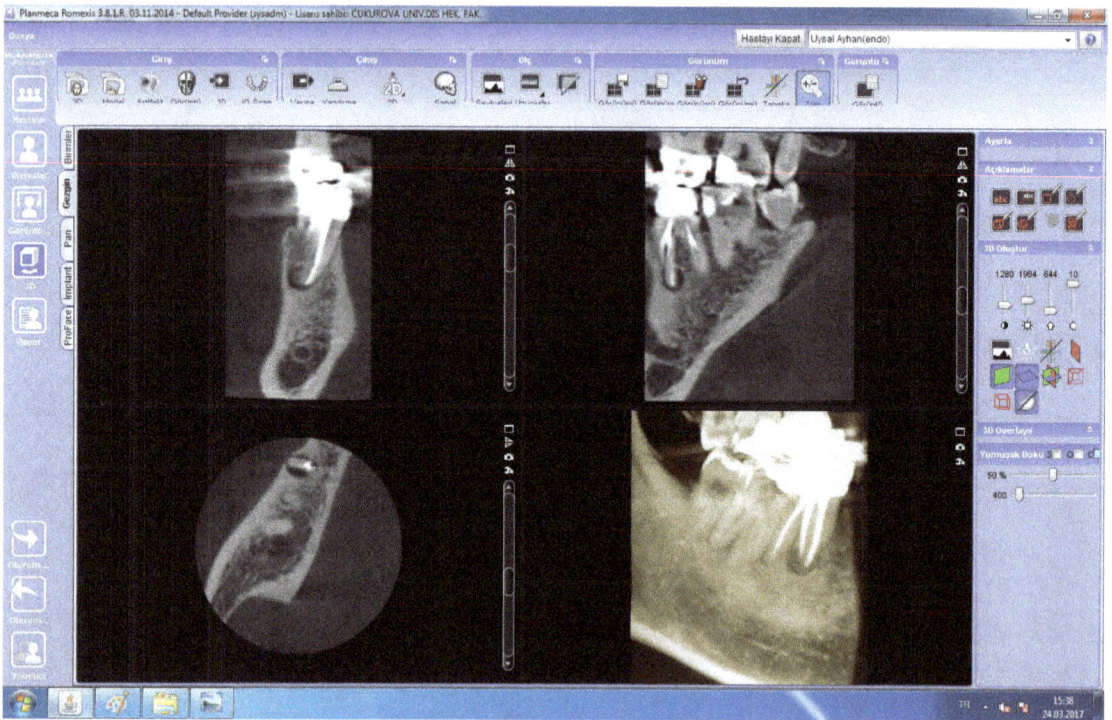

Figure 20. The example of CBCT imaging acquired for detailed assessment of mandibular first molar tooth after endodontic treatment.

In conclusion, according to the contemporary literature, the decision to perform a CBCT examination in endodontics should be kept in limited due to its low accuracy in diagnosis. However, utilization of CBCT may give more benefits in planning endodontic surgery.

3.5. Otolaryngology

Depending on the FOV used, CBCT images may show partial or the entire nasal cavity, paranasal sinuses, airway, cervical vertebrae, and temporal bone. In fact, specific ear, nose, and throat imaging programs have been increasingly included in CBCT systems, suggesting that CBCT may at some point entirely replace medical CT imaging in certain otolaryngology-related applications [64]. In terms of otolaryngology, CBCT imaging can be used to assess airway, paranasal sinus pathologies, nasal polyps, temporal and frontal bone anatomy, middle ear, and cochlear implantation [9, 65–68]. As an imaging guidance, CBCT can be used to treat lymphatic leakage after thyroidectomy [69]. The CBCT-based percutaneous image-guided technique may provide mini invasivity and identification of the anatomy and site of the leakage. An example of CBCT imaging used for detailed assessment of maxillary sinus volume is shown in **Figure 21**.

3.6. Forensic medicine

One of the contemporary application fields of CBCT for maxillofacial imaging is forensic medicine. Age estimation of individuals is an important aspect of forensic science. The CBCT can also be used as new method of age estimation by measuring the pulp-to-tooth area ratio

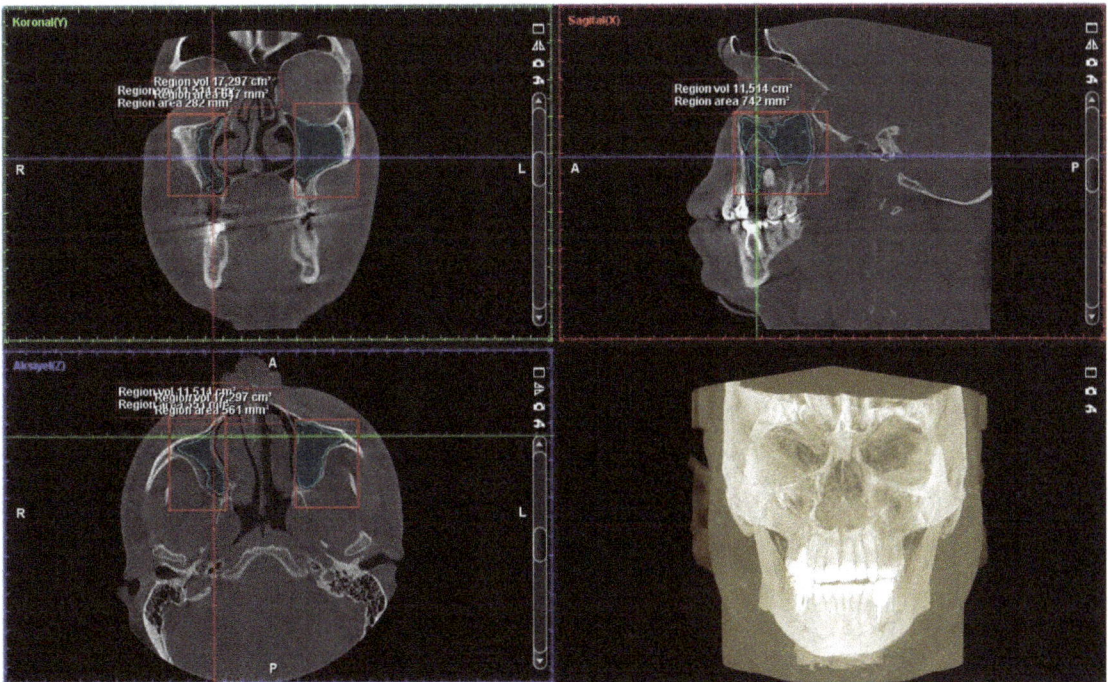

Figure 21. An example of CBCT imaging showing measurement of maxillary sinus volume.

in 3D images in living individuals [70, 71]. The forensic age estimation can also be performed using CBCT-derived analysis of spheno-occipital synchondrosis [72].

Moreover, the CBCT-derived anthropometric measurements on mandibular images can be used for sex estimation in forensic settings [73]. Besides age and sex estimation, CBCT can be used in forensic science for identification of unknown human bodies through frontal sinus 3D superimposition technique [74].

4. Conclusion

In the present chapter, a review of literature related to the clinical applications of CBCT technique for oral and maxillofacial imaging was undertaken with illustrated sample cases. Tremendous advancements have been acquired after the introduction of CBCT imaging technology especially for oral and maxillofacial practice. The contributions of CBCT for maxillofacial imaging have been demonstrated in several studies for diagnosis, treatment planning, evaluation of treatment outcome, and research purposes. The widespread use of CBCT in maxillofacial region represents the most important advance in diagnostic radiology without disadvantages of multi-slice CT especially including high radiation dose and increased cost. In most of the cases in OMF region, CBCT takes the place of multi-slice CT. Dentists and clinicians dealing with this field should have the knowledge of working principles, requirements, appropriate indications, clinical benefits, drawbacks, and hazardous effects of CBCT technology for proper utilization. In literature, there were inconsistencies and discrepancies about the CBCT device settings, properties, radiation doses, image acquisition protocol, and estimation of bone density which confuse the readers. The most common clinical applications of CBCT were in OMF surgery including implantology and impacted teeth. The subjective image quality was higher in multi-slice CT than in older CBCT units. However, the recent CBCT units showed opposite results. Moreover, new CBCT units with flat panel detectors seem to be less prone to metal artifacts. The CBCT provides less radiation than multi-slice CT but more than panoramic X-ray. Thus, it is crucial that the ALARA principle ("As Low As Reasonably Achievable" radiation dose) should be respected.

Author details

Ufuk Tatli[1]* and Burcu Evlice[2]

*Address all correspondence to: dr.ufuktatli@gmail.com

1 Department of Oral and Maxillofacial Surgery, Faculty of Dentistry, Çukurova University, Adana, Turkey

2 Department of Oral and Maxillofacial Radiology, Faculty of Dentistry, Çukurova University, Adana, Turkey

References

[1] Brenner DJ, Hall EJ. Computed tomography—An increasing source of radiation exposure. The New England Journal of Medicine. 2007;**357**:2277-2284. DOI: 10.1056/NEJMra072149

[2] Hatcher DC, Dial C, Mayorga C. Cone beam CT for pre-surgical assessment of implant sites. Journal of the California Dental Association. 2003;**31**:825-833

[3] Arai Y, Tammisalo E, Iwai K, Hashimoto K, Shinoda K. Development of a compact computed tomographic apparatus for dental use. Dentomaxillofacial Radiology. 1999;**28**:245-248. DOI: 10.1038/sj/dmfr/4600448

[4] Mozzo P, Procacci C, Tacconi A, Martini PT, Andreis IA. A new volumetric CT machine for dental imaging based on the cone-beam technique: Preliminary results. European Radiology. 1998;**8**:1558-1564

[5] Scarfe WC, Farman AG. Cone beam computed tomography. In: White SC, Pharoah MJ, editors. Oral Radiology: Principles and Interpretation. 6th ed. St. Louis: Mosby Elsevier; 2009. pp. 225-243

[6] Scarfe WC, Farman AG. What is cone-beam CT and how does it work? Dental Clinics of North America. 2008;**52**:707-730. DOI: 10.1016/j.cden.2008.05.005

[7] White SC, Pharoah MJ. The evolution and application of dental maxillofacial imaging modalities. Dental Clinics of North America. 2008;**52**:689-705. DOI: 10.1016/j.cden.2008.05.006

[8] Pauwels R, Araki K, Siewerdsen JH, Thongvigitmanee SS. Technical aspects of dental CBCT: State of the art. Dentomaxillofacial Radiology. 2015;**44**:20140224. DOI: 10.1259/dmfr.20140224

[9] De Vos W, Casselman J, Swennen GR. Cone-beam computerized tomography (CBCT) imaging of the oral and maxillofacial region: A systematic review of the literature. International Journal of Oral and Maxillofacial Surgery. 2009;**38**:609-625. DOI: 10.1016/j.ijom.2009.02.028

[10] Akarslan ZZ, Peker I. Advances in radiographic techniques used in dentistry. In: Virdi MS, editor. Emerging Trends in Oral Health Sciences and Dentistry. Rijeka: InTech; 2015. pp. 763-799. DOI: 10.5772/59129

[11] Machado GL. CBCT imaging—A boon to orthodontics. The Saudi Dental Journal. 2015;**27**:12-21. DOI: 10.1016/j.sdentj.2014.08.004

[12] Isoda K, Ayukawa Y, Tsukiyama Y, Sogo M, Matsushita Y, Koyano K. Relationship between the bone density estimated by cone-beam computed tomography and the primary stability of dental implants. Clinical Oral Implants Research. 2012;**23**:832-836. DOI: 10.1111/j.1600-0501.2011.02203.x

[13] Kamburoğlu K. Use of dentomaxillofacial cone beam computed tomography in dentistry. World Journal of Radiology. 2015;7:128-130. DOI: 10.4329/wjr.v7.i6.128

[14] Tyndall DA, Price JB, Tetradis S, Ganz SD, Hildebolt C, Scarfe WC, American Academy of Oral and Maxillofacial Radiology. Position statement of the American Academy of Oral and Maxillofacial Radiology on selection criteria for the use of radiology in dental implantology with emphasis on cone beam computed tomography. Oral Surgery, Oral Medicine, Oral Pathology and Oral Radiology. 2012;113:817-826. DOI: 10.1016/j.oooo.2012.03.005

[15] Holberg C, Steinhäuser S, Geis P, Rudzki-Janson I. Cone-beam computed tomography in orthodontics: Benefits and limitations. Journal of Orofacial Orthopedics. 2005;66:434-444. DOI: 10.1007/s00056-005-0519-z

[16] Hashimoto K, Kawashima S, Kameoka S, Akiyama Y, Honjoya T, Ejima K, Sawada K. Comparison of image validity between cone beam computed tomography for dental use and multidetector row helical computed tomography. Dentomaxillofacial Radiology. 2007;36:465-471. DOI: 10.1259/dmfr/22818643

[17] Schulze D, Heiland M, Thurmann H, Adam G. Radiation exposure during midfacial imaging using 4- and 16-slice computed tomography, cone beam computed tomography systems and conventional radiography. Dentomaxillofacial Radiology. 2004;33:83-86. DOI: 10.1259/dmfr/28403350

[18] Oztunç H, Evlice B, Tatli U, Evlice A. Cone-beam computed tomographic evaluation of styloid process: A retrospective study of 208 patients with orofacial pain. Head & Face Medicine. 2014;10:5. DOI: 10.1186/1746-160X-10-5

[19] Orhan K, Kusakci Seker B, Aksoy S, Bayindir H, Berberoğlu A, Seker E. Cone beam CT evaluation of maxillary sinus septa prevalence, height, location and morphology in children and an adult population. Medical Principles and Practice. 2013;22:47-53. DOI: 10.1159/000339849

[20] Sinanoglu A, Orhan K, Kursun S, Inceoglu B, Oztas B. Evaluation of optic canal and surrounding structures using cone beam computed tomography: Considerations for maxillofacial surgery. The Journal of Craniofacial Surgery. 2016;27:1327-1330. DOI: 10.1097/SCS.0000000000002726

[21] Erdogan Ö, Uçar Y, Tatlı U, Sert M, Benlidayı ME, Evlice B. A clinical prospective study on alveolar bone augmentation and dental implant success in patients with type 2 diabetes. Clinical Oral Implants Research. 2015;26:1267-1275. DOI: 10.1111/clr.12450

[22] Turkyilmaz I, Sennerby L, McGlumphy EA, Tözüm TF. Biomechanical aspects of primary implant stability: A human cadaver study. Clinical Implant Dentistry and Related Research. 2009;11:113-119. DOI: 10.1111/j.1708-8208.2008.00097.x

[23] Farré-Pagés N, Augé-Castro ML, Alaejos-Algarra F, Mareque-Bueno J, Ferrés-Padró E, Hernández-Alfaro F. Relation between bone density and primary implant stability. Medicina Oral Patologia Oral y Cirugia Bucal. 2011;16:e62–e67. DOI: 10.4317/medoral.16.e62

[24] Naitoh M, Hirukawa A, Katsumata A, Ariji E. Evaluation of voxel values in mandibular cancellous bone: Relationship between cone-beam computed tomography and multislice helical computed tomography. Clinical Oral Implants Research. 2009;**20**:503-506. DOI: 10.1111/j.1600-0501.2008.01672.x

[25] Nomura Y, Watanabe H, Honda E, Kurabayashi T. Reliability of voxel values from cone-beam computed tomography for dental use in evaluating bone mineral density. Clinical Oral Implants Research. 2010;**21**:558-562. DOI: 10.1111/j.1600-0501.2009.01896.x

[26] Pauwels R, Nackaerts O, Bellaiche N, Stamatakis II, Tsiklakis K, Walker A, Bosmans H, Bogaerts R, Jacobs R, Horner K. Variability of dental cone beam CT grey values for density estimations. The British Journal of Radiology. 2013;**86**:20120135. DOI: 10.1259/bjr.20120135

[27] Salimov F, Tatli U, Kürkçü M, Akoğlan M, Oztunç H, Kurtoğlu C. Evaluation of relationship between preoperative bone density values derived from cone beam computed tomography and implant stability parameters: A clinical study. Clinical Oral Implants Research. 2014;**25**:1016-1021. DOI: 10.1111/clr.12219

[28] Tatli U, Salimov F, Kürkcü M, Akoğlan M, Kurtoğlu C. Does cone beam computed tomography-derived bone density give predictable data about stability changes of immediately loaded implants?: A 1-year resonance frequency follow-up study. The Journal of Craniofacial Surgery. 2014;**25**:e293–e299. DOI: 10.1097/SCS.0000000000000727

[29] Jawad Z, Carmichael F, Houghton N, Bates C. A review of cone beam computed tomography for the diagnosis of root resorption associated with impacted canines, introducing an innovative root resorption scale. Oral Surgery, Oral Medicine, Oral Pathology and Oral Radiology. 2016;**122**:765-771. DOI: 10.1016/j.oooo.2016.08.015

[30] Subramanian G, Kalyoussef E, Blitz-Goldstein M, Guerrero J, Ghesani N, Quek SY. Identifying MRONJ-affected bone with digital fusion of functional imaging (FI) and cone-beam computed tomography (CBCT): Case reports and hypothesis. Oral Surgery, Oral Medicine, Oral Pathology and Oral Radiology. 2017;**123**:e106–e116. DOI: 10.1016/j.oooo.2016.11.007

[31] Johari M, Ghavimi MA, Mahmoudian H, Javadrashid R, Mirakhor Samani S, Fouladi DF. A comparable study of the diagnostic performance of orbital ultrasonography and CBCT in patients with suspected orbital floor fractures. Dentomaxillofacial Radiology. DOI: 10.1259/dmfr.20150311

[32] Thor A. Preoperative planning of virtual osteotomies followed by fabrication of patient specific reconstruction plate for secondary correction and fixation of displaced bilateral mandibular body fracture. Craniomaxillofacial Trauma and Reconstruction. 2016;**9**:188-194. DOI: 10.1055/s-0036-1572492

[33] Veldhoen S, Schöllchen M, Hanken H, Precht C, Henes FO, Schön G, Nagel HD, Schumacher U, Heiland M, Adam G, Regier M. Performance of cone-beam computed tomography and multidetector computed tomography in diagnostic imaging of the midface: A comparative study on phantom and cadaver head scans. European Radiology. 2017;**27**:790-800. DOI: 10.1007/s00330-016-4387-2

[34] Peltola EM, Mäkelä T, Haapamäki V, Suomalainen A, Leikola J, Koskinen SK, Kortesniemi M, Koivikko MP. CT of facial fracture fixation: An experimental study of arte-fact reducing methods. Dentomaxillofacial Radiology. 2017;46:20160261. DOI: 10.1259/dmfr.20160261

[35] Honda K, Bjørnland T. Image-guided puncture technique for the superior temporoman-dibular joint space: Value of cone beam computed tomography (CBCT). Oral Surgery, Oral Medicine, Oral Pathology, Oral Radiology and Endodontics. 2006;102:281-286. DOI: 10.1016/j.tripleo.2005.10.042

[36] Benlidayi ME, Tatli U, Kurkcu M, Uzel A, Oztunc H. Comparison of bovine-derived hydroxyapatite and autogenous bone for secondary alveolar bone grafting in patients with alveolar clefts. Journal of Oral and Maxillofacial Surgery. 2012;70:e95–e102. DOI: 10.1016/j.joms.2011.08.041

[37] Gander T, Bredell M, Eliades T, Rücker M, Essig H. Splintless orthognathic surgery: A novel technique using patient-specific implants (PSI). Journal of Craniomaxillofacial Surgery. 2015;43:319-322. DOI: 10.1016/j.jcms.2014.12.003

[38] Holm M, Jost-Brinkmann PG, Mah J, Bumann A. Bone thickness of the anterior pal-ate for orthodontic miniscrews. The Angle Orthodontist. 2016;86:826-831. DOI: 10.2319/091515-622.1

[39] Tozlu M, Germeç Cakan D, Ulkur F, Ozdemir F. Maxillary buccal cortical plate inclination at mini-screw insertion sites. The Angle Orthodontist. 2015;85:868-873. DOI: 10.2319/070914-480.1

[40] Kwon SY, Kim Y, Ahn HW, Kim KB, Chung KR, Kim Sunny SH. Computer-aided design-ing and manufacturing of lingual fixed orthodontic appliance using 2D/3D registration software and rapid prototyping. International Journal of Dentistry. 2014;2014:164164. DOI: 10.1155/2014/164164

[41] Wriedt S, Jaklin J, Al-Nawas B, Wehrbein H. Impacted upper canines: Examination and treatment proposal based on 3D versus 2D diagnosis. Journal of Orofacial Orthopedics. 2012;73:28-40. DOI: 10.1007/s00056-011-0058-8

[42] Cevidanes LH, Heymann G, Cornelis MA, DeClerck HJ, Tulloch JF. Superimposition of 3-dimensional cone-beam computed tomography models of growing patients. American Journal of Orthodontics and Dentofacial Orthopedics. 2009;136:94-99. DOI: 10.1016/j.ajodo.2009.01.018

[43] Almeida RC, Cevidanes LH, Carvalho FA, Motta AT, Almeida MA, Styner M, Turvey T, Proffit WR, Phillips C. Soft tissue response to mandibular advancement using 3D CBCT scanning. International Journal of Oral and Maxillofacial Surgery. 2011;40:353-359. DOI: 10.1016/j.ijom.2010.11.018

[44] van Vlijmen OJ, Bergé SJ, Swennen GR, Bronkhorst EM, Katsaros C, Kuijpers-Jagtman AM. Comparison of cephalometric radiographs obtained from cone-beam computed tomography scans and conventional radiographs. Journal of Oral and Maxillofacial Surgery. 2009;67:92-97. DOI: 10.1016/j.joms.2008.04.025

[45] Joshi V, Yamaguchi T, Matsuda Y, Kaneko N, Maki K, Okano T. Skeletal maturity assessment with the use of cone-beam computerized tomography. Oral Surgery, Oral Medicine, Oral Pathology and Oral Radiology. 2012;113:841-849. DOI: 10.1016/j.oooo.2011.11.018

[46] Vizzotto MB, Liedke GS, Delamare EL, Silveira HD, Dutra V, Silveira HE. A comparative study of lateral cephalograms and cone-beam computed tomographic images in upper airway assessment. European Journal of Orthodontics. 2012;34:390-393. DOI: 10.1093/ejo/cjr012

[47] Ogawa T, Enciso R, Shintaku WH, Clark GT. Evaluation of cross-section airway configuration of obstructive sleep apnea. Oral Surgery, Oral Medicine, Oral Pathology, Oral Radiology and Endodontics. 2007;103:102-108. DOI: 10.1016/j.tripleo.2006.06.008

[48] Cossellu G, Biagi R, Sarcina M, Mortellaro C, Farronato G. Three-dimensional evaluation of upper airway in patients with obstructive sleep apnea syndrome during oral appliance therapy. The Journal of Craniofacial Surgery. 2015;26:745-748. DOI: 10.1097/SCS.0000000000001538

[49] Zimmerman JN, Lee J, Pliska BT. Reliability of upper pharyngeal airway assessment using dental CBCT: A systematic review. European Journal of Orthodontics. DOI: 10.1093/ejo/cjw079

[50] Acar B, Kamburoğlu K. Use of cone beam computed tomography in periodontology. World Journal of Radiology. 2014;6:139-147. DOI: 10.4329/wjr.v6.i5.139

[51] Bayat S, Talaeipour AR, Sarlati F. Detection of simulated periodontal defects using cone-beam CT and digital intraoral radiography. Dentomaxillofacial Radiology. DOI: 10.1259/dmfr.20160030

[52] Walter C, Kaner D, Berndt DC, Weiger R, Zitzmann NU. Three-dimensional imaging as a pre-operative tool in decision making for furcation surgery. Journal of Clinical Periodontology. 2009;36:250-257. DOI: 10.1111/j.1600-051X.2008.01367.x

[53] Ozturan S, Oztunc H, Keles Evlice B. Assessment of the soft tissue volumetric changes following acellular dermal matrix grafts with cone beam computerized tomography. Quintessence International. 2015;46:171-178. DOI: 10.3290/j.qi.a32826

[54] Pinheiro LR, Scarfe WC, Augusto de Oliveira Sales M, Gaia BF, Cortes AR, Cavalcanti MG. Effect of cone-beam computed tomography field of view and acquisition frame on the detection of chemically simulated peri-implant bone loss in vitro. Journal of Periodontology. 2015;86:1159-1165. DOI: 10.1902/jop.2015.150223

[55] Golubovic V, Mihatovic I, Becker J, Schwarz F. Accuracy of cone-beam computed tomography to assess the configuration and extent of ligature-induced peri-implantitis defects. A pilot study. Oral and Maxillofacial Surgery. 2012;16:349-354. DOI: 10.1007/s10006-012-0320-2

[56] Kühl S, Zürcher S, Zitzmann NU, Filippi A, Payer M, Dagassan-Berndt D. Detection of peri-implant bone defects with different radiographic techniques—A human cadaver study. Clinical Oral Implants Research. 2016;27:529-534. DOI: 10.1111/clr.12619

[57] Kamburoğlu K, Yılmaz F, Gulsahi K, Gulen O, Gulsahi A. Change in periapical lesion and adjacent mucosal thickening dimensions one year after endodontic treatment: Volumetric cone-beam computed tomography assessment. Journal of Endodontics. 2017;**43**:218-224. DOI: 10.1016/j.joen.2016.10.023

[58] Tyndall DA, Kohltfarber H. Application of cone beam volumetric tomography in endodontics. Australian Dental Journal. 2012;**57**:72-81. DOI: 10.1111/j.1834-7819.2011.01654.x

[59] Saberi E, Mollashahi NF, Movasagh Z, Moghaddam AA, Mohammadi A. Value of CBCT in vertical root fracture detection in endodontically-treated teeth. Minerva Stomatologica. 2017;**66**:69-74. DOI: 10.23736/S0026-4970.17.03972-3

[60] Haghanifar S, Moudi E, Mesgarani A, Bijani A, Abbaszadeh N. A comparative study of cone-beam computed tomography and digital periapical radiography in detecting mandibular molars root perforations. Imaging Science in Dentistry. 2014;**44**:115-119. DOI: 10.5624/isd.2014.44.2.115

[61] Ramos Brito AC, Verner FS, Junqueira RB, Yamasaki MC, Queiroz PM, Freitas DQ, Oliveira-Santos C. Detection of fractured endodontic instruments in root canals: Comparison between different digital radiography systems and cone-beam computed tomography. Journal of Endodontics. 2017;**43**:544-549. DOI: 10.1016/j.joen.2016.11.017

[62] Kurt SN, Üstün Y, Erdogan Ö, Evlice B, Yoldas O, Öztunc H. Outcomes of periradicular surgery of maxillary first molars using a vestibular approach: A prospective, clinical study with one year of follow-up. Journal of Oral and Maxillofacial Surgery. 2014;**72**:1049-1061. DOI: 10.1016/j.joms.2014.02.004

[63] Low KM, Dula K, Bürgin W, von Arx T. Comparison of periapical radiography and limited cone-beam tomography in posterior maxillary teeth referred for apical surgery. Journal of Endodontics. 2008;**34**:557-562. DOI: 10.1016/j.joen.2008.02.022

[64] Miracle AC, Mukherji SK. Conebeam CT of the head and neck, part 2: Clinical applications. American Journal of Neuroradiology. 2009;**30**:1285-1292. DOI: 10.3174/ajnr.A1654

[65] Güldner C, Diogo I, Leicht J, Mandapathil M, Wilhelm T, Teymoortash A, Jahns E. Reduction of radiation dosage in visualization of paranasal sinuses in daily routine. International Journal of Otolaryngology. 2017;**2017**:3104736. DOI: 10.1155/2017/3104736

[66] Güldner C, Diogo I, Bernd E, Dräger S, Mandapathil M, Teymoortash A, Negm H, Wilhelm T. Visualization of anatomy in normal and pathologic middle ears by cone beam CT. European Archives of Oto-Rhino-Laryngology. 2017;**274**:737-742. DOI: 10.1007/s00405-016-4345-2

[67] Razafindranaly V, Truy E, Pialat JB, Martinon A, Bourhis M, Boublay N, Faure F, Ltaïef-Boudrigua A. Cone beam CT versus multislice CT: Radiologic diagnostic agreement in the postoperative assessment of cochlear implantation. Otology & Neurotology. 2016;**37**:1246-1254. DOI: 10.1097/MAO.0000000000001165

[68] Al Abduwani J, ZilinSkiene L, Colley S, Ahmed S. Cone beam CT paranasal sinuses versus standard multidetector and low dose multidetector CT studies. American Journal of Otolaryngology. 2016;**37**:59-64. DOI: 10.1016/j.amjoto.2015.08.002

[69] Ierardi AM, Pappalardo V, Liu X, Wu CW, Anuwong A, Kim HY, Liu R, Lavazza M, Inversini D, Coppola A, Floridi C, Boni L, Carrafiello G, Dionigi G. Usefulness of CBCT and guidance software for percutaneous embolization of a lymphatic leakage after thyroidectomy for cancer. Gland Surgery. 2016;**5**:633-638. DOI: 10.21037/gs.2016.12.13

[70] Rai A, Acharya AB, Naikmasur VG. Age estimation by pulp-to-tooth area ratio using cone-beam computed tomography: A preliminary analysis. Journal of Forensic Dental Sciences. 2016;**8**:150-154. DOI: 10.4103/0975-1475.195118

[71] Pinchi V, Pradella F, Buti J, Baldinotti C, Focardi M, Norelli GA. A new age estimation procedure based on the 3D CBCT study of the pulp cavity and hard tissues of the teeth for forensic purposes: A pilot study. Journal of Forensic and Legal Medicine. 2015; **36**:150-157. DOI: 10.1016/j.jflm.2015.09.015

[72] Sinanoglu A, Kocasarac HD, Noujeim M. Age estimation by an analysis of spheno-occipital synchondrosis using cone-beam computed tomography. Legal Medicine (Tokyo, Japan). 2016;**18**:13-19. DOI: 10.1016/j.legalmed.2015.11.004

[73] Gamba Tde O, Alves MC, Haiter-Neto F. Mandibular sexual dimorphism analysis in CBCT scans. Journal of Forensic and Legal Medicine. 2016;**38**:106-110. DOI: 10.1016/j.jflm.2015.11.024

[74] Beaini TL, Duailibi-Neto EF, Chilvarquer I, Melani RF. Human identification through frontal sinus 3D superimposition: Pilot study with Cone Beam Computer Tomography. Journal of Forensic and Legal Medicine. 2015;**36**:63-69. DOI: 10.1016/j.jflm.2015.09.003

9

The Use of Computed Tomography to Explore the Microstructure of Materials in Civil Engineering: From Rocks to Concrete

Miguel A. Vicente, Jesús Mínguez and
Dorys C. González

Abstract

Computed tomography (CT) is a nondestructive technique, based on absorbing X-rays, that permits the visualisation of the internal microstructure of material. The field of application is very wide. This is a well-known technology in medicine, because of its enormous advantages, but it is also very useful in other fields. Computed tomography is used in palaeontology to study the internal structure of the bones from ancient hominids. In addition, this technology is being used by engineers to analyse the microstructure of materials. Materials engineers use this technology to analyse or develop new materials. Mechanical engineers use CT scans to study the internal defects of materials. Geotechnical engineers use CT scans to study several aspects of the rocks and minerals (cracks, voids, etc). This technology is also very useful to study de microstructure of concrete, especially in case of the new concretes (ultra-high performance concrete, fiber reinforced concrete, etc). In this chapter, an extended state-of-the-art of the most relevant research, related to the use of computed tomography to explore the microstructure of materials in civil and mechanical engineering, is exposed. The main objective of this chapter is that the reader can discover new applications of the computed tomography, different from conventional ones.

Keywords: CT scan, rocks, high performance concrete, fiber-reinforced high performance concrete

1. Introduction to computed tomography (CT) scan technology

Ever since Wilhelm Röntgen discovered X-rays in 1895, these rays have been used in many scientific fields. One property of this type of radiation is that it can travel through matter, losing energy on the way, in accordance with the law of Beer that equates intensity I with a mono-chromatic X-ray travelling through an object in terms of the following expression (Eq. (1)).

$$I = I_0 \cdot exp\{-\int \mu(s)ds\} \tag{1}$$

where I_0 is the initial intensity of the ray and $\mu(s)$ the linear attenuation coefficient along its trajectory.

The aforementioned linear attenuation coefficient, μ, fundamentally depends on the density, ρ, of the material at each point through which the ray travels. The quotient μ/ρ is approximately proportional to Z^3 in the standard range used in the computed tomography (CT) scans, where Z is the atomic number of the element.

CT is a nondestructive technique used to analyze the internal microstructure of materials based on the above-mentioned property of X-rays. The tomography equipment is composed of an emitter, which emits a ray at a given intensity, and a detector, which registers the reception intensity of the ray. In the analysis, the object revolves in front of the apparatus, consisting of the emitter, emitting rays in all directions on the plane, and the detector. Postprocessing of the signal to produce attenuation-corrected images, which coincide with the measurement of attenuation, means that the density of each point of the specimen under study may be determined. This process is repeated for different sections of the specimen, thereby obtaining tri-dimensional (tomographic) information. Alternatively, a conic beam of X-rays can be emitted that are collected on a flat detector. In this case, only the specimen has to revolve, and relative displacement between the emitter-detector apparatus and the specimen is unnecessary (**Figure 1**):

In all cases, the practical result is a tri-dimensional image, in grey scale, in which each grey area corresponds to a particular density value. Clearer tones represent higher densities, and darker tones represent lower densities.

The use of this technique commenced in medicine, during the last century, around the 1970s, as a non-invasive technique to explore the internal parts of patients, to display the inside of the body (organs, tissue, bones, etc.) and to detect abnormal structures that can indicate some pathology.

Over recent years, the technique has been discarded in medicine; however, it has been used in a more intense way in other scientific fields, especially science and engineering, where all variants of computerized tomography are increasingly employed.

In the 1980s, high-resolution tomographic equipment emerged commonly called micro CT scan. This new equipment used new sources of emissions, in the form of gamma rays and synchrotron radiation. At present, synchrotron radiation is the most widely used in modern equipment because of its high resolution and sharpness.

There are substantial differences between a CT scan for medical purposes and a CT scan in research and in the industrial sector. In the former case concerning medical equipment, the specimen or patient remains immobile, and it is the emitter-receptor apparatus that moves and revolves. However, it is the specimen that is moved and turned in an industrial or research CT scan.

Moreover, the equipment used in medicine presents very low intensity values because of the effects of high radiation on human health. These levels of radiation result in lower resolution and sharpness (**Figures 2 and 3**):

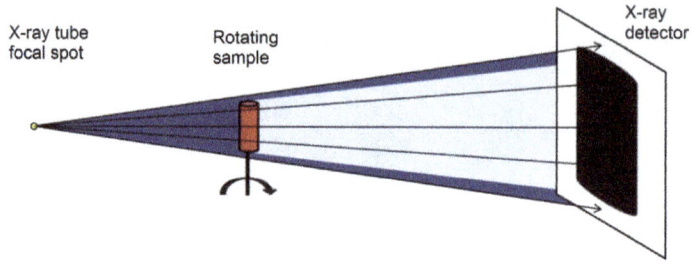

Figure 1. The principle of the working of a CT scan [1].

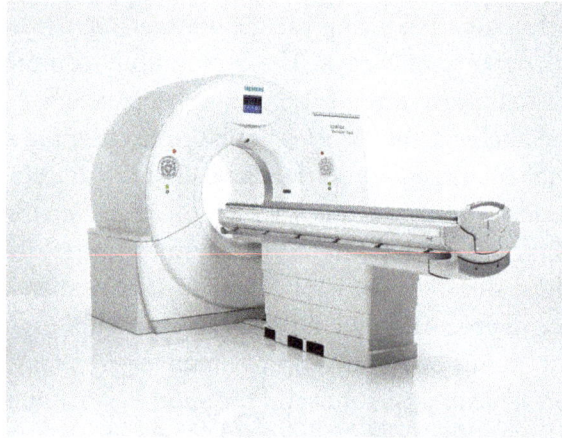

Figure 2. An example of medical CT scan. Courtesy of Siemens.

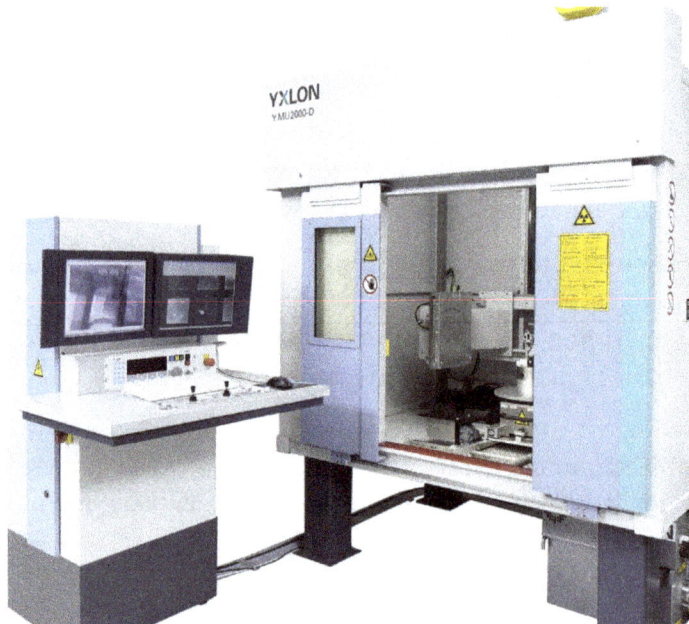

Figure 3. An example of medical CT scan. Courtesy of YXLON.

2. Use of CT scan technology in paleontology

Paleontology is one of the first scientific fields in which the use of computerized tomography started outside of medicine. Obviously, the technique of analyzing the bones of hominids and dinosaurs hardly differs from the technique used with humans and animals that are alive.

Numerous research papers have published studies in this field in which the CT scan is a very valuable instrument.

The fossilization process of an organism takes place over thousands of years, during which time loss and fragmentation of bones and other hard parts of the skeleton, decomposition, and so on occur. In addition, breakage occurs during their manipulation and study, which can imply an enormous loss. The primary objective of paleontological investigation is the reconstruction of skeletons and, from that point, to interpret many other biological and environmental characteristics, and so on.

The CT scan is a very useful tool here because it permits exact tridimensional images and, by means of software for the post-processing of images, can reconstruct skeletons without any need to manipulate the pieces. In addition, the information collected by the CT scan can serve as the basis for the regeneration of exact replicas using 3D printers [2–6].

In other cases, it may be physically impossible to remove the rocky sediment that hardens around the fossil. In that case, the CT scan can virtually eliminate it, revealing the "clean" piece [7] (**Figure 4**):

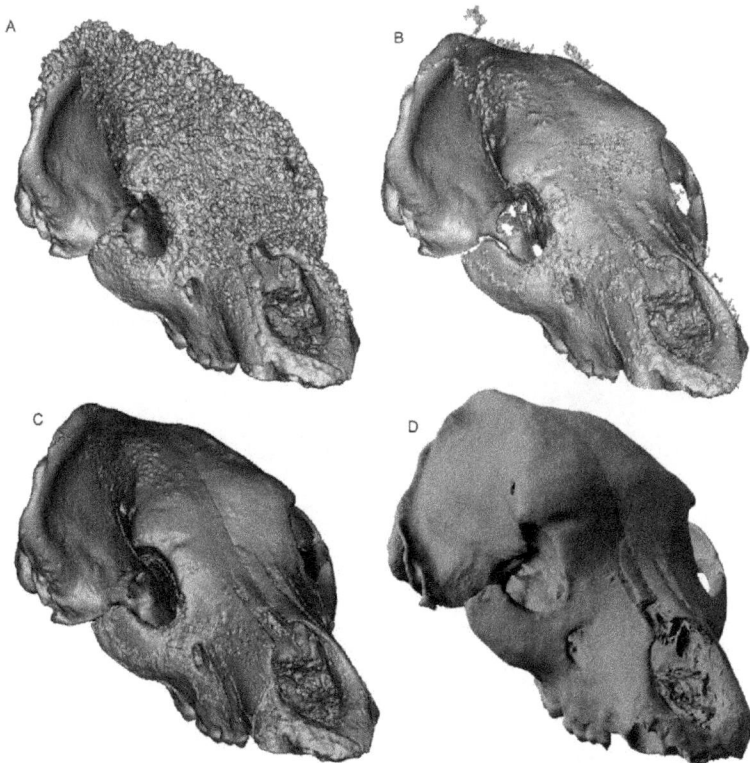

Figure 4. Virtual reconstruction and cleaning [7].

In other cases, the CT scan can determine the biomechanical parameters of the fossils [8] and detect disease and pathologies [9].

Recently, some research works have been published, in which possible alterations to the sample, due to the radiation emitted by the CT-Scan in the course of dating studies, are analyzed [10, 11].

3. Use of CT scan technology in heritage and ancient relics

Relics and ancient artifacts, to some extent, share the characteristics of fossils, explained in the earlier section. In the first place, these objects are of singular value, so they have to be handled with great care. In many cases, they are pieces that have remained buried for thousands of years and may be covered by layers of rocky sediment that is strongly attached, the mechanical removal of which implies a serious problem for the piece.

In these cases, the use of CT scan technology is of enormous interest. In the first place, the archaeological piece may be separated from the surrounding sediment as a virtual replica. In this way, the piece may be examined with the naked eye and studied without damaging it. Moreover, on the basis of the information obtained by the CT scan, exact replicas of the piece may be produced, using 3D printers. This option allows researchers to manipulate the replicas and to study them without the dangers, and the limitations involved in handling the original piece. It is also of interest for museums, as they can exhibit the replicas, for keeping the original piece safe in storage [12–16]. (**Figure 5**).

In other cases, the pieces are extremely delicate, such as paintings [17] and mummies [18]. In both cases, an analysis by means of CT scan technology preserves the integrity of the piece.

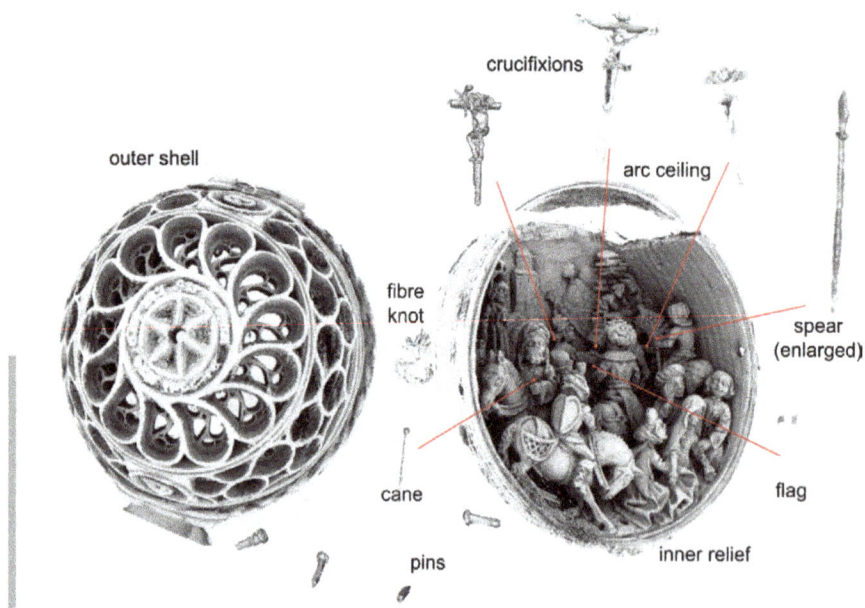

Figure 5. An example of rendering a prayer nut [12].

4. Use of CT scan technology in asphalt mixtures

Asphalt mixtures are widely used in the construction of road pavements and airports, because of the advantages that they contribute, among which are high strength, easy manufacturing and maintenance, low noise emission, and so on.

From the structural point of view, asphalt mixtures are heterogeneous materials, composed of aggregates, asphalt, and porous networks. Their mechanical properties show high levels of dispersion, given that those properties depend on many factors, such as the form and the distribution of the aggregate, the asphalt content, the pore content, pore distribution, and so on.

Comparative numeric models, as close as possible to the real specimens, need to be developed, in order to understand the behavior of the asphalt mixtures better. In this sense, the CT scan is of great assistance, as it generates the exact geometry of the internal structure of the asphaltic mixture and subsequently a finite elements model (FEM) with which the real capacity may be estimated against certain external actions. Comparing the numerical results with the tests carried out on the real specimen, it is possible to advance in the calibration of these models that predict the behavior of the material to improve its properties [19–23] (**Figure 6**).

In the case of special asphalts, it may be of great interest to know the exact distribution of certain compounds, with a view to understand their effectiveness. This situation applies to both additives for pavement restoration [24] and fiber-reinforced asphalts [24]. In many cases, with the assistance of the CT scan, correlations are sought between the mechanical behavior of the asphalt mix and its internal microstructure [25–28].

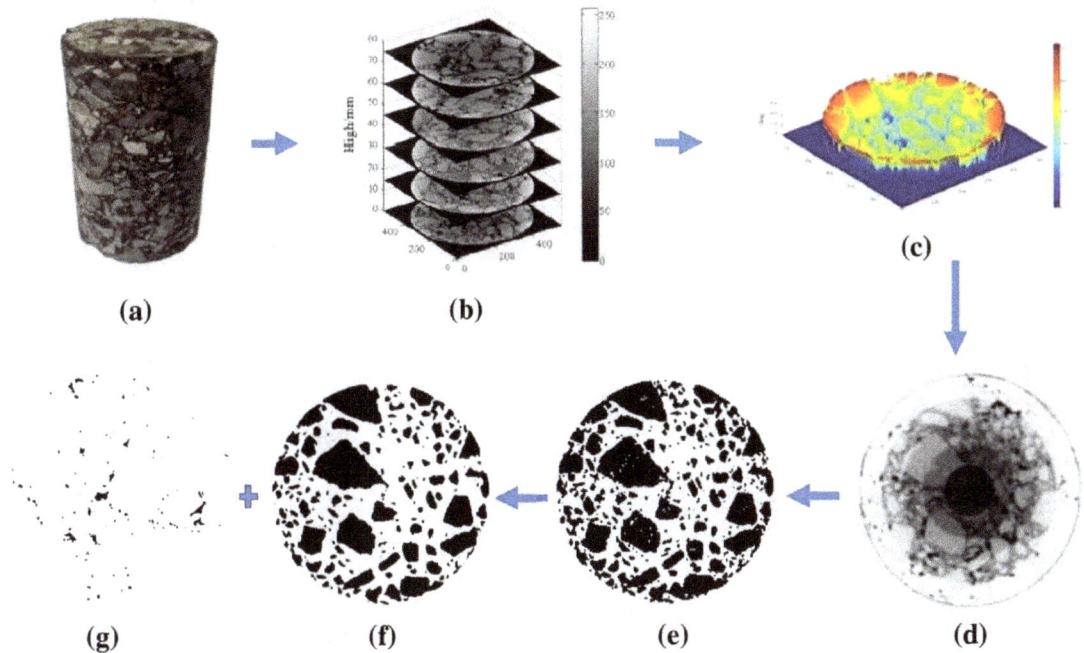

Figure 6. Extraction of the area of interest using CT scan technology [19].

5. Use of CT scan technology in rock mineralogy

Since the 1980s, research has taken place in which CT scan technology has been applied to the analysis of the internal microstructures of rocks.

Rocks are heterogeneous materials containing pores and fissures and consisting of various materials, with different mechanical properties and of varying density. On many occasions, the structural behavior of a rock is strongly conditioned by its microstructure, especially in reference to pores and fissures.

Rock, as a structural material, is present in a range of civil engineering works, among which tunnels and dams are prominent. In tunnels, the mechanical characteristics of the rocks, their porosity, and their degree of internal fracturing strongly condition their stability, their convergence, and so on.

Something similar occurs in the case of dams, especially arch dams. These structural elements are cemented to rock faces, and their structural safety is strongly dependent on the mechanical behavior of the rocks. The existence of failure planes or excessive internal fissuring might mean that the dam is not stable against the loads that it transfers, or it is not sufficiently watertight to ensure the retention of the water in the reservoir.

The foundations of large bridges, generally very deep foundations constructed with piles, usually reach down to the bedrock. Once again, the geological and mechanical characteristics of the rock clearly determine the structural safety of the bridge.

The possibilities offered by CT scanning in the field of geo-mineralogy are enormous [1, 29–31]. In all of these cases, CT scan technology has been successfully used to understand the microstructure of the bedrock and its behavior in reaction to certain physical and mechanical processes (**Figure 7**).

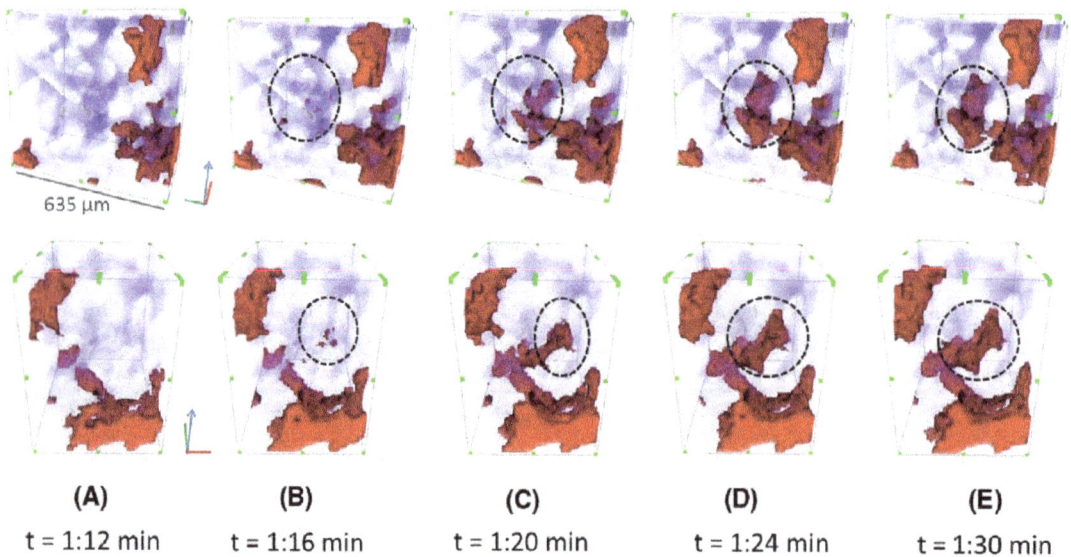

| (A) | (B) | (C) | (D) | (E) |
| t = 1:12 min | t = 1:16 min | t = 1:20 min | t = 1:24 min | t = 1:30 min |

Figure 7. Example of the possibilities of CT scan technology in rocks [29]. This time, the sequence shows a pore filling event.

Porosity, linked to water absorption capacity, is a very important parameter in rocks, as demonstrated by the high number of scientific publications in this field. At present, the most relevant investigations are currently applying CT scan technology to evaluate porosity, regardless of whether it has structural consequences [32, 33]. Other investigative works have analyzed mechanical behavior and its connection with the mineralogical microstructure [34].

One of the variants of this theme is the study of petrous elements for their use in construction. A theme of great interest is the study of porosity in limestone used, for example, in façades and pedestrian pavements, as well as for the rehabilitation of historic buildings and as a masonry element. In all of these cases, determination of the porosity of limestone is essential when determining whether it is convenient for use in a particular climate. In the case of environments subjected to freezing-thawing cycles, a high porosity substantially reduces the working life of the limestone.

On this point, it is worth highlighting the studies developed by Dewanckele et al. [35] and Boone et al. [36], in which the behavior of porous limestone was analyzed against erosive processes and water absorption. To do so, CT scanning was used to analyze how the internal structure of the limestone evolves due to the aforementioned processes (**Figure 8**).

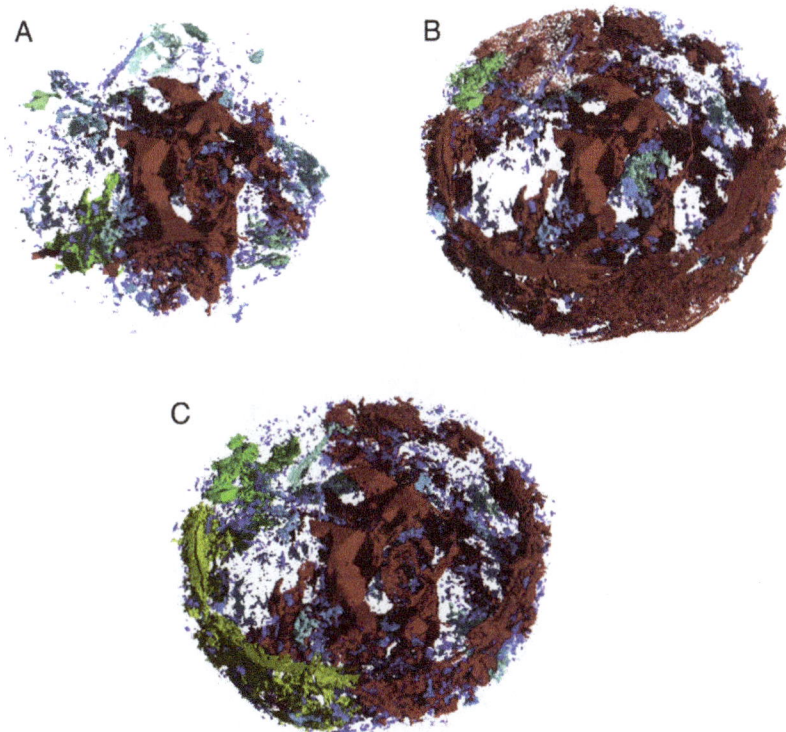

Figure 8. The example of rendering volumes of the changing pores in limestone [35]. The pores are color coded from red (large) to blue (small). Drawing A belongs to unweathered state, drawing B belongs to 6 days of weathering process, and drawing C belongs to 21 days of weathering process.

6. Use of CT scan technology in metals

Metals are widely used materials in the industrial sector. At present, innumerable types of simple metals and alloys are used, each one of them with specific properties, useful for the function that they have to perform: very light or carrying heavy loads, electrical conductivity or otherwise, high and low thermal transmissivity, tenacity and fracture strength, abrasion resistance, hardness, mechanical capacity, corrosion resistance, and so on.

Metals are used in all fields of industrial engineering, without exception. Metal manufacturing processes are very varied, ranging from smelting and casting to more modern systems of stamping and injection. In general, the metals used in different fields present optimal properties for the function they will serve, with the optimal design of parts in terms of material consumption.

The use of CT scan technology is quite widespread in the industrial sector, especially in those sectors that develop elements of high added value (aeronautical, aerospatial, automotive sectors, etc). One very common line of investigation, in which CT scan technology plays a relevant role, is the study of defects produced during the manufacturing process, with a view to their improvement [37–40]. In some cases, comparisons have been established between the microstructure of the material and its mechanical behavior [41–44]. In these cases, the information obtained by means of CT scanning is used for the generation of the tridimensional FEM models for the numerical simulation of the expected results and their subsequent comparison with the values measured in the tests. Here, the advantage of CT scanning is that it permits the construction of exact numerical models, which not only includes the different phases that constitute the piece but also the pores, defects, fissures, and so on in their exact position (**Figure 9**).

Within this line of investigation, it is worth highlighting welded joints and their analysis [45]. Welding is the most extensive process, whenever possible, for joining together two metallic parts. The way in which the welding is done is fundamental to the final quality of the joint.

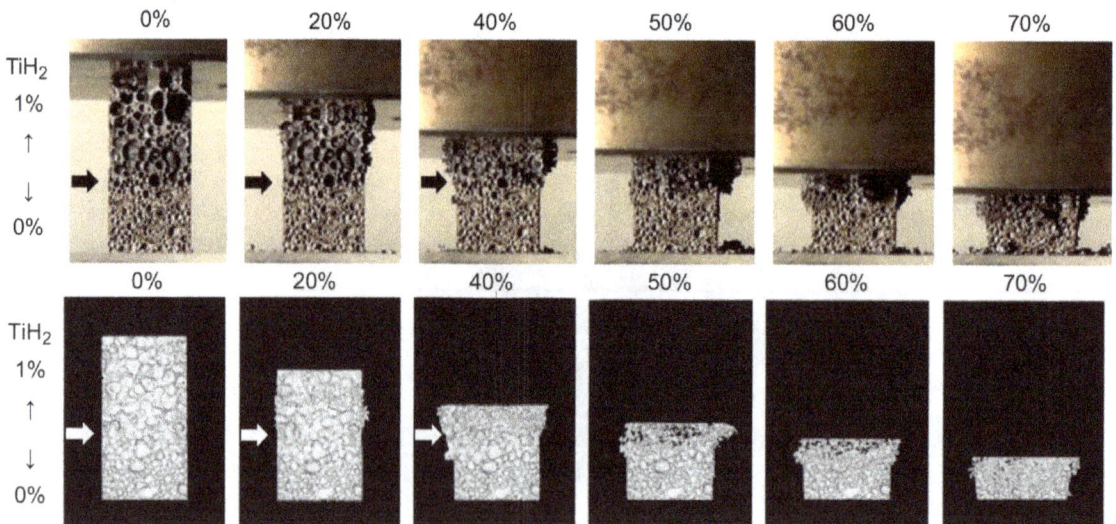

Figure 9. The example of an analysis of mechanical behavior of metal under compression and CT scan analysis [44]. (a) Sequential deformation recorded with a video camera and (b) sequential deformation "recorded" with a CT scan.

In this sense, as in the earlier case, the defects produced in the weld can be evaluated during welding with CT scan technology helping to improve the process.

One particular case of metals, used from a structural point of view, is composite metals, generally composed of a bland or foamy metallic matrix to which fibers or particles are usually added to improve their rigidity and strength [46]. In these cases, the microstructure of the composite material may be analyzed with CT scan technology, evaluating the distribution of the reinforcement, its orientation in the case of fibers, and so on.

7. Use of CT scan technology in composites

Composite materials are widely used in engineering. They are generally composed of a matrix and reinforcement that is generally of particles or fibers. The reinforcement has the role of modifying the natural properties of the matrix, with the objective of achieving a material of the desired characteristics.

In general, in a composite material, three phases may be distinguished: matrix, reinforcement, and pores or cracks.

The behavior of the composite materials strongly depends on the distribution and the orientation of the reinforcement (the latter solely in the case of fibers) as well as the location in the pores and cracks.

Of great interest in this field, CT scan technology permits the evaluation of the microstructure of the composite material [47–52]. In many cases, the combined use of CT scan and mechanical or thermal characterization tests of the composite material allows relations to be established between the microstructure and its macroscopic response [53–57] (**Figure 10**).

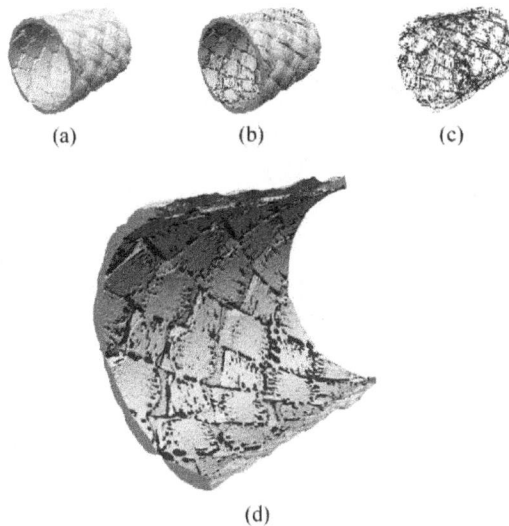

Figure 10. The example of analysis of the microstructure of a composite [47]. (a) 3D braid geometry, (b) 3D braid geometry with imperfections, (c) 3D distribution imperfections, and (d) detailed view.

As commented in earlier sections, a CT scan is the basis for the generation of exact FEM models, from which numerical simulations of all kinds may be performed [58, 59].

8. Use of CT scan technology in concrete

Concrete is one of the most widely used materials in the construction of infrastructure and buildings. One of the reasons for its extensive use is the relatively low price of extracting petrous materials from the environment. Another reason is the possibility of molding its geometry as it is poured in the fresh (fluid) state. The composition of concrete is highly heterogeneous as its matrix is composed of different materials: cement, sand, and rough aggregate. The dosages of those elements are modified to obtain optimum mechanical capacities. Additionally, other types of materials are used to improve the performance of the concrete such as fibers and additives to modify the internal structure of the material.

Internally, what is generated is a matrix composed of aggregate fines and hydrated cement that cover the coarse aggregate (**Figure 11**).

It is noteworthy that there are a multitude of parameters with a role in the final characteristic. The dosages of the different components are based on experimentation due to the different typologies or aggregates, sand, and cement that are available on the market. As an example, if in one region, the rocky material in the surrounding environment is granite, the aggregate will be based on this material.

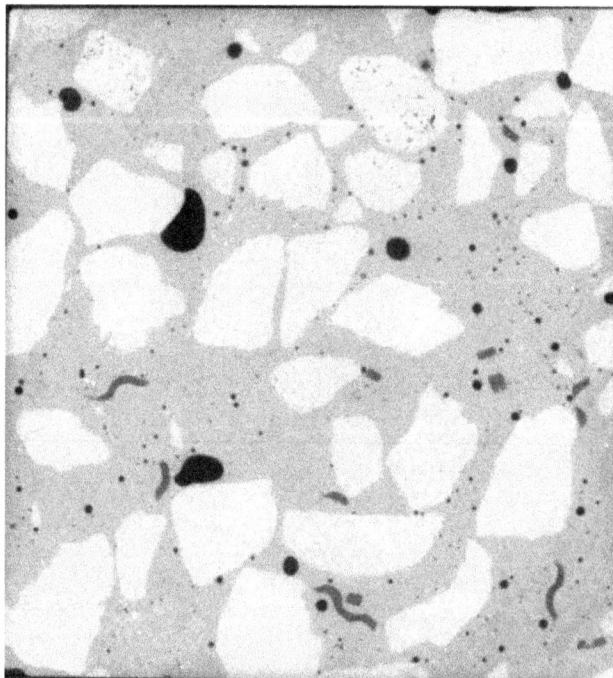

Figure 11. Polypropylene fiber-reinforced concrete specimen. Aggregates (in white), cement matrix (in soft grey), polypropylene fibers (in dark grey), and porous (in black) can be identified. Courtesy of the University of Burgos (Spain).

Moreover, concretes with additional qualities are under development in which fibers are added to their mixtures. There is at present a large quantity of fiber typologies in the market, so that at present, there is a broad process of investigation aimed at generating an optimal concrete in accordance with the desired performance.

Besides, public administrations are considering sustainability criteria that imply the development of research that aims to produce concrete that incorporates recycled materials, so as to reduce the carbon footprint and the environmental impact.

Therefore, in view of the above, it may be said that even though concrete is a priori a relatively rough and ready technology, constant development and improvements in performance, as well as new applications in construction elements are topics that are in the investigative projects of universities and research centers throughout the world.

New tools that provide the researcher with information to supplement the results of conventional tests have been incorporated to analyze concrete in this process of innovation for the determination of mechanical characteristics.

One of these tools that can be used to analyze the internal matrix of concretes and mortars is the computed tomography scan. The researcher is capable of analyzing unaltered samples of concrete in a non-destructive way, for example, in order to determine whether certain geometric patterns exist that can in turn classify the physical characteristics of the sample.

Next, some of the practical applications of computerized tomography to concretes are described.

8.1. Application to the analysis of the internal matrix

Among the applications of the CT scan technology for the analysis of a concrete matrix, there are some experimental studies focused on recycled concretes [60]. In these studies, concretes with equal percentages of 50% recycled aggregate (RCA) and 50% natural aggregates were analyzed. The objective of the use of tomography is to evaluate the interfaces between both types of concretes. In addition, the porosity of each type of matrix is analyzed (**Figure 12**).

The identification of pores provides information on these internal gaps that the matrix presents. This information may relate to the size of the pores and their distribution within the specimen. Information may also be extracted on the sphericity of the pores that is compared with a perfect sphere and finally, the spatial position of these pores within the matrix [61] (**Figure 13**).

The application of superabsorbent polymers (SAP) for the development of high performance concretes with the aim of reducing hydration-related problems of the cementitious matrix generates variations in the distribution of the pores within the concrete matrix and its porosity. These changes lead to modifications in the physical properties of the component [62].

Images of the spatial distribution of the pores may be obtained by means of computerized topography image analysis and the use of post-processing tools including volumes, numbers of pores, positions within the specimen, and sphericity indexes.

In this way, researchers can determine how the porosity map of the specimen is modified for different types of SAP additions (**Figure 14**).

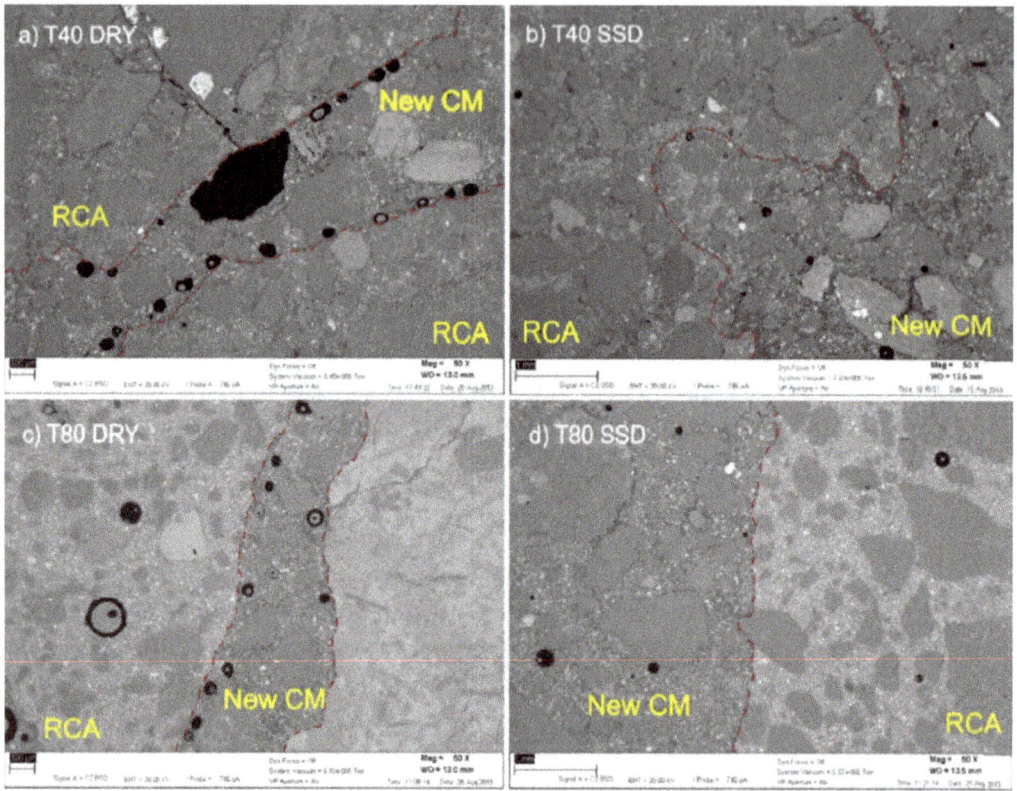

Figure 12. Interface paste-aggregate and porosity between matrices with recycled aggregates and natural aggregates [60].

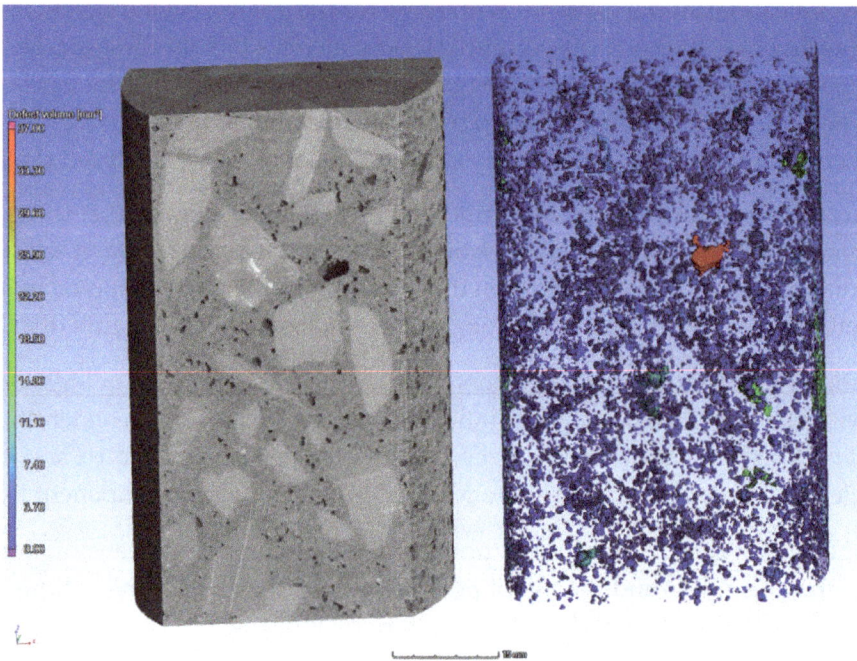

Figure 13. Identification and classification of pores in sizes [61].

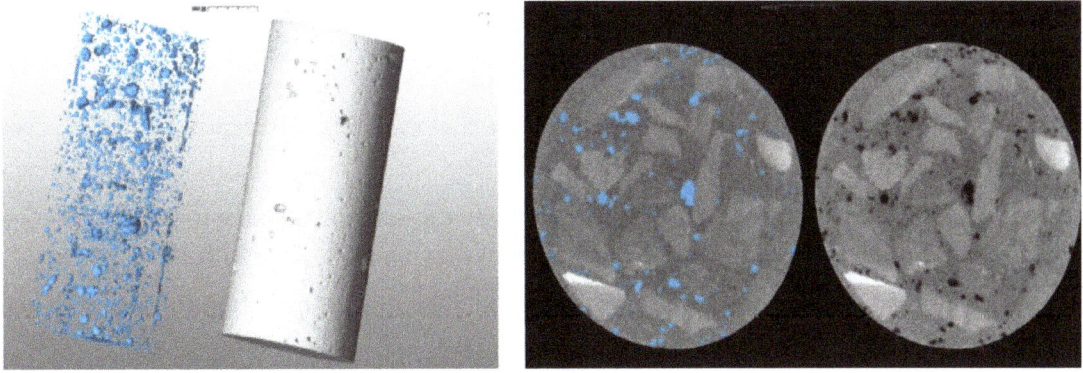

Figure 14. Identification of pores inside concrete matrix [62].

In addition to the pores, the distribution of polymeric components is established. In the following image, the way each of the components of the polymer is obtained following segmentation and their grouping is shown (**Figure 15**).

8.2. Applications to visualize fiber distribution

The addition of fibers improves the characteristics of concretes used in many different applications. The clearest and most widely used application is for the improvement of mechanical performance. The fibers withstand traction forces that the concrete is incapable of withstanding. As with all petrous materials, concrete presents a very good capacity to withstand compressive forces, while its resistance to traction stress is relatively low.

Hence, the need to add strengthening elements, in the form of fibers to resist traction forces, is necessary.

By way of an example, fibers are in a phase of expansion in their application to self-compacting concretes. The distribution and quantity of fibers represent a fundamental role in the final stress-resistant capacities of the concrete element [63].

Another factor that influences the mechanical capacities of fiber-reinforced concretes is fiber orientation within the matrix in relation to the traction planes of the component.

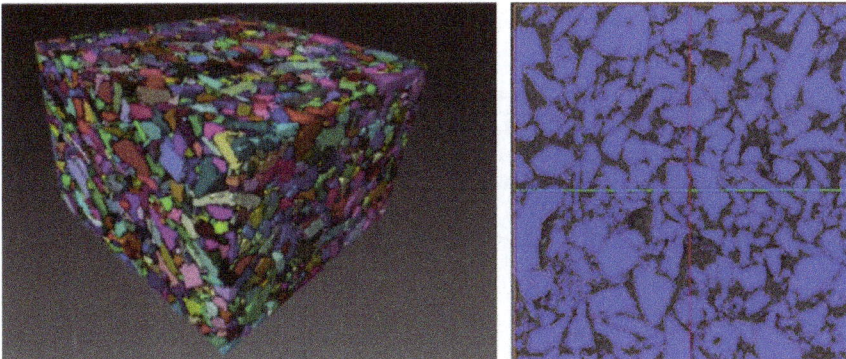

Figure 15. Segmentation and packing of the concrete matrix [61].

There are different segmentation techniques for the determination of fiber orientation [64, 65] (**Figure 16**). In all cases, they begin with a common process divided into different phases:

1. In the first phase, it is necessary to separate those materials that correspond to the concrete matrix by means of a grey-scale threshold.

2. In the second phase, the voxels that correspond to the same fiber have to be separated, in an attempt to separate those groups of fibers that may be in contact with other groups.

3. Once each fiber has been identified and separated, it is possible to obtain the orientation of each fiber and to identify its position in space.

Another application of computerized axial tomography consists of analyzing the way in which the fibers may be distinguished during the manufacturing process of pre-fabricated elements and how that affects the reinforcement bars in the element [66] (**Figures 17** and **18**).

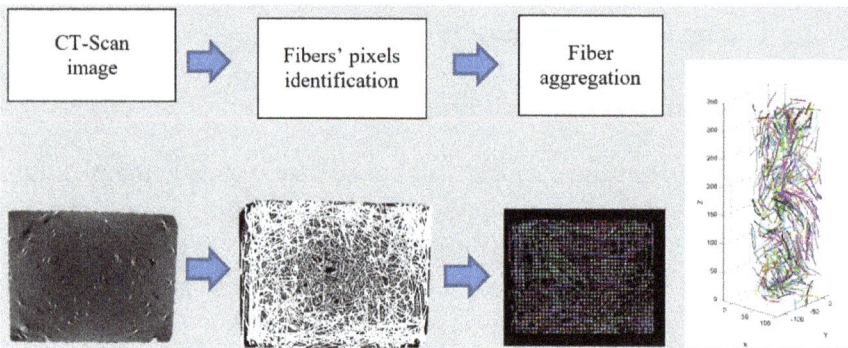

Figure 16. Procedure to identify fibers. The courtesy of the University of Burgos (Spain).

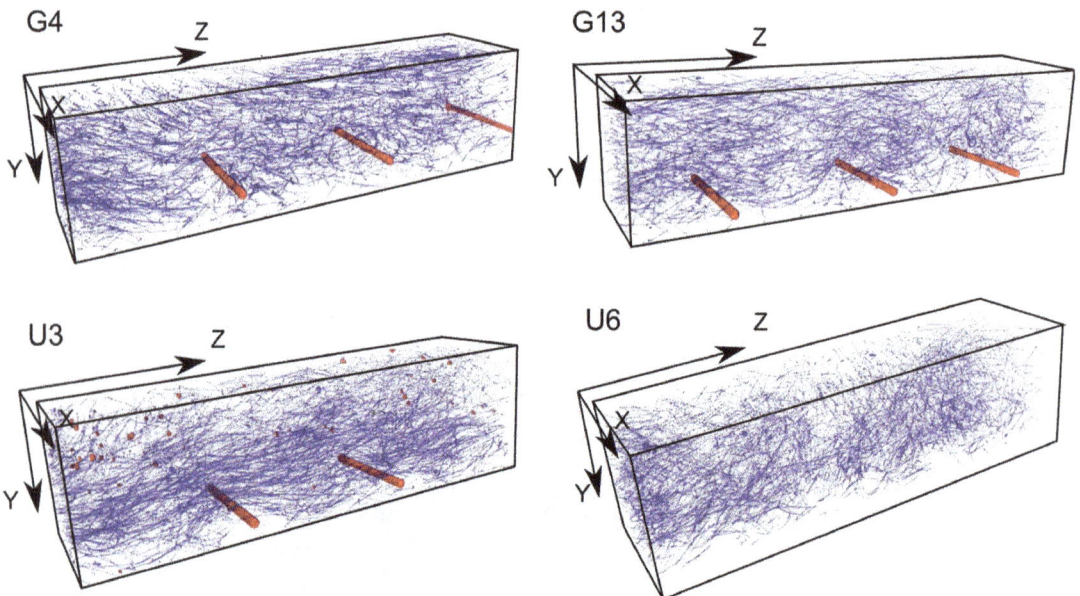

Figure 17. Fiber distribution around longitudinal rebars [66].

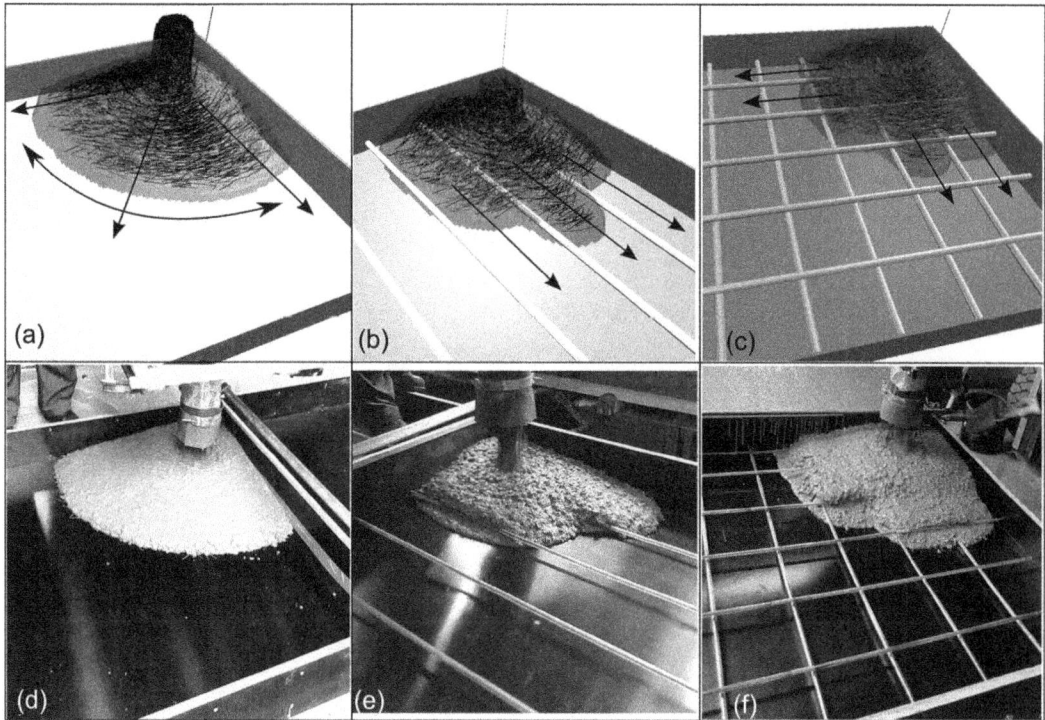

Figure 18. Schema of the fiber distribution and orientation during casting process [66].

8.3. Applications on internal analysis and cracking

The technology of the CT scan allows researchers to conduct analyses of concrete at a macro-level to identify the damage that may be generated in its matrix due to physical and chemical factors.

As described in the above sections, three-dimensional maps may be generated with this tool, which help the researcher to understand the internal mechanics of the concrete. There is at present no other real alternative that can reach the sub-millimetric level of detail of which tomography is capable.

In the case of the practical application carried out by Kim, Yun, and Park [67], CT scan technology was used to analyze samples of concrete and mortar at high temperatures. The objective was to determine how variations in temperature affected the behavior of the internal pores of the material until their collapse. In the following image, the fissures that developed when the concrete was subjected to 1000°C are shown (**Figures 19** and **20**):

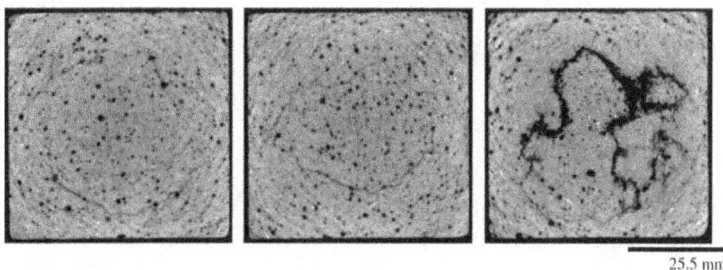

25.5 mm

Figure 19. Fracture development at 1000°C [67].

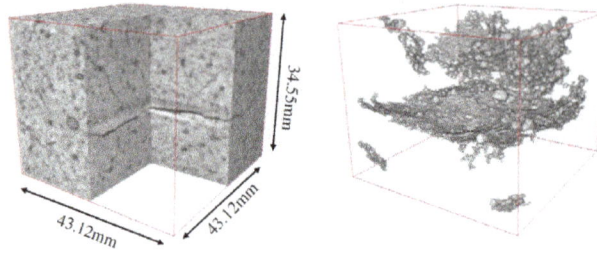

Figure 20. Imaging of fractures that developed at 1000°C [67].

It was determined that the appearance of fissuring began at a temperature of 600°C, and that this damage fundamentally began to occur in the zones close to the edges of the specimen, in the external zones, progressing as the temperature increased towards critical values until it reached a point of collapse.

Other studies related to fracture mechanics have analyzed how the fissuring of an element evolves when subjected to a flexural-traction test by using scanned images, in order to create a finite element model and a model of discrete damage adjusted to the physical interactions detected in the images [68] (**Figure 21**).

Finally, the following paragraphs describe research work that has been developed to determine the damage produced under cyclic loading in concrete specimens. Different specimens subjected to fatigue cycles at stress levels of 60, 70, 80, and 90% of resistance to static compression were analyzed.

The specimens were introduced before and after subjecting them to fatigue in the CT scan AC. The fissures within the concrete and their development were compared. A 3DMA algorithm was used to calculate the "burn number" of the pores and fissures, a number that represents the distance of the voxels under analysis to the external surface of the pore. So, for example, the external voxels are assigned a value equal to zero. As the scan progresses into the interior of the pore or fissure, a higher value than the burn number is obtained [69]. Those voxels, in general within the value of 1, represented fissures of 1 voxel in width (**Figure 22**).

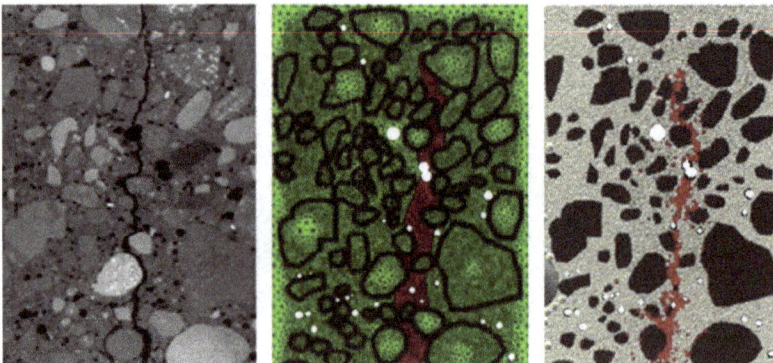

Figure 21. Results of three studies: real (left), using CT-Scan (middle), and FEM (right) [68].

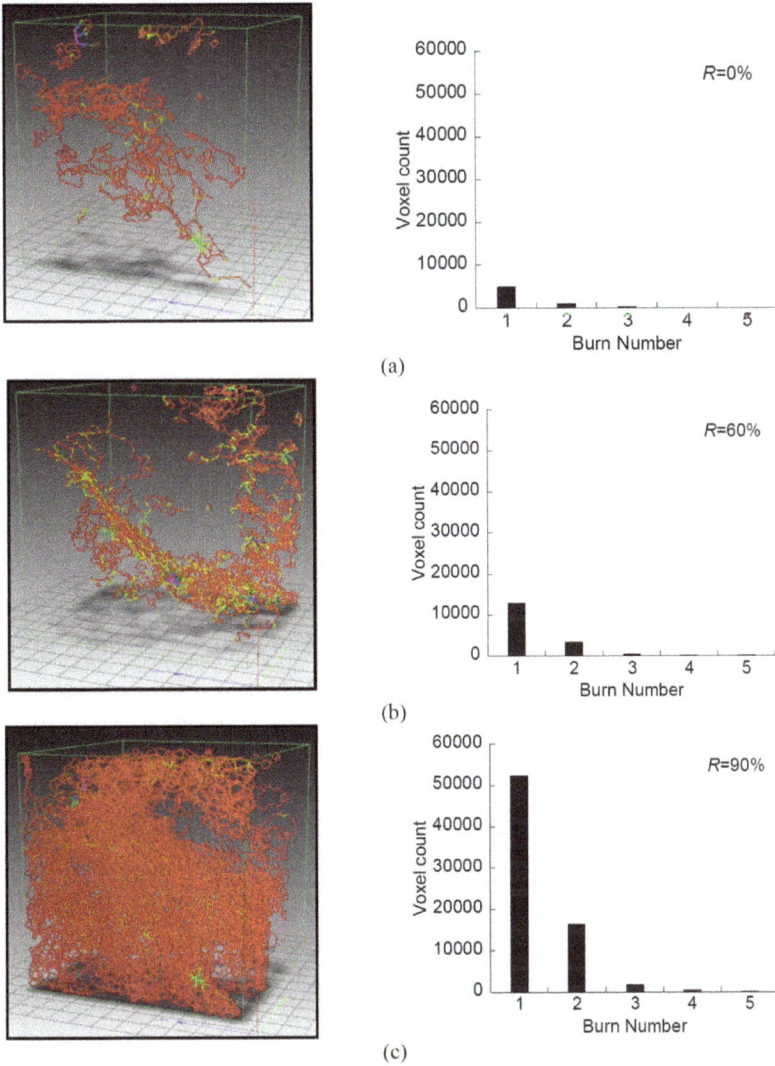

Figure 22. Spatial representation of damage (burn number) to different stress levels [69].

Following the tests, a growth in the internal damage was observed as the stress levels of the uniaxial cyclic loading increased.

9. Conclusions

CT scan technology is a powerful research tool, with wide use capabilities in many scientific fields, and not only in medicine.

In this chapter, a general review has been carried out by different fields of science and engineering in which CT scan technology is currently being used successfully. As can be seen, the possibilities of this technology are very large and allow relevant advances in the knowledge of the materials.

In the future, new equipment will be more powerful and more precise, which will allow us to see better the internal microstructure of our materials, which will help us to know them better and improve them, obtaining solutions adapted to each need.

Author details

Miguel A. Vicente*, Jesús Mínguez and Dorys C. González

*Address all correspondence to: mvicente@ubu.es

Department of Civil Engineering, University of Burgos, Spain

References

[1] Cnudde V, Boone MN. High-resolution X-ray computed tomography in geosciences: A review of the current technology and applications. Earth-Science Reviews. 2013;**123**:1-17

[2] Lautenschlager S. Reconstructing the past: Methods and techniques for the digital restoration of fossils. Royal Society Open Science. 2016;**3**:160342:1-18

[3] Tafforeau R, Boistel R, Boller E, Bravin A, Brunet M, Chaimanee Y, Cloetens P, Feist M, Hoszowska J, Jaeger JJ, Kay RF, Lazzari V, Marivaux L, Nel A, Nemoz C, Thibault X, Vignaud P, Zabler S. Applications of X-ray synchroton microtomography for non-destructive 3D studies of paleontological specimens. Applied Physics A. 2006;**83**(2):195-202

[4] Lautenschlager S. Cranial myology and bite force performance of Erlikosaurus andrewsi: A novel approach for digital muscle reconstructions. Journal of Anatomy. 2013;**222**(2):260-272

[5] Quam R, Lorenzo C, Martínez I, Gracia-Téllez A, Arsuaga JL. The bony labyrinth of the middle Pleistocene Sima de los Huesos hominins (Sierra de Atapuerca, Spain). Journal of Human Evolution. 2016;**90**(2):260-272

[6] López-Polín L, Ollé A, Cáceres I, Carbonell E, Bermúdez de Castro JM. Pleistocen human remains and conservation treatment: The case of a mandible from Atapuerca (Spain). Journal of Human Evolution. 2008;**90**:1-15

[7] Santos E, García N, Carretero JM, Arsuaga JL, Tsoukala E. Endocranial traits of the Sima de los Huesos (Atapuerca, Spain) and Petralona (Chalkidiki, Greece) Middle Pleistocene ursids. Phylogenetic and biochronological implications. Anales de Paléontologie. 2013;**100**(4):297-309

[8] Lorkiewicz-Muszynska D, Przystanska A, Kociemba W, Sroka A, Rewekant A, Zaba C, Paprzycki W. Body mass estimation in modern population using anthropometric measurements from computed tomography. Forensic Science International. 2013;**231**(1-3):405. e1-405.e6

[9]   Ceperuelo D, Lozano M, Duran-Sindreu F, Mercadé M. Supernumerary fourth molar and dental pathologies in a Chalcolithic individual from the El Mirador Cave site (Sierra de Atapuerca, Burgos, Spain). HOMO-Journal of Comparative Human Biology. 2015;**66**(1):15-26

[10] Duval M, Martín-Francés L. Quantifying the impact of μCT-scanning of human fossil teeth on ESR age results. American Journal of Physical anthropology. 2017;**00**:1-8

[11] Immel A, Le Cabec A, Bonazzi M, Herbig A, Temming H, Schuenemann VJ, Bos KI, Langbein F, Harvati K, Bridault A, Pion G, Julien MN, Krotova O, Conard NJ, Münzel SC, Drucker DG, Viola B, Hublin JJ, Tafforeau P, Krause J. Effect of X-ray irradiation on ancient DNI in sub-fossil bones—guidelines for safe X-ray imaging. Scientific Reports. 2016;**6**:32969:1-14

[12] Zhang X, Blass J, Botha C, Reischig P, Bravin A Dik J. Process for the 3D virtual reconstruction of a microcultural heritage artifact obtained by synchrotron radiation CT technology using open source and free software. Journal of Cultural Heritage. 2012;**13**:221-225

[13] Lehmann EH, Vontobel, P, Deschler-Erb E, Soares, M. Non-invasive studies of objects from cultural heritage. Nuclear Instruments and Methods in Physics Research Section A. 2005;**542**:68-75

[14] Zhang K, Bao H. Research on the Application of Industrial CT for Relics Image Reconstruction. In: Asia-Pacific Conference on Information Processing. 2009. pp. 404-408

[15] Abel RL, Parfitt S, Ashton N, Lewis SG, Beccy-Scott C. Digital preservation and dissemination of ancient lithic technology with modern micro-CT. Computers & Graphics. 2011;**35**:878-884

[16] Morigi MP, Casali F, Bettuzzi M, Bianconi D, Brancaccio R, D'Errico V. Application of X-ray computed tomography to cultural heritage diagnostics. Applied Physics A. 2010;**100**:653-661

[17] Morigi MP, Casali F, Bettuzzi M, Bianconi D, Brancaccio R, Cornacchia S, Pasinia A, Rossi A, Aldrovandi A, Cauzzi D. CT Investigation of two paintings on wood tables by Gentile da Fabriano. Nuclear Instruments and Methods in Physics Research Section A. 2007;**580**:735-738

[18] Cesarini F, Martina MC, Ferraris A, Grilletto R, Boano R, Marochetti EF, Donadoni AM, Gandini G. Whole-body three-dimensional multidetector CT of 13 Egyptian human mummies. American Journal of Roentgenology. 2003;**180**:597-606

[19] Hu J, Qian Z, Wang D, Oeser M. Influence of aggregate particles on mastic and air-voids in asphalt concrete. Construction and Building Materials. 2015;**93**:1-9

[20] Liu P, Wang D, Oerser M, Alber S, Ressel W, Canon Falla G. Modelling and evaluation of aggregate morphology on asphalt compression behavior. Construction and Building Materials. 2017;**133**:196-208

[21] Yin A, Yang X, Zeng G, Gao H. Experimental and numerical investigation of fracture behavior of asphalt mixture under direct shear loading. Construction and Building Materials. 2015;**86**:21-32

[22] Chen XH, Wang DW. Fractal and spectral analysis of aggregate surface profile in polishing process. Wear. 2011;**271**(11-12):2746-2750

[23] Wang D, Wang H, Bu Y, Schulze C, Oeser M. Evaluation of aggregate resistance to wear with Micro-Deval test in combination with aggregate imaging techniques. Wear. 2015;**338-339**:288-296

[24] Zhang Y, Verwaal W, Van de Ven, MFC, Molenaar AAA, Wu SP. Using high-resolution industrial CT scan to detect the distribution of rejuvenation products in porous asphalt concrete. Construction and Building Materials. 2015;**100**:1-10

[25] Norambuena-Contreras J, Serpell R, Valdés Vidal G, González A, Schlangen E. Effects of fibres addition on the physical and mechanical properties of asphalt mixtures with crack-healing purposes by microwave radiation. Construction and Building Materials. 2016;**127**:369-382

[26] Jing Hu, Qian Z, Xue Y, Yang Y. Investigation on fracture performance of lightweight epoxy asphalt concrete based on microstructure characteristics. Journal of Materials in Civil Engineering. 2016;**28**(9):04016084:1-8

[27] Wang H, Zhang R, Chen Y, You Z, Fang J. Study on microstructure of rubberized recycled hot mix asphalt base X-ray CT technology. Construction and Building Materials. 2016;**121**:177-184

[28] Rinaldini E, Schuetz P, Partl MN, Tebaldi G, Poulikakos LD. Investigating the blending of reclaimed asphalt with virgin materials using rheology, electron microscopy and computer tomography. Composites: Part B. 2014;**67**:579-587

[29] Bultreys T, Boone MA, Boone MN, De Schryver T, Masschaele B, Hoorebeke LV, Cnudde V. Fast laboratory-based in micro-computed tomography for pore-scale research: Illustrative experiments and perspectives on the future. Advances in Water Resources. 2016;**95**:341-351

[30] De Kock T, Boone MA, De Schryver T, Van Stappen J, Derluyn H, Masschaele B, De Schutter G, Cnudde V. A pore-scale study of fracture dynamics in rock using X-ray micro-CT under ambient freeze-thaw cycling. Environmental Science & Technology. 2015;**49**:2867-2874

[31] Bultreys T, De Boever W, Cnudde V. Imaging and image-based fluid transport modelling at the pore scale in geological materials: A practical introduction to the current state-of-the-art. Earth-Science Reviews. 2016;**155**:93-128

[32] Lin Q, Al-Khulaifi Y, Blunt MJ, Bijeljic B. Quantification of sub-resolution porosity in carbone rocks by applying high-salinity contrast brine using X-ray microtomography differential imaging. Materials Characterization. 2014;**97**:150-160

[33] Bultreys T, Van Hoorebeke L, Cnudde V. Simulating secondary water flooding in heterogeneous rocks with variable wettability using an image-based, multiscale pore network model. Water Resources Research. 2016;**52**:6833-6850

[34] Charalampidou EM, Hall SA, Stanchits S, Viggiani G, Lewis H. Experimental character-ization of shear and compaction band mechanisms in porous sandstone by a combina-tion of AE and 3D-DIC. EDP Web of Conferences. 2010;**6**:22009:1-7

[35] Dewanckele J, De Kock T, Fronteau G, Derluyn H, Vontobel P, Dierick M, Van Hoorebeke L, Jacobs P, Cnudde V. Neutron radiography and X-ray computed tomography for quan-tifying wathering and water uptake processes inside porous limestone used as building material. Materials Characterization. 2014;**88**:86-99

[36] Boone MA, De Kock T, Bultreys T, De Schutter G, Vontobel P, Van Hoorebeke L, Cnudde V. 3D mapping of water in oolithic limestone at atmospheric and vacuum saturation using X-ray micro-CT differential imaging. Advances in Water Resources. 2016;**96**:306-366

[37] Yand S, Zhang R, Qu X. X-ray analysis of powed-binder separation during SiC injection process in L-shaped mould. Journal of European Ceramic Society. 2015;**35**:61-67

[38] Yand S, Zhang R, Qu X. Optimization and evaluation of metal injection molding by using X-ray tomography. Materials Characterization. 2015;**104**:107-115

[39] Wicke M, Luetje M, Bacaicoa I, Brueckner-Foit A. Characterization of casting pores in Fe-rich Al-Si-Cu alloys by microtomography and finite elements analysis. Procedia Structural Integrity. 2016;**2**:2643-2649

[40] Szkodo M, Bien A, Antoszkiewicz M. Effect of plasma sprayed and laser re-melted Al_2O_3 coatings on hardness and wear properties of stainless steel. Ceramics International. 2016;**42**:11275-11284

[41] Dahdah N, Limodin N, El Bartali A, Witz JF, Seghir R, Charkaluk E, Buffiere JY. Influence of the casting process in high temperature fatigue of A319 aluminium alloy investi-gated by in situ X-ray tomography and digital volume correlation. Procedia Structural Integrity. 2016;**2**:3057-3064

[42] Nemcko MJ, Wilkinson DS. On the damage and fracture of commercially pure magne-sium using X-ray microtomography. Material Science & Engineering A. 2016;**676**:146-155

[43] Chan LC, Lu XZ, Yu KM. Multiscale approach with RSM for stress-strain behaviour prediction of micro-void-considered metal alloy. Materials & Design. 2015;**83**:129-137

[44] Hangai Y, Takahashi K, Yamaguchi R, Utsunomiya T, Kitahara S, Kuwazuru O, Yoshikawa N. Nondestructive observation of pore structure deformation behaviour of functionally graded aluminum foam by X-ray computed tomography. Materials Science & Engineering A. 2012;**556**:678-684

[45] Kuryntsev SV, Gilmutdinov AK. The effect of laser beam wobbling mode in weld-ing process for structural steels. The International Journal of Advanced Manufacturing Technology. 2015;**81**(9):1683-1691

[46] Leitlmeier D, Degischer HP, Flankl HJ. Development of a foaming process for particu-late reinforced aluminum melts. Advanced Engineering Materials. 2002;**4**(10):735-740

[47] Melenka GW, Lepp E, Cheung BKO, Carey JP. Micro-computed tomography analysis of tubular braided composites. Composite Structures. 2015;**131**:384-396

[48] Grammatikos SA, Kordatos EZ, Matikas TE, David C, Paipetis AS. Current injection phase thermography for low-velocity impact damage identification in composite laminates. Materials and Design. 2014;**55**:429-441

[49] Shen H, Nutt S, Hull D. Direct observation and measurement of fibre architecture in short fiber-polymer composite foam through micro-CT imaging. Composites Science and Technology. 2004;**64**:2113-2120

[50] Hayashi T, Kobayashi T, Takahashi J. Quantification of the void content of composite materials using soft X-ray transmittance. Journal of Thermoplastic Composite Materials. 2016;**00**:1-19

[51] Nikishkov Y, Airoldi L, Makeev A. Measurement of voids in composites by X-ray computed tomography. Composites Science and Technology. 2013;**89**:89-97

[52] McCombe GP, Rouse J, Trask RS, Withers PJ, Bond IP. X-ray damage characterisation in self-healing fibre reinforced polymers. Composites: Part A. 2012;**43**:613-620

[53] Wang Y, Burnett TL, Chai Y, Soutis C, Hogg PJ, Withers PJ. X-Ray computed tomography study of kink bands in unidirectional composites. Composite Structures. 2017;**160**:917-924

[54] Yu B, Bradley RS, Soutis C, Hogg PJ, Withers PJ. 2D and 3D imaging of fatigue failure mechanisms of 3D woven composites. Composites: Part A. 2015;**77**:37-49

[55] Grammatikos SA, Jones RG, Evernden M, Correia JR. Thermal cycling effects on the durability of a pultruded GFRC material for off-shore civil engineering structures. Composite Structures. 2016;**153**:297-310

[56] Jespersen KM, Zangenberg J, Lowe T, Withers PJ. Fatigue damage assessment of unidirectional non-crimp fabric reinforced polyester composite using X-ray computed tomography. Composites Science and Technology. 2016;**136**:94-103

[57] Stamopoulos AG, Tserpes KI, Prucha P, Vavrik D. Evaluation of porosity effects on the mechanical properties of carbon fiber-reinforced plastic unidirectional laminates by X-ray computed tomography and mechanical testing. Journal of Composite Materials. 2016;**50**(15):2087-2098

[58] Sencu RM, Yang Z, Wang YC, Withers PJ, Rau C, Parson A, Soutis C. Generation of micro-scale finite element models from synchrotron X-ray CT images for multidirectional carbon fibre reinforced composites. Composites: Part A. 2016;**91**:85-95

[59] Czabaj MW, Riccio ML, Whitacre WW. Numerical reconstruction of graphite/epoxy composite microstructure based on sub-micron resolution X-ray computed tomography. Composites Science and Technology. 2014;**105**:174-182

[60] Leite MB, Monteiro PJM. Microstructural analysis of recycled concrete using X-ray microtomography. Cement and Concrete Research. 2016;**81**:38-48

[61] du Plessis A, Olawuyi BJ, Boshoff WP, le Roux SG. Simple and fast porosity analysis of concrete using X-ray computed tomography. Materials and Structures. 2016;49(1):553-562

[62] Olawuyi BJ, Boshoff WP. Influence of SAP content and curing age on air void distribution of high performance concrete using 3D volume analysis. Construction and Building Materials. 2017;135:580-589

[63] Ponikiewski T, Katzer J, Bugdol M, Rudzki M. Steel fibre spacing in self-compacting concrete precast walls by X-ray computed tomography. Materials and Structures. 2015;48:3863-3874

[64] Herrmann H, Pastorelli E, Kallonen A, Suuronen JP. Methods for fibre orientation analysis of X-ray tomography images of steel fibre reinforced concrete (SFRC). Journal of Materials Science. 2016;51(8):3772-3783

[65] Vicente MA, Gonzalez DC, Mínguez J. Determination of dominant fibre orientations in fibre-reinforced high-strength concrete elements based on computed tomography scans. Nondestructive Testing and Evaluation. 2014;29:164-182

[66] Zirgulis G, Svec O, Geiker MR, Cwirzen A, Kanstad T. Influence of reinforcing bar layout on fibre orientation and distribution in slabs cast from fibre-reinforced self-compacting concrete (FRSCC). Journal of Materials Science. 2016;17(2):245-256

[67] Kim KY, Yun TS, Park KP. Evaluation of pore structures and cracking in cement paste exposed to elevated temperatures by X-ray computed tomography. Cement and Concrete Research. 2013;50:34-40

[68] Skarzynski L, Nitka M, Tejchman J. Modelling of concrete fracture at aggregate level suing FEM and DEM based on X-ray μCT images of internal structure. Engineering Fracture Mechanics. 2015;147:13-35

[69] Obara Y, Tanikura I, Jung J, Shintani R, Watanabe S. Evaluation of micro-damage of concrete specimens under cyclic uniaxial loading by X-ray CT method. Journal of Advanced Concrete Technology. 2016;14(8):433-443

10

Treatment Planning in Brachytherapy HDR Based on Three-Dimensional Image

Marcin Sawicki

Abstract

Treatment planning in High Dose Rate (HDR) brachytherapy based on three-dimensional (3D) imaging allows for prearranging and realization optimal treatment process. This process consists of procedure planning, the choice of applicators, adjusting the appropriate implantation technique, and planning of three-dimensional distribution of dose in computerized treatment planning system. 3D images used in treatment planning in HDR brachytherapy allows for choosing the most appropriate application technique. This in turn allows for the best area coverage by reference dose with simultaneous protection of critical organs. Treatment planning on 3D images assures individual planning of dose dispersion in target area. Several techniques will be presented based on 3D imaging in location such as lung, skin cancer, breast, and prostate cancer. For each location, relative cases will be provided where different applicators and techniques were applied. These examples are going to present images from before and after performed application along with the pictures from computer treatment planning system. In each of described locations, relative advice and rules of conducting accurate application will be provided.

Keywords: HDR brachytherapy, treatment planning, 3D, three-dimensional images

1. Introduction

HDR brachytherapy is a radiotherapy method in which a source of ionizing radiation is administered directly into the tumor area or to its nearest surroundings. Dissemination of this method, nowadays, is associated with the possibility of using radiation sources with relatively low dimension. Small size of capsules made administration of catheter possible in the areas where previously it would have not been possible or would have involved a number of inconveniences for the patient as well as considerable risks of complications, e.g., bronchial carcinoma. This unique method also provides the possibility to determine the exact location of catheter in the tumor area for applying several visualization methods.

The purpose of the following chapter is to introduce practical application of HDR brachytherapy based on the three-dimensional (3D) computed tomography method. This publication is for those who are interested in applying and using 3D images in HDR brachytherapy and are searching for practical treatment examples based on this method. The purpose of this section is to spread treatment HDR brachytherapy treatment planning based on 3D images. The majority of brachytherapy departments still base their treatment on 2D imaging in spite of relatively popular CT scanners.

This chapter aims to familiarize the reader with treatment planning based on CT imaging to draw attention to the benefits coming from this method not only for the treatment planning but also for the patient. It is a practical guide based on brachytherapy department experiences located in Subcarpathian Cancer Center.

This chapter includes CT images presenting brachytherapy treatment in different stages of treatment planning. It is going to introduce a course of planning process in different locations as well as the application methods used in correspondence to the location of the treatment. With each location, relevant suggestions and recommendations will be provided, which would improve the whole treatment planning process.

This chapter is mainly addressed to radiotherapy specialists but also residents, physical medics, radiologists, and everyone who is interested in the topic of applying CT imaging in HDR brachytherapy.

First section deals with what the approach of brachytherapy is and what imaging methods it uses. Also, the differences emerging from using different imaging methods and locations where 3D imaging was used will be described as well as the methods applied to enhance the treatment planning procedure. It will illustrate the guidelines we use in our department when treating different tumor locations along with the necessary equipment relevant in the 3D imaging method.

Second section will demonstrate, in detail, its applications in various locations. In this chapter, I am going to demonstrate the utilization of HDR brachytherapy in treatment of breast, prostate, skin, and lung cancers. Depending on the tumor location, one or more examples will be provided. For each case, there will be one accepted treatment plan presented. Each case includes a wide range of materials in the form of CT images and computed planning system, each of them will be described under the angle of planning and conducting in most optimal application, based on the experience of our department. I am going to present several planning stages, starting from CT scans on different application levels to the demonstration of images and results of computer treatment planning system (TPS).

2. Treatment planning in brachytherapy HDR

Brachytherapy HDR is administration of a source of ionizing radiation into the immediate vicinity of the tumor. Because of the high gradient dose, the administered application allows for reduction of ionizing radiation in the critical organs area with simultaneous coverage of tumor area with reference dose. Treatment planning process can be based on two- and three-dimensional imaging. In case of 2D imaging, distribution of dosage around the **catheter** would conventionally be calculated on X-ray pictures taken in two different projections. This reconstruction allows us to determine the dose around the guide or guides [1]. We do not have the exact information about the dose in the target and the critical organs in the immediate vicinity to catheter. When planning a treatment, CT images provide actual information about the location of the applicator, target, and organ at risk (OAR). Images from computer tomography are electronic cross-sections (scans) of a patient body, which includes cancerous areas. The distance between those scans is adjusted accordingly to achieve best-possible three-dimensional reconstruction of the patient's body. It is necessary to calculate and determine the dose on the clear scans from the CT. The dosage calculation area here is the patient's body. Second, radiation area is determined along with critical organs and structures. Using the linear method, involving manual or automatic contouring of selected areas in each scan, ionizing areas are determined as well as critical organs and structures. Ionizing area in brachytherapy is defined by a three-step process:

- Gross tumor volume (GTV)—macroscopic tumor area defined by diagnostic methods.

- Clinical target volume (CTV)—clinical area for radiation.

- Planning target volume (PTV)—1 cm safety margin top-bottom in regard to CTV and additional 1 cm resulting from uncertain location of catheter or possible applicator movements caused, i.e., transporting the patient.

As a result of reconstruction, you get a three-dimensional image of target volume and critical organs. Application of computer treatment planning methods enables a precise dosage calculation. Dosage distribution is determined using formalism TG-43 or Monte Carlo method. Individual treatment plan is verified before the treatment starts. Designated dosage, active length, dwell times, and source activity are being confirmed. Once all these data have been verified, the treatment plan begins to be realized.

The main purpose of treatment planning based on computed tomography images is to determine the best-possible dosage in the therapeutic area, simultaneously decreasing its volume in organs and critical structures. Such adjustment can be accomplished by treatment planning enhancement [2–6].

This process depends on defining the location and appropriate dwell time to achieve the desired dose distribution in the patient's body. Introduction of new 3D methods that are applied in treatment planning triggered studies on optimization algorithms using data from three-dimensional imaging. One example is graphical optimization. Thanks to the information from target volume and surrounding it structures, optimization algorithm provided a possibility to target the area of interest with reference dose while protecting tissues surrounding implant. Graphical optimization allows change of shape of the isodose in any way. Applying such set of applicators enables the reduction of organ at risk (OARs) dose. Utilizing 3D imaging allows us to define the exact application place as well as determine the type and correct amount of applicators.

2.1. Lung cancer

In case of lung cancer, HDR brachytherapy treatment planning is conventionally based on two-dimensional imaging. More and more brachytherapy departments get access to computer tomography, which provide three-dimensional imaging. In our brachytherapy department, the entire treatment process is based on three-dimensional imaging. Dosage distribution in treatment planning based on 2D imaging is conventionally set in reference points of axis. Reference points are identified in constant proximity from the reconstructed applicator axis, which usually is 1 cm. The applicators curvature is an important factor taken into consideration while calculating dose distribution in 3D-based treatment. Dose disperse is set on the target area taking into consideration critical organs. Equipment routinely used for administering bronchial applicators in our department is a bronchovideoscope.

Before the treatment begins, the patient has computed tomography. Then, radiotherapist familiarizes themselves with the patient's history and then determines the area for administering the ionizing radiation.

In cases where the tumor area allows for applying the catheter into the tumor, usually only one applicator is used. In situations where the tumor location does not allow for the direct application of a catheter into the tumor area, several applicators are applied into the immediate surroundings of therapeutic area. Usage of one applicator in the tumor area does not allow for optimal coverage by the reference dose. It is caused by unsymmetrical shape of the target in the reference to the applicator. By such implantation, applicator can be the reason for a quantity that exceeds reference dose many times over. To achieve the best coverage of the tumor area, it is best to use several applicators. Applicators, as long as the clinical situation allows, are placed to be inside the tumor and in the external target area. Such treatment allows the reduction of high contact dose, which is the case when using only one applicator, as well as a considerable dose reduction in OARs.

Once application is completed, markers are injected to each of the catheters. Markers role is to visualize the catheter in which stepping source is going to maneuver. The next step is to execute CT imaging, and it is advised to perform imaging of the entire inspiration stage. Its purpose is to mineralize movement of markers during the treatment. When images indicate patients major movements while breathing, it is necessary to repeat the procedure as there is a possibility of artifacts occurring, e.g., in form of blurred images. Changes in applicator location in reference to the target caused by the patient's movement do not have a significant effect on dose dispersion in the patients system [7]. Scans are performed every 2.5 mm. In case, scans are performed below 2.5 mm proximity, the quality of images is significantly impaired.

Once CT images are accepted by radiotherapist and medical physicist, they are being sent to the computerized system of treatment planning. Radiotherapist marks each image for PTV and OARs areas. In lung cancer area, the critical organs are esophagus, heart, and spinal cord. In our department, we contour the actual image of target and critical organs on the images from computed tomography. Dose is specified for the entire PTV area. Most recent American Brachytherapy Society guidelines suggest 3D imaging for lung cancer treatment planning while applying HDR brachytherapy [8].

During the next stage, medical physicist performs reconstruction of applicators trajectory. Selection of the optimal source step and stop place in the in the nearest proximity from PTV. Then, the treatment plan is being optimized. Generally, treatment plan is optimized onto dose reference points usually situated 1 cm from catheter axis [9]. Reference dose should be calculated for the target area. This process is greatly influenced by the number of applicators. In our department, it is usually between two and four. The number of catheters administered depends mainly on patient's condition, location, and the volume of therapeutic area. When possible, bronchial applicators are implemented into the terminal bronchioles. Such allocation prevents catheter from sliding out what can stem from patient's couch movements caused by the presence of excrescence in patient's airways.

Routinely, treatment plans are optimized by graphical optimization. It is crucial to examine the dose dispersion in patient's system after each modification based on graphic optimization. After the development process is completed, plan is evaluated. Radiotherapist analyzes volume dose histogram (DVH). Evaluation of target coverage by reference dose in 85, 100, and 115% volume, as well as the dose in most important critical volume structures, was done. In instances of heart, spinal cord, and esophagus, the dose examined was 0.1, 1, and 2 cm^3 volume in each of those structures. After initial DVH, the dose dispersion is determined on each cross-section (image). After the plan is accepted, it is sent to the Treatment Control Station.

2.1.1. Case

In this case, patient is diagnosed with an inoperable non–small cell right lung cancer. Before the treatment begins, the patient has computed tomography (**Figure 1**). Overall patient's condition and the location of changes allowed the introduction of three bronchial applicators. All applicators were in the immediate proximity to tumor area. **Figure 2** shows scans with volume target contoured in computerized treatment planning systems (TPS). Illustration from computerized planning system depicts three-dimensional reconstruction of bronchial applicators, PTV, OARs, and dose distribution (**Figure 3**). Reconstruction on several planes and DVH is presented in **Figure 4**. The patient was treated with 18 Gy dose in three fractions.

2.1.2. Case

Second situation presents a patient with an inoperable non–small cell right lung cancer. Before the treatment begins, the patient has computed tomography. Overall patient's condition and the location of changes allowed the introduction of three bronchial applicators. Two applicators (nr1 and nr2) were introduced through the PTV area and planted in bronchial tubes. Applicator nr3 was placed where the bronchial tubes light has been blocked by the neoplastic changes. Very often, such applicator placement causes dilatation of bronchial tube, making it possible to introduce applicator through this area during next fraction. This, furthermore, improves the coverage on tumor area. **Figure 5** shows scans with volume target contoured in TPS. Illustration from computerized planning system depicts three-dimensional reconstruction of bronchial applicators, PTV, OARs, and dose distribution (**Figure 6**). Reconstruction on several planes and DVH is presented in **Figure 7**. The patient was treated with 18 Gy dose in three fractions. In **Figure 8**, cancer photo was captured during the application.

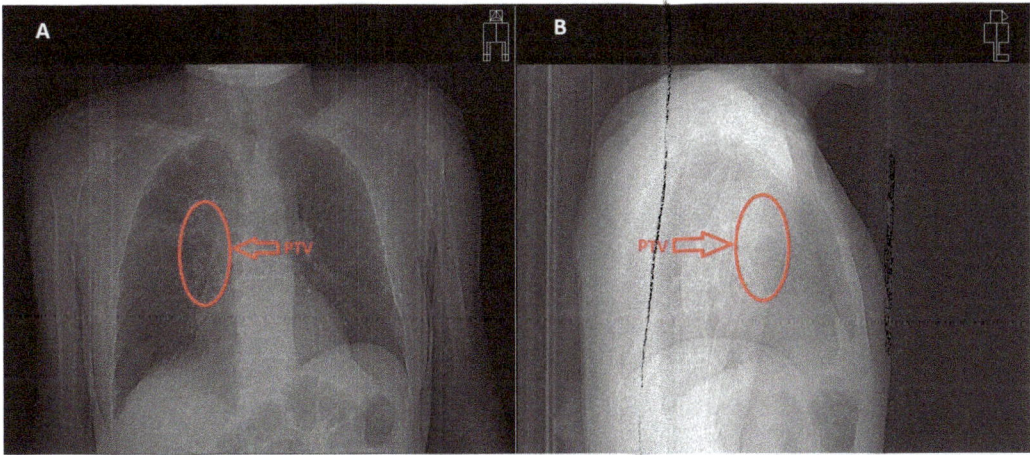

Figure 1. CT image of the front (A) and side (B) of the patient with marked PTV.

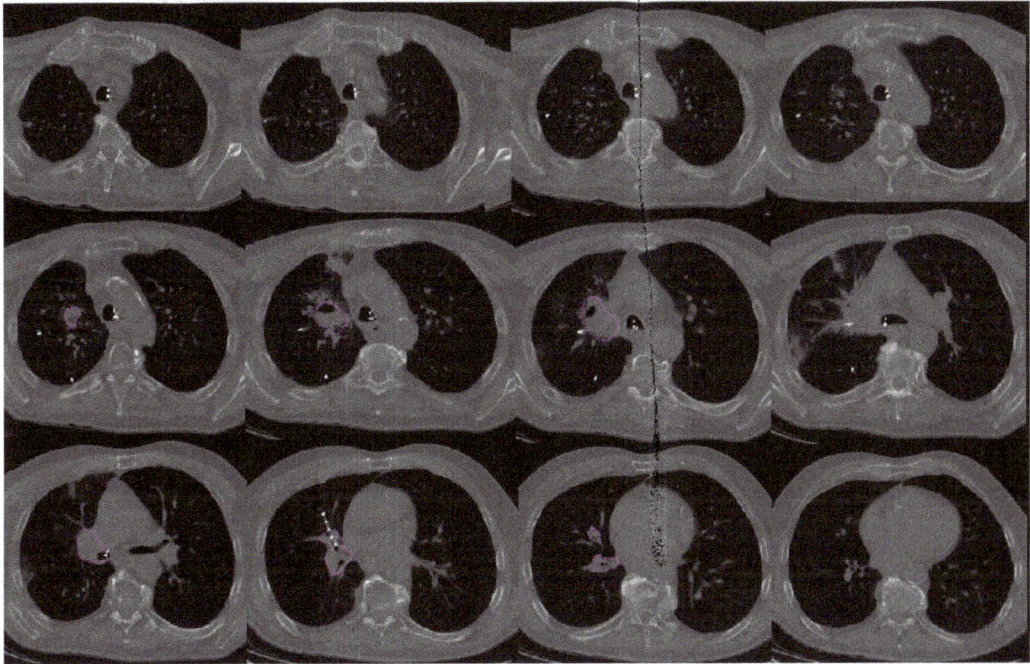

Figure 2. Images of the TPS with PTV.

2.2. Skin cancer

In the case of skin cancer, depending on its size and location, we can differentiate several types of applicators. With small and superficial skin changes, usually Leipzig applicators are being used. When dealing with long and flat changes, i.e., on the leg, then usually Freiburg flap is applied. The advantage of this applicator derives from the parallel positioning of catheters and consistent length at which they are situated. The distance of the catheters from the surface is also consistent. This type of applicator is also characterized

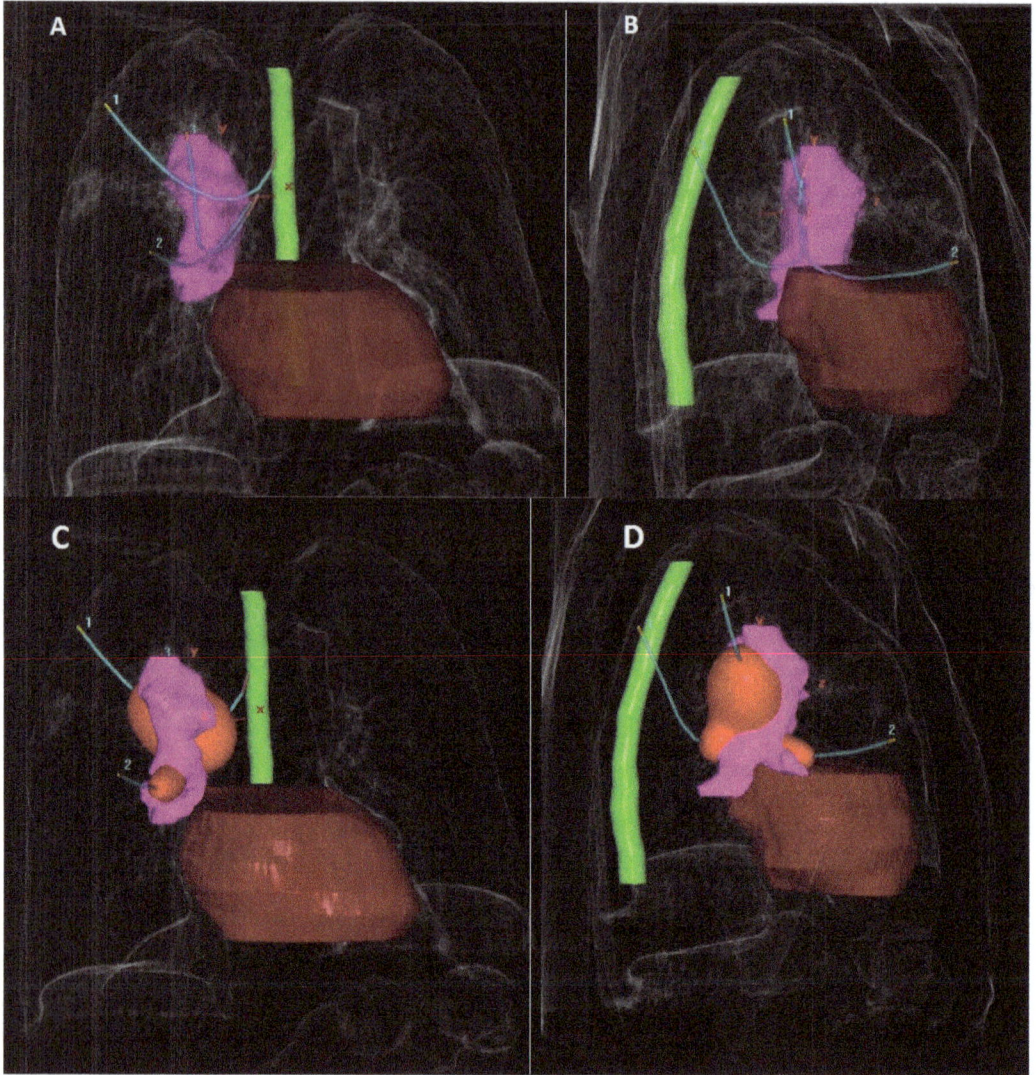

Figure 3. 3D reconstruction (A, C: front; B, D: side) of PTV applicators and OARs and 3D dose reference distribution.

by the high repetitiveness during the following irradiation fractions. The only requirement is the correct marking of applicator placement on the patient's skin. Very often, the place in which cancer is situated, i.e., in nose, ear, or cheek area, doesn't allow for application of standard applicators. In this case, it is very difficult to determine with the use of standard applicator. Using of standard applicator will not allow for ensuring optimal dose distribution in the PTV area. It is caused by inability to adjust catheter location in reference to the target [10].

Applicator adjustment during the following irradiation fractions is influenced by a considerable inaccuracy margin caused by a limited applicator placement repetitiveness in regard to patient's body. In cases when changes are located in close proximity to risk organs, applicator reconstruction can be planned so that it can decrease irradiation dose in those organs. The dose can also be reduced by appropriate arrangement of catheters in the applicator.

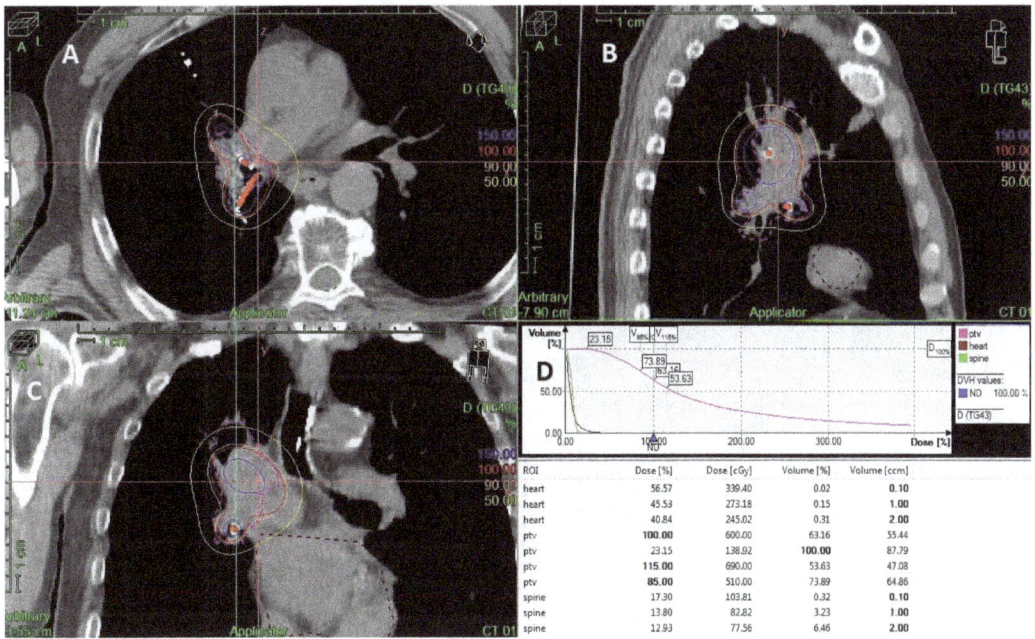

Figure 4. CT images and reconstruction on several planes (A, B, and C) and DVH (D).

ROI	Dose [%]	Dose [cGy]	Volume [%]	Volume [ccm]
heart	56.57	339.40	0.02	0.10
heart	45.53	273.18	0.15	1.00
heart	40.84	245.02	0.31	2.00
ptv	100.00	600.00	63.16	55.44
ptv	23.15	138.92	100.00	87.79
ptv	115.00	690.00	53.63	47.08
ptv	85.00	510.00	73.89	64.86
spine	17.30	103.81	0.32	0.10
spine	13.80	82.82	3.23	1.00
spine	12.93	77.58	6.46	2.00

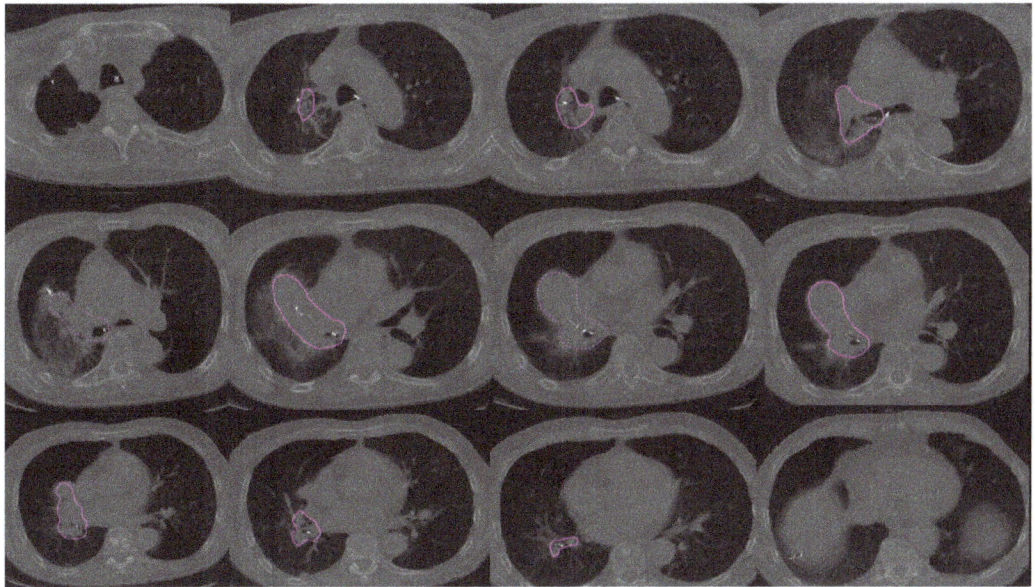

Figure 5. Images of the TPS with PTV.

In cases of shallow changes, situated in immediate proximity to applicators surface, catheters can be placed slightly further away from the target to avoid high dosage besides the PTV area. However, if the cancerous region is situated underneath the layer of skin and skin itself is OAR, the applicators will be moved toward the skin surface, inside the silicone

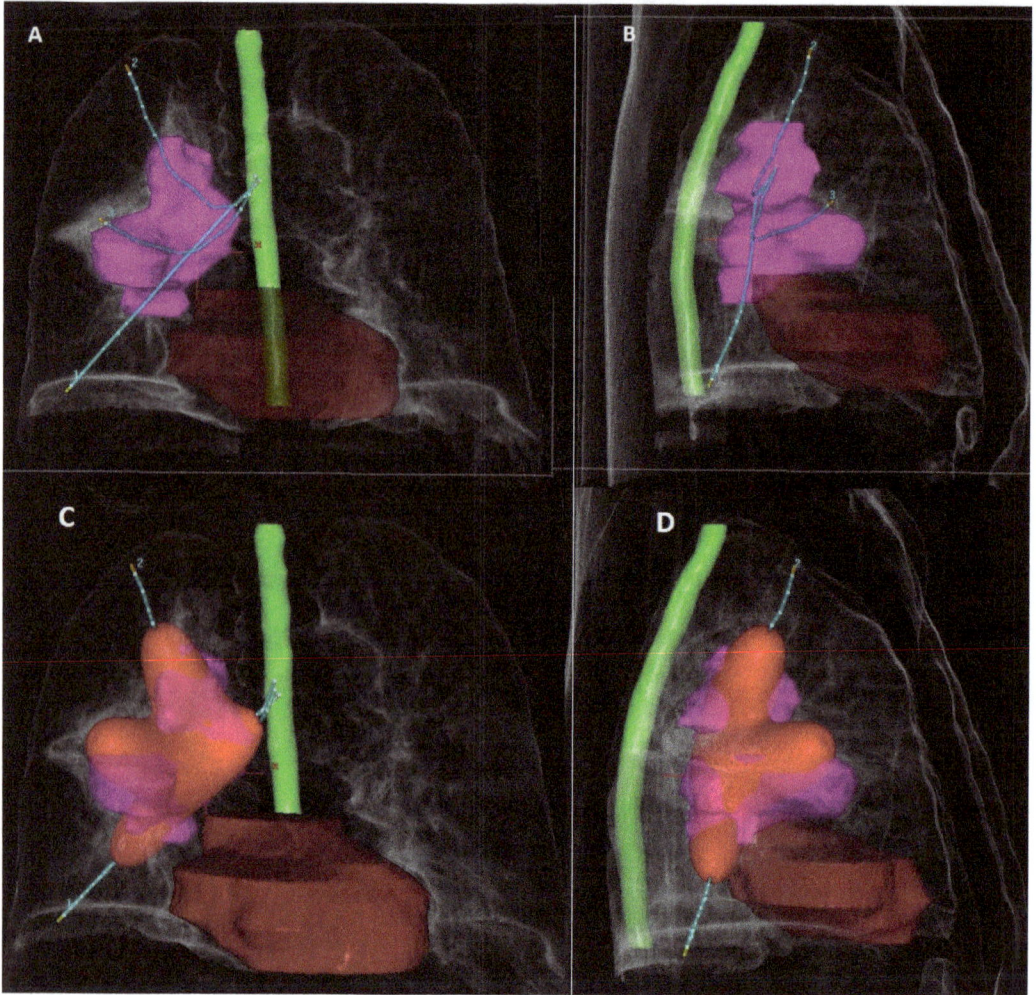

Figure 6. 3D reconstruction (A, C: front; B, D: side) of PTV applicators OARs and 3D dose reference distribution.

mask. Such applicator distribution is the reason for the high dose, and catheters being the source do not reach to skin region. Another way to dose distribution, and therefore protection for critical organs, is the adoption of shields. Their task is to absorb (reduce) the dose, for I192 the half value is 2.5 mm for lead (HVL pb). Shields can be in the form of led strips in different thickness. Such shield can be produced in workshop of teleradiotherapy department. Shield adjustment takes place on provided patient's gypsum cast. Shields are fixed in a silicone mask with the exception of the three-dimensional computer tomography imaging. LED shields are the source of artifacts during CT imaging, hence disturbing the treatment process. Because the individual shields are removed for the CT imaging, they are not visible on patient's scans sent to the computerized system of treatment planning. The dose that reaches critical organs protected by shields is calculated based on the thickness of applied shield. It is necessary to conduct *in vivo* dosimetry before the first irradiation to verify the prearranged dosage. Dosimetry can be conducted through applying the MOSFET detector. In cases where it is necessary to determine the dosage absorbed by an individual

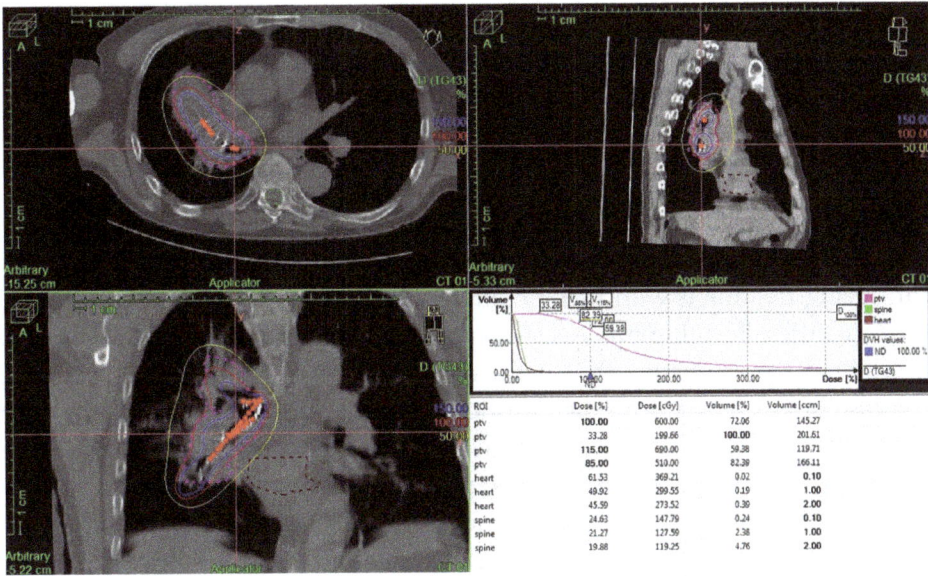

Figure 7. CT images and reconstruction on several planes (A, B, and C) and DVH (D).

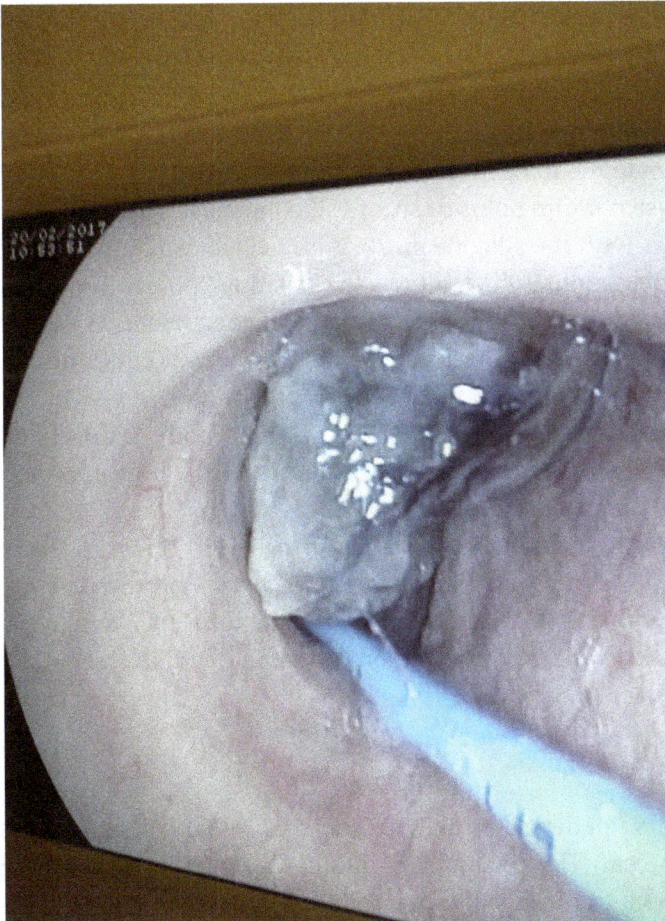

Figure 8. Lung cancer photo.

shield, Micro-MOSFET detectors are very effective, and because of their small-scale dimensions, they can be placed between irradiative area and the shield itself. In cases where cancerous changes are located in the area of nose or cheeks, it is advised to place such shields around patient's eyes. Such placement prevents the shield from moving while during the treatment process.

Another method of manufacturing individual applicators is the usage thermoplastic mask. Usage of the orfit masks is widely spread in teleradiotherapy. They are applied to immobilize the patient during treatment with help of external bundles. They are characterized by very good tracing qualities. Forming process takes place on patient's body. High level of its reproducibility is advantageous during the treatment process. They can be used to immobilize any location. In case of brachytherapy, such properties as reproducibility of patient's curvatures are very desirable. This is one of the reasons why I became interested in applying this type of material in the HDR brachytherapy treatment process. The concept and theory are quite similar to silicone masks. However, there are some relevant differences between these two types of individual applicators. First, it is the use of the material itself. With the orfit mask, we get a premade product that has to be heated. When heat treated, it becomes very malleable, and after applying it onto the given surface, it easily adapts to its shape. It is setting just within few minutes. If the reproduction is not satisfying, the material can be reheated and formed again. Once it reaches ambient temperature, the mask is ready to use. Another difference lays in the way catheters are mounted to the surface of the individual applicator. With the silicone mask, applicators are inside, and with the Orfit mask, they can be freely mounted onto it. So in situation where the applicators need to be close to the surface of the skin, we can immobilize catheters by sewing them to the mask. When they have to be further away from the surface of the orfit mask, we can use paraffin bolus or secure silicone mask. With shields, the workflow procedure is the same as with the silicone mask. Because we use thermoplastic material, we can contour the shield placement, which allows the position control throughout every treatment fraction. The last difference between the orfit and silicone masks is the manner of mounting it onto the patient. The silicone mask uses patient's natural curvatures for the appropriate setting. In large areas, it is easy to adjust the applicator; however, in cases with flat areas, it is necessary to mark reference points on the patient's body. Additionally, for the mask to adhere properly through irradiation process, it is advisable to use immobilizing bands. The orfit mask is fixed to the base on which the patent is laid. It is mounted to specialized brackets and that is why mask adjustment is the same during every fraction. Immobilizing bands are no more necessary nor is the marking of reference points on the patient's body. Routinely, silicone masks are ready in 4 to 5 days after taking the imprint. When adopting the use of the orfit mask, first fraction can be performed on the same day that the patient is accepted to the brachytherapy department.

2.2.1. Case

The first case presents a patient with skin cancer (squamous cell carcinoma). Cancer is located in the vicinity of the ear. The patient was qualified for treatment with the applicator individual (silicone mask). In the silicone mask were placed seven applicators. The patient was treated with 40 Gy in 10 fractions once a day. **Figure 9** shows scans with volume target contoured in TPS. Illustration from computerized planning system depicts three-dimensional reconstruction applicators, PTV, and dose distribution (**Figure 10**). Reconstruction on several planes and DVH is presented in **Figure 11**. Patient treated with silicone mask is presented in **Figure 12**.

2.2.2. Case

The second case presents a patient with skin cancer (basal cell carcinoma). Cancer is located in the vicinity of the nose. The patient was qualified for treatment with the applicator individual (orfit mask). In the silicone mask were placed four applicators. The patient was treated with 50 Gy in 10 fractions once a day. The patient had a shield on both eyes. Before the treatment begins, the patient has computed tomography to verify the mask fit to the patient (**Figure 13**). **Figure 14** shows scans with volume target contoured in TPS. Illustration from TPS depicts three-dimensional reconstruction applicators, PTV, OARs, and dose distribution (**Figure 15**). Reconstruction on several planes and DVH is presented in **Figure 16**. Patient treated with the orfit mask is presented in **Figure 17**.

2.2.3. Case

The third case presents a patient with skin cancer (basal cell carcinoma). Cancer is located in the vicinity of the nose. The patient was qualified for treatment with the applicator individual

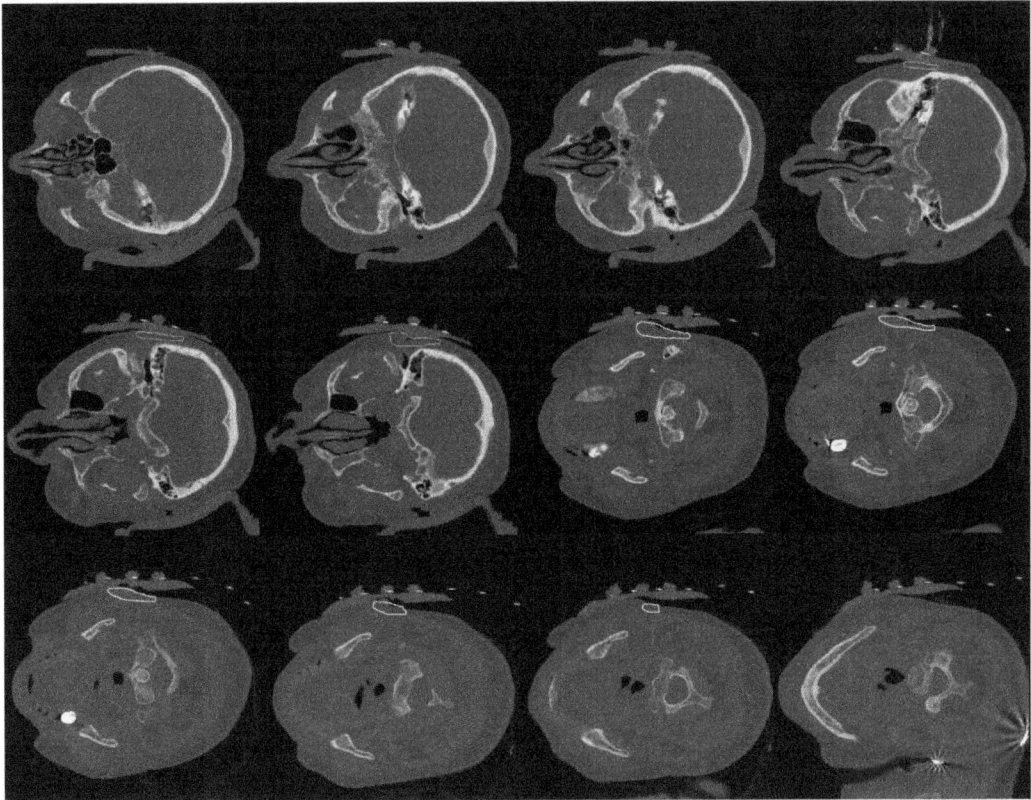

Figure 9. Images of the TPS with PTV.

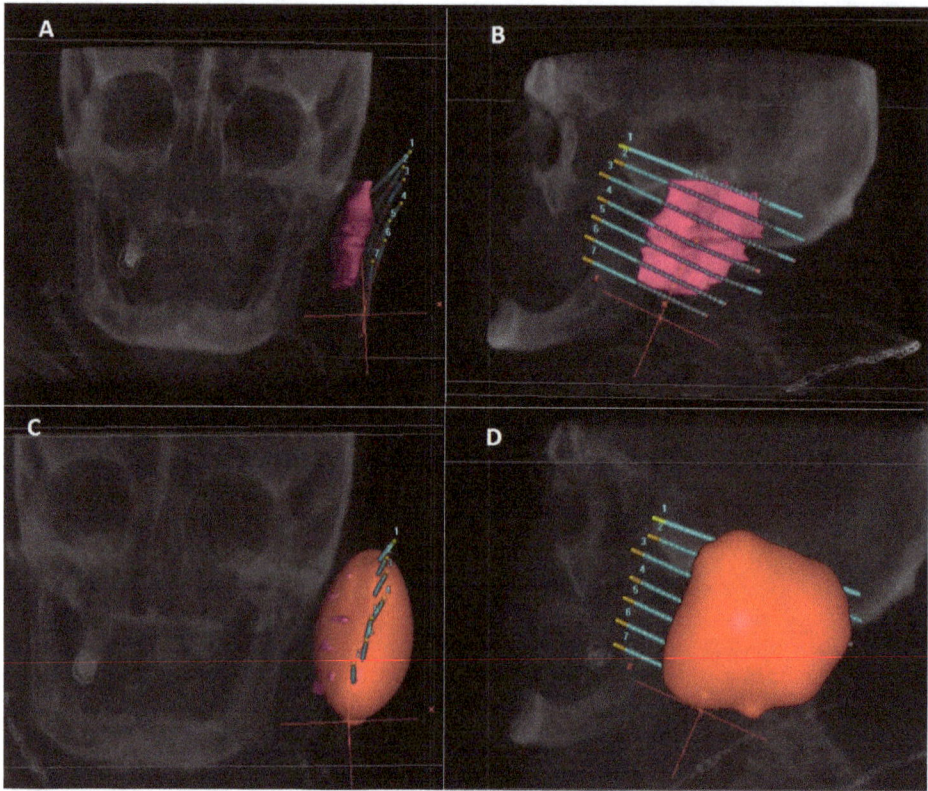

Figure 10. 3D reconstruction (A, C: front; B, D: side) of PTV applicators and 3D dose reference distribution.

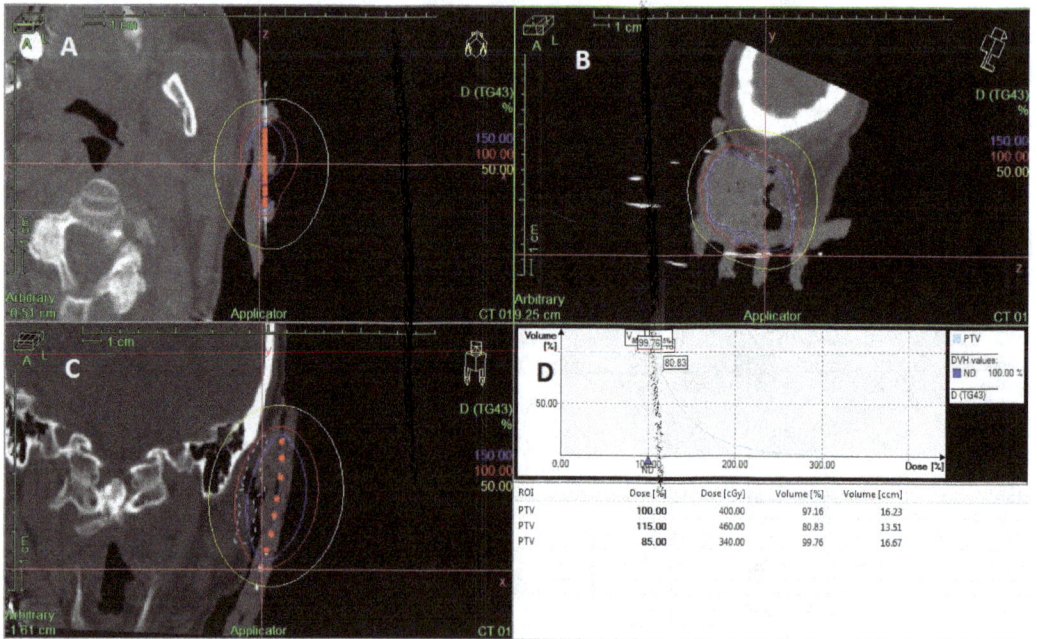

Figure 11. CT images and reconstruction on several planes (A, B, and C) and DVH (D).

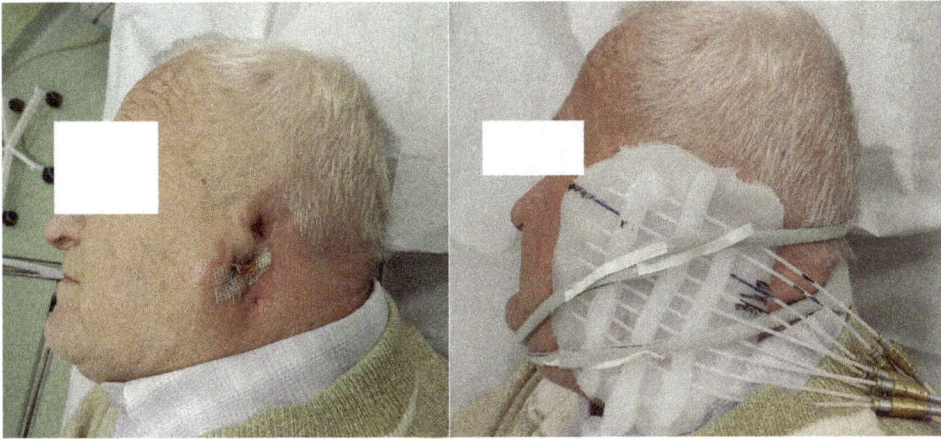

Figure 12. Patient treated with the silicone mask.

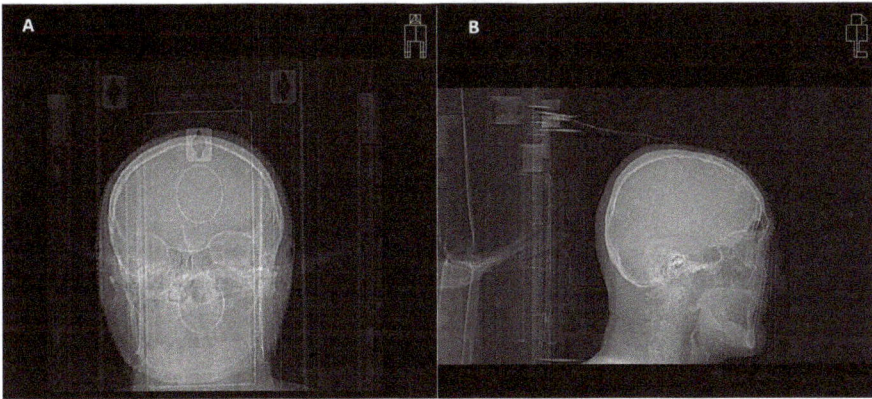

Figure 13. CT image of the front (A) and side (B) of the patient with an orfit mask.

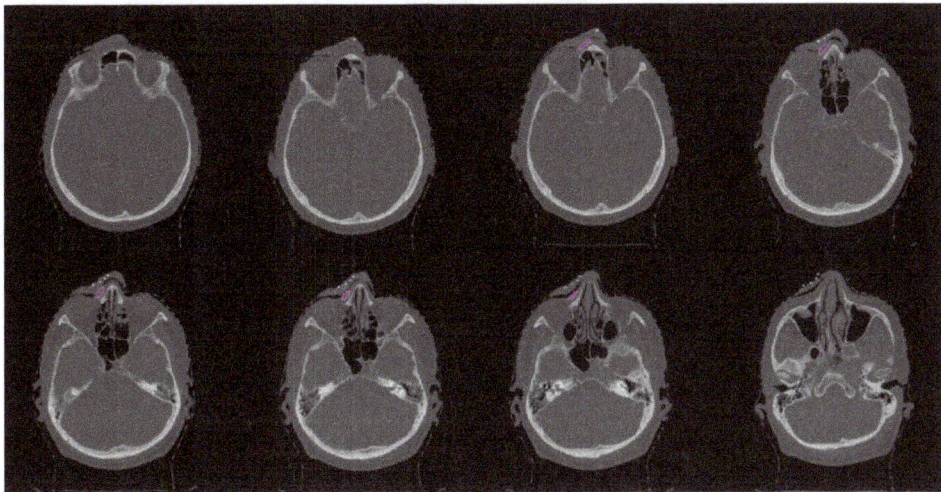

Figure 14. Images of the TPS with PTV.

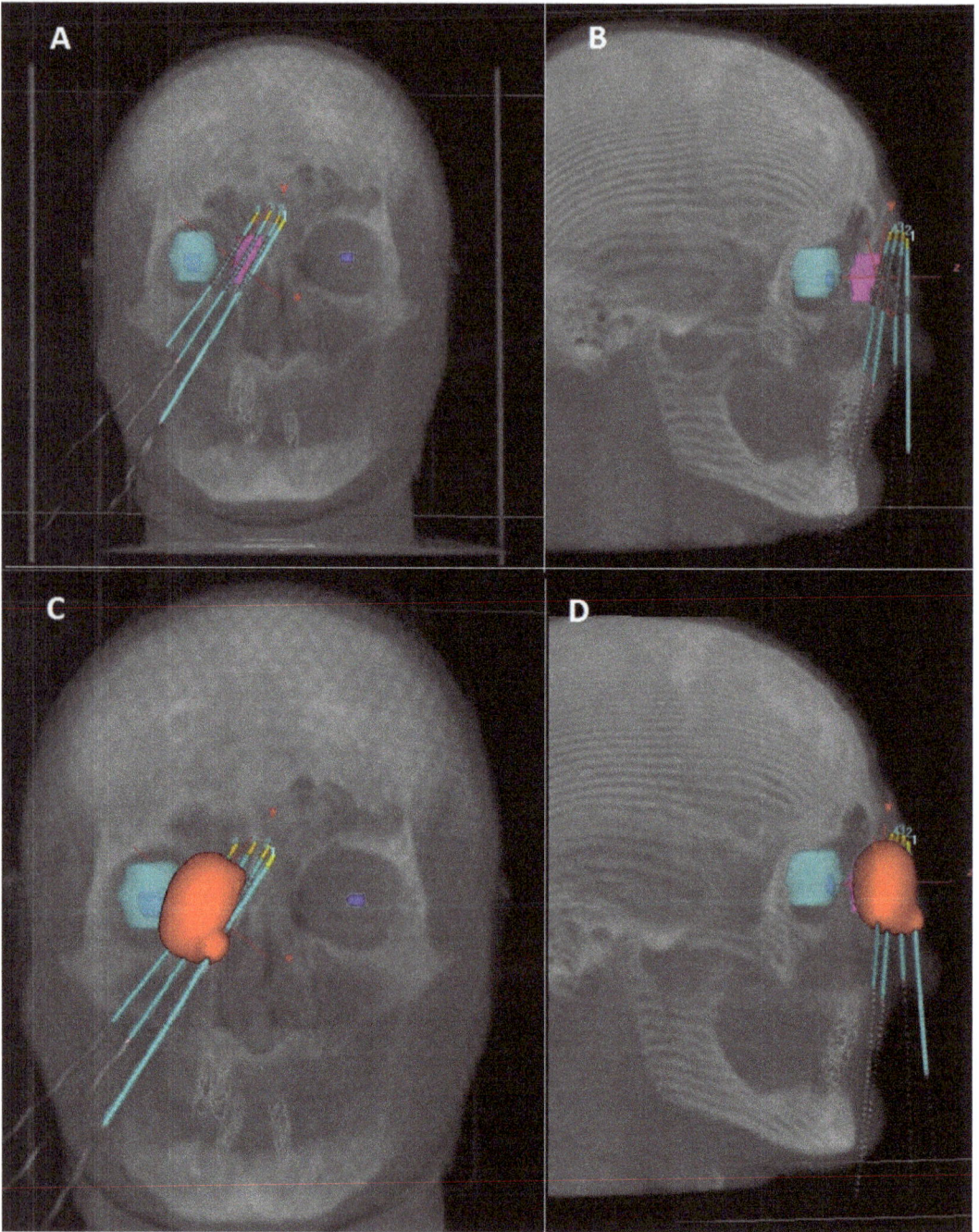

Figure 15. 3D reconstruction (A, C: front; B, D: side) of PTV applicators OARs and 3D dose reference distribution.

(Orfit mask). In the silicone mask were placed eight applicators. The patient was treated with 50 Gy in 10 fractions once a day. The patient had individual shield on one eye and standard shield on the other eye (**Figure 18**). Before the treatment begins, the patient has computed tomography to verify the mask fit to the patient (**Figure 19**). **Figure 20** shows scans with

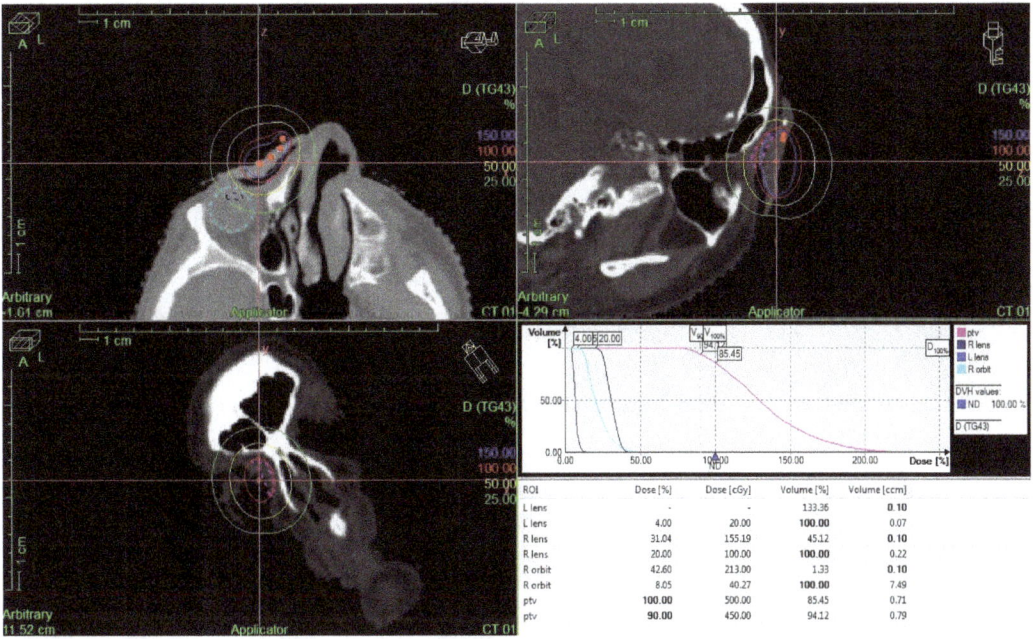

Figure 16. CT images and reconstruction on several planes (A, B, and C) and DVH (D).

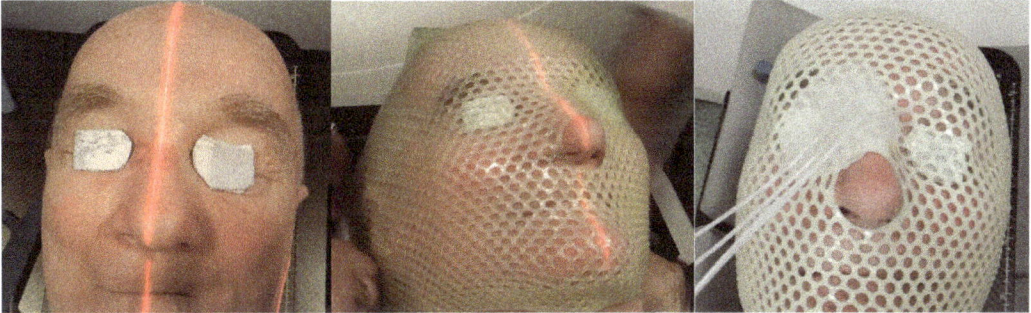

Figure 17. Patient treated with an orfit mask.

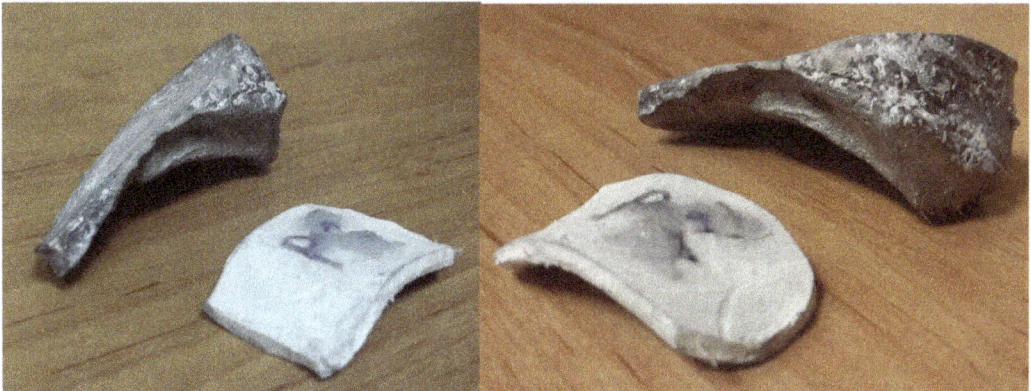

Figure 18. Picture of shield.

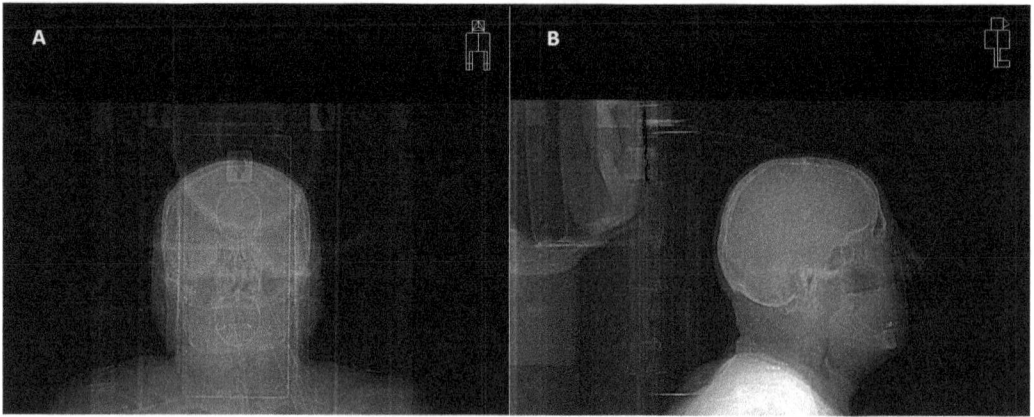

Figure 19. CT image of the front (A) and side (B) of the patient with an orfit mask.

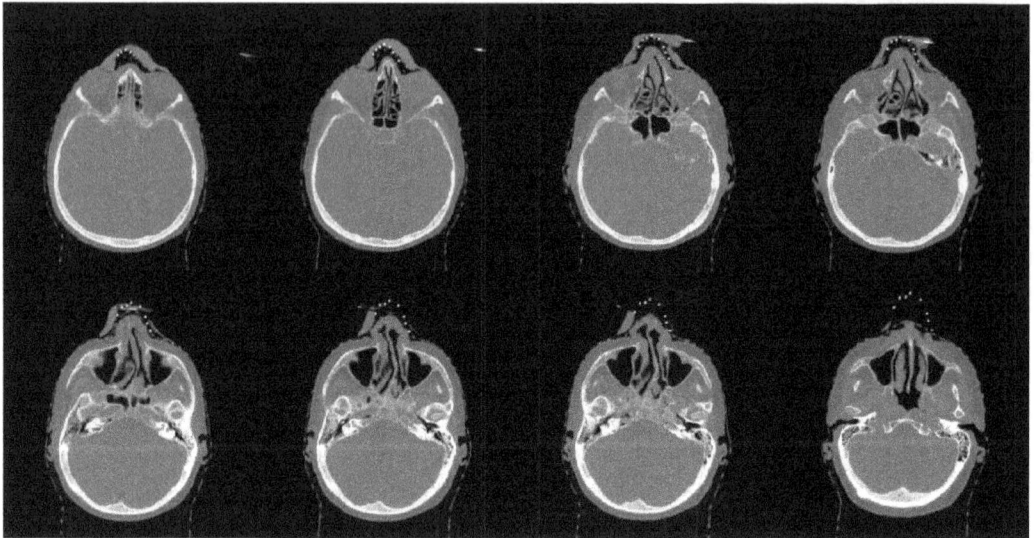

Figure 20. Images of the TPS with PTV.

volume target contoured in TPS. Illustration from TPS depicts three-dimensional reconstruction applicators, PTV, OARs, and dose distribution (**Figure 21**). Reconstruction on several planes and DVH is presented in **Figure 22**. Patient treated with the orfit mask is presented in **Figure 23**

2.3. Breast cancer

With breast cancer, brachytherapy can be applied as a method associated with teleradiotherapy after breast-conserving surgery. It is realized in form of boost. It can also be applied as an independent form of post-surgical treatment (Accelerated Partial Breast Irradiation) as an alternative to the external beam radiotherapy.

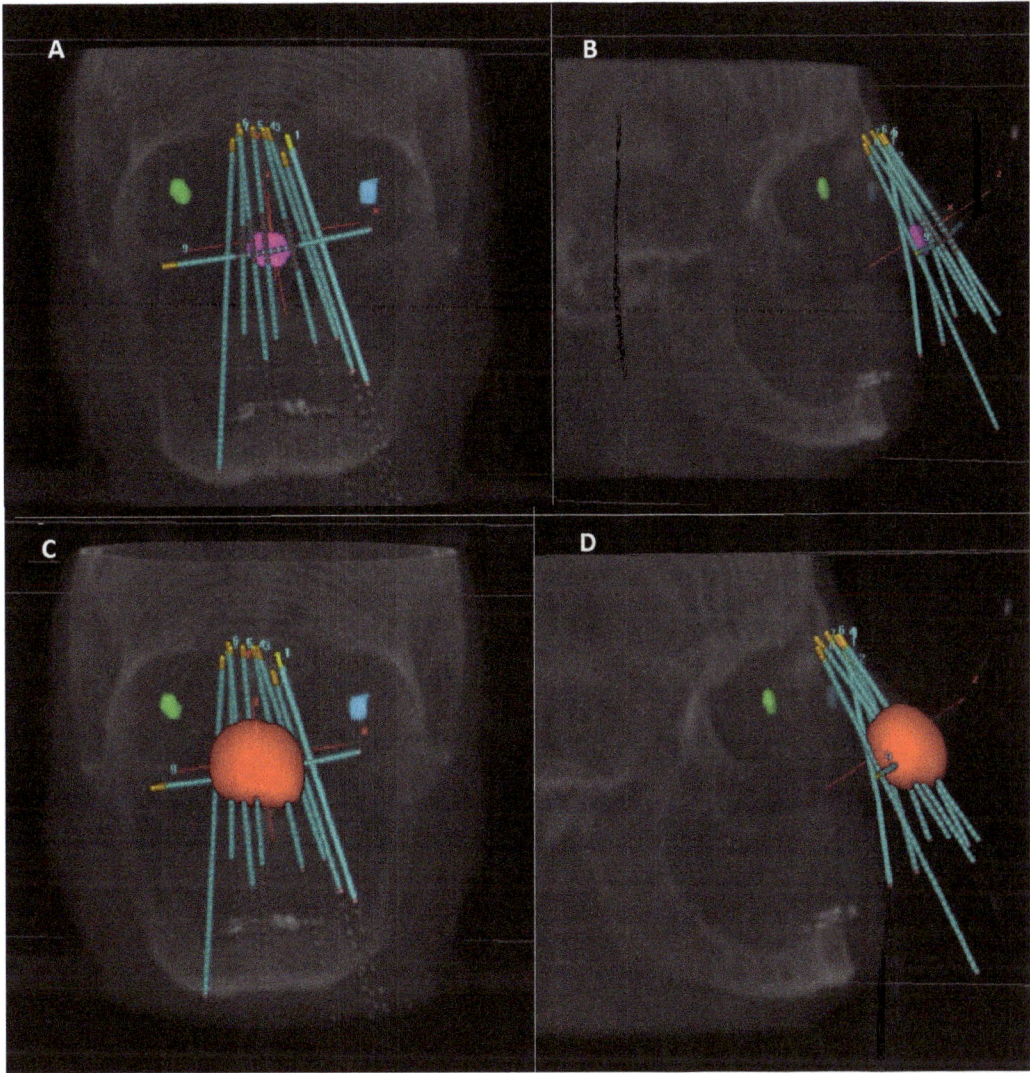

Figure 21. 3D reconstruction (A, C: front; B, D: side) of PTV applicators OARs and 3D dose reference distribution.

Before breast brachytherapy treatment begins, after radical dissection, it is necessary to perform tumor bed imaging. Computed tomography is the advised method to apply. Before CT examination, it is necessary to place markers on the post-surgical scar. The presence of this marker does not have a significant effect on the quality of images from CT. It is possible to use specialized markers for CT which, because of the material they are made of, is not the source of artifacts. Markers placed on the scar allow more precise tumor bed localization and therefore more precise applicator administration into the tumor bed area. The process for locating of tumor area is facilitated by surgical clips. They are easily identifiable in CT examination. Their presence allows for exact defining of targets location. We can adopt two techniques with the boost. One technique takes advantage of a frame so-called a template; another one on the other hand uses metal needles. The choice of a given technique depends mainly on target

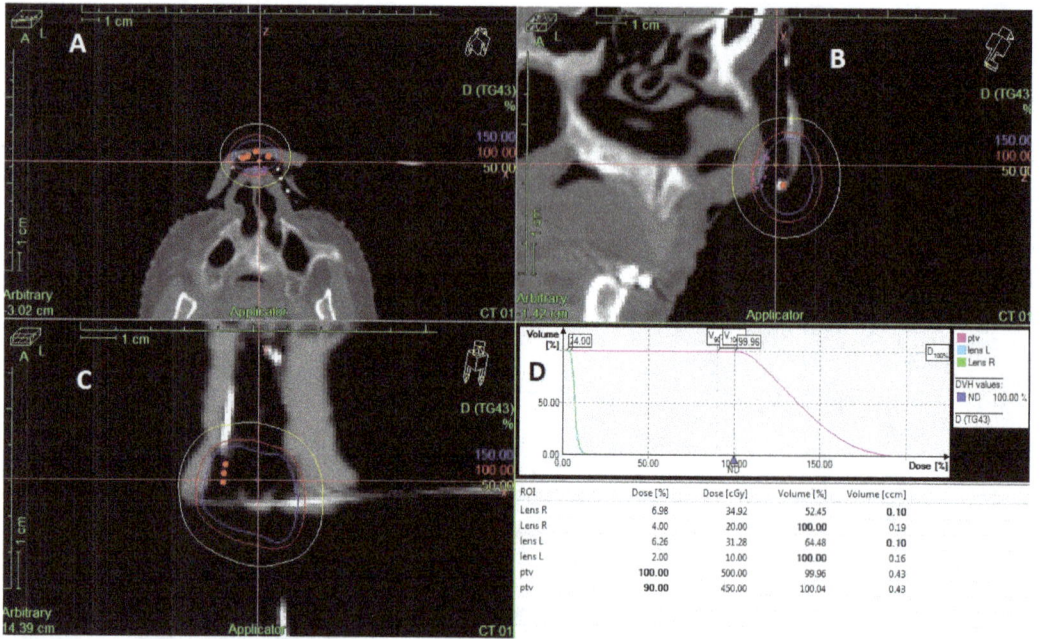

Figure 22. CT images and reconstruction on several planes (A, B, C) and DVH (D).

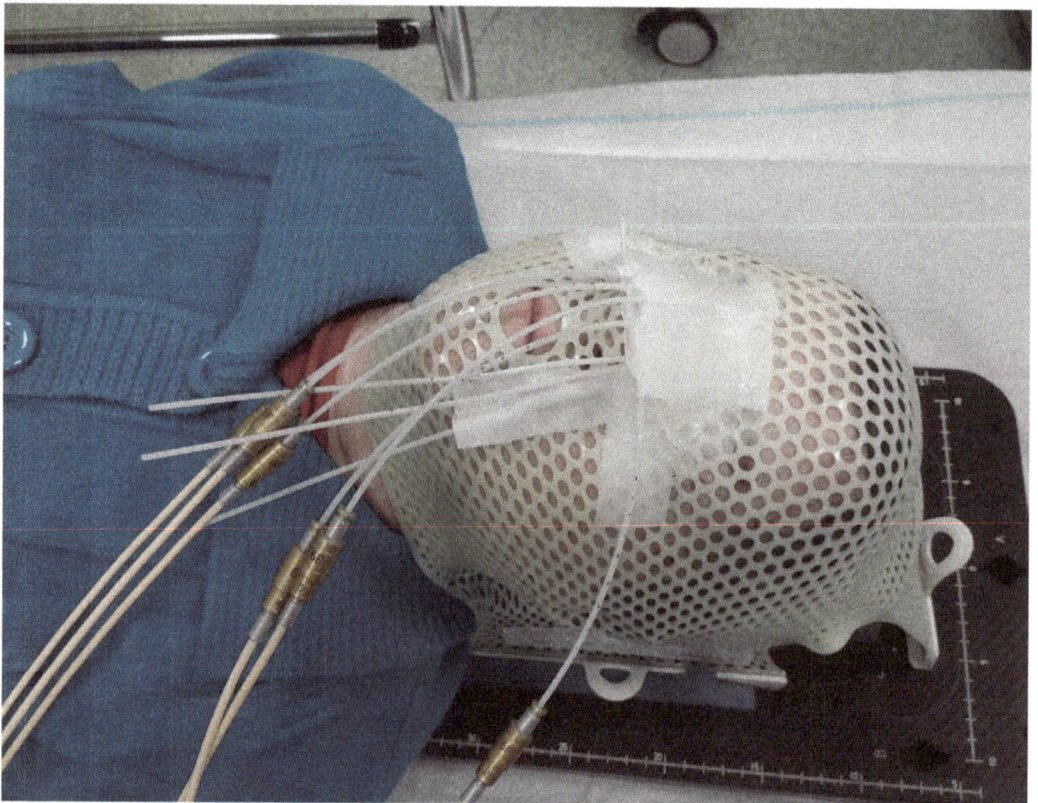

Figure 23. Patient treated with an orfit mask.

location and patient's anatomical structure. If a patient has got big breasts and the tumor bed is located in the central area of the breast, then we use the template. This template consists of two plates and a connector which mounts those plates parallel within specified proximity. The plates have openings through which applicators are put through. The number and the arrangement of the plains are the same on both plates. The distance between openings on plates is between 10 and 18 mm. The choice of the appropriate template depends on the size, positioning of the tumor bed, and patient's anatomical structure. By using templates, the position of needles is parallel. By applying the template, depending on patient's breast size, we can change its form. The breast is squeezed by the plates what can result in differences in implantation geometry. This kind of obstacle can be avoided by performing three-dimensional imaging with already applied template. In cases where the application geometry is not satisfactory, it is possible to use a different template. Where the implant geometry is not satisfactory after application deriving from the used template, there is no possibility to change it without removing applicators.

Second technique, so-called free hand, differs from the one already mentioned as in this case, the needles are applied without using templates. This technique requires extensive experience from the person performing the treatment. Location of needles is not determined by the plates so they can run non parallel. Such distribution can provoke difficulties in obtaining the required spatial distribution of isodose in the target area. Creating of an acceptable computerized treatment plan by physicist requires wide experience in this type of application. It is simply because it is possible that some areas can occur with higher or lower dosage than the reference dosage prepared for PTV areas. This method can be successfully applied with small and average breasts. Arbitrariness in needle maneuvering in the breast allows for higher degree of risk organs protection. After applying templates, skin, as its being squeezed by plates, can move to closer proximity to the PTV area. This can cause telangiectasias in the skin area. When applicators are applied free hand, tumor beds do not change their location in reference to the skin. In cases where tumor bed is positioned in small proximity to the chest wall, it is possible to introduce applicators directly into bed area while applying the free-hand technique. Where templates are used, structure of the plate reduces the possibility of introducing applicators in the PTV area. After deciding on palliation technique based on previously performed imaging, we can proceed to needle implantation. During application, it is possible to perform low-dose CT in order to regulate applicator's trajectory through tumor bed area. After application is completed, it is necessary to secure the needles from moving out by applying clips onto them. It is particularly important when taking advantage of this technique, but it also secures the needles from relocation while attaching transfer tubes. It is crucial to remove mandrins from the needles as they are the source of numerous artifacts in computer tomography imaging. They significantly affect the image quality especially because they are in the PTV area.

In case of brachytherapy as an independent form of treatment, we can use several different applicators. As with the boost, we can apply plate/template techniques. The difference between boost procedures and unassisted treatment lies mainly in the number of fractions. Boost is applied in one of the fractions whereas Accelerated Partial Breast Irradiation (APBI) in eight fractions. Because of that, all metal needles have been replaced with plastic guides, which remain in patient's body through the whole treatment process. The guides are closed up with clips on the one end, whereas on the other end, we can find a connector that mounts introduced needle. Plastic needle is present in patient's body only during irradiation; they are being removed once irradiation has been completed. Because those needles are made of plastic, it is necessary to introduce dedicated markers to make them visible in CT imaging. Another method applied is so-called balloon method which takes advantage of SAVI applicator. This applicator consists of several channels with in its central part and rest in its circumferential area. To be able to apply this applicator, the patient has to be operated for open cavity surgery. After introducing applicator into tumor bed, it is being adjusted by dilating channels located on its boarders (circumferentially). Applicator is monitored by ultrasonography (USG) while being introduced; then, thee-dimensional imaging is performed. Before CT examination, it is important to mark one of the channels on patient's body to be able to verify applicator's location in reference to the tumor bed. Verification should be taken place before each and every irradiation fraction. The applicator is introduced into patient's body for the whole time of treatment process. Breast cancer treatment process based on three-dimensional images allows you to determine the dosage for the actual PTV area. Taking advantage of computer tomography made it possible to search for new types of applicators, which, in course, allows to cover the desirable target area and protection of critical organs. TPS images present marked the target and all risk organs. Reference dose is specified for the whole PTV area, and risk organs in this case are skin area and the wall of the chest. In case of boost, the dosage equals 10 Gy, and in case of APBI/SAVI, it is 4 Gy 8 times twice a day [11].

2.3.1. Case

The first case presents a patient with breast cancer. The patient is after conservative treatment. Treatment is realized in the form of boost after external beam radiotherapy. The patient was treated with 10 Gy in 1 fraction. Before the treatment begins, the patient has computed tomography (**Figure 24**).The patient was treated with template. In the tumor bed were placed five applicators. **Figure 25** shows scans with volume target contoured in TPS. Illustration from computerized planning system depicts three-dimensional reconstruction applicators, PTV, and dose distribution (**Figure 26**). Reconstruction on several planes and DVH is presented in **Figure 27**.

2.3.2. Case

The second case presents a patient with breast cancer. Patient is after breast-conserving surgery. Treatment is realized in the form of boost after external beam radiotherapy. The patient was treated with 10 Gy in 1 fraction. Before the treatment begins, the patient has computed tomography (**Figure 28**). The patient was treated with the free-hand technique. In the tumor bed were placed eight applicators. **Figure 29** shows scans with volume target contoured in TPS. Illustration from computerized planning system depicts three-dimensional reconstruction applicators, PTV, and dose distribution (**Figure 30**). Reconstruction on several planes and DVH is presented in **Figure 31**. Patient with breast cancer treated using the free-hand technique is presented in **Figure 32**.

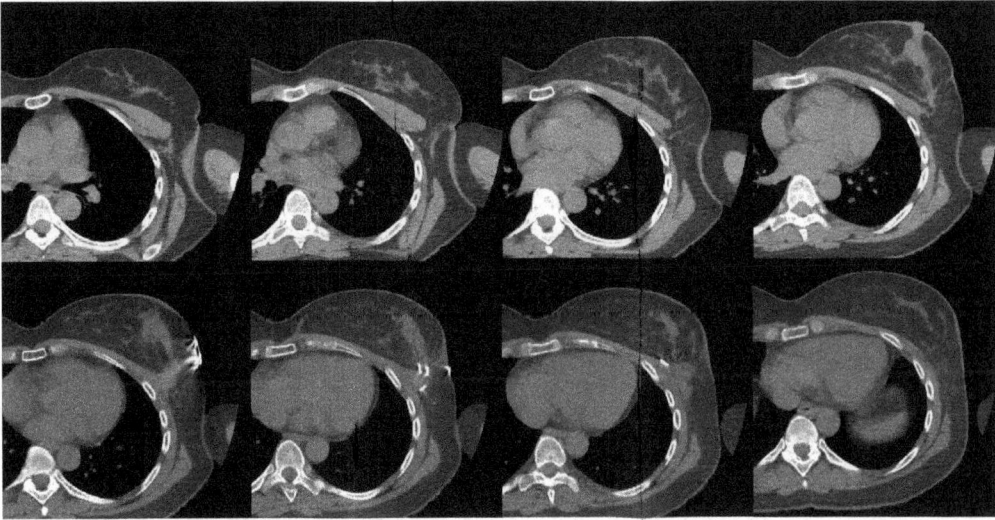

Figure 24. CT image before application with a marked scar.

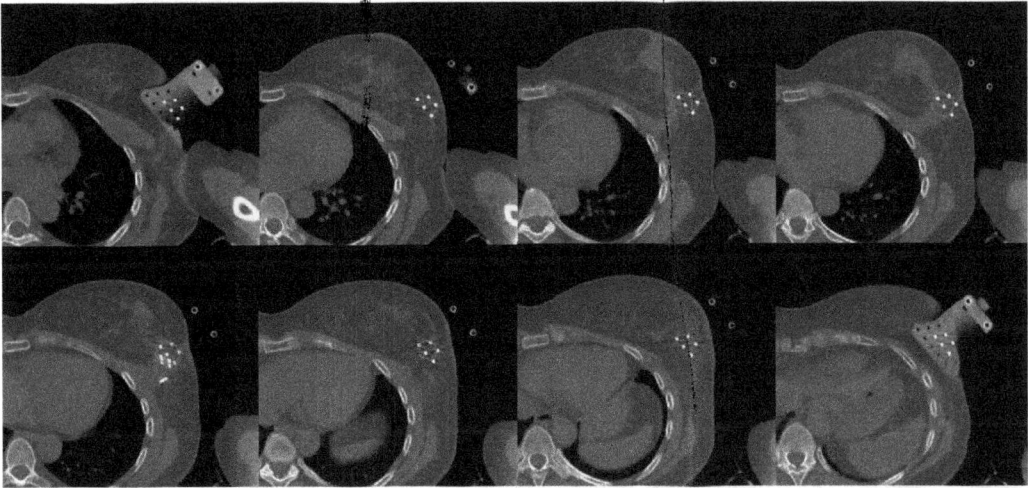

Figure 25. Images of the TPS with PTV.

2.3.3. Case

The third case presents a patient with breast cancer. Patient is after breast-conserving surgery. Treatment is realized in the form of post-surgical treatment (Accelerated Partial Breast Irradiation). The patient was treated with 32 Gy in eight fractions twice a day. Before the treatment begins, the patient has computed tomography (**Figure 33**). In the tumor bed were placed 12 applicators. **Figure 34** shows scans with volume target contoured in TPS. Illustration from computerized planning system depicts three-dimensional reconstruction applicators, PTV, and dose distribution (**Figure 35**). Reconstruction on several planes and DVH is presented in **Figure 36**.

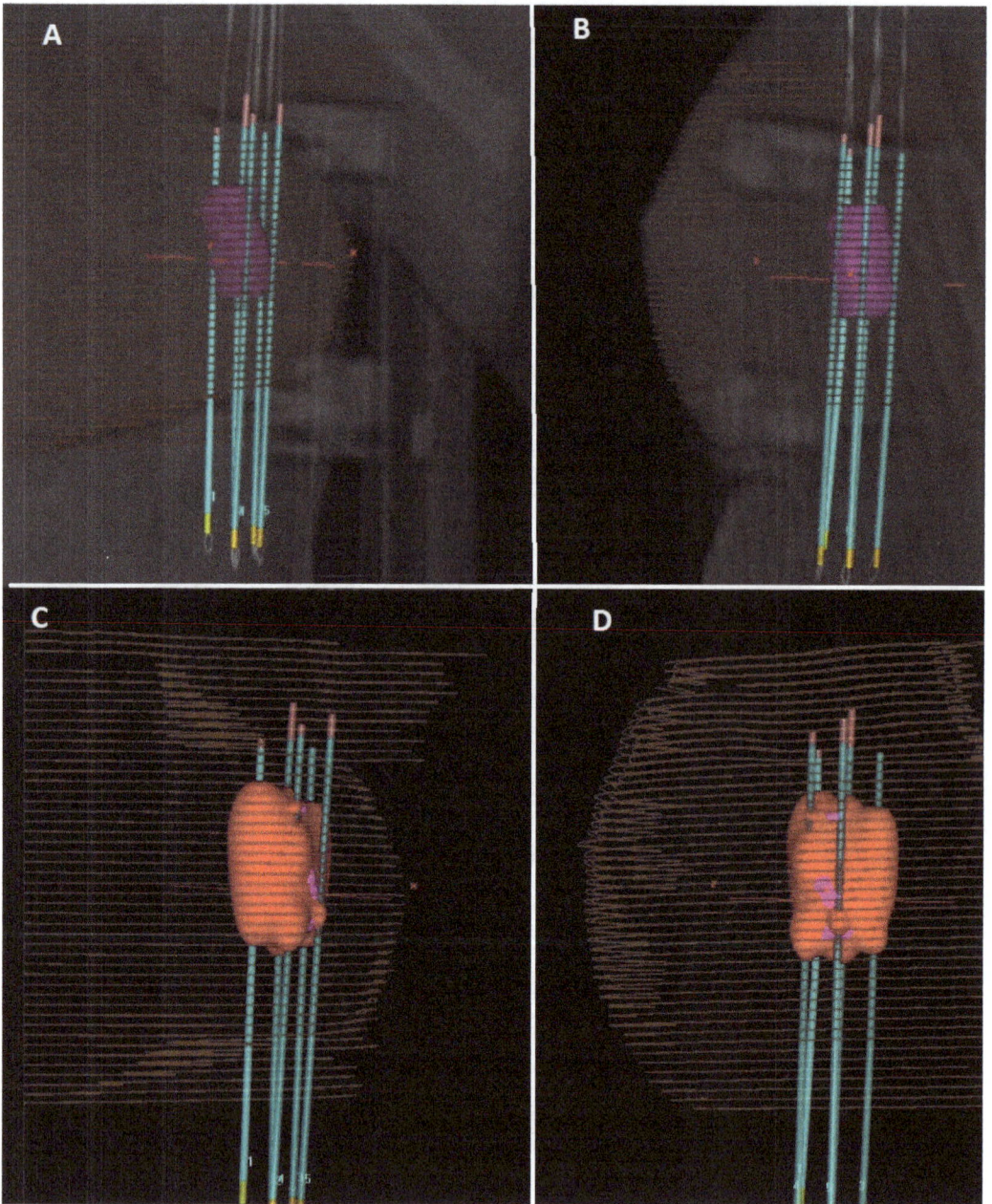

Figure 26. 3D reconstruction (A, C: front; B, D: side) of PTV applicators OARs and 3D dose reference distribution.

2.3.4. Case

The fourth case presents a patient with breast cancer. Patient is after breast-conserving surgery. Treatment is realized in the form of post-surgical treatment (Accelerated Partial Breast Irradiation). The patient was treated with 34 Gy in 10 fractions twice a day. Patient was treated by using applicator SAVI. Before the treatment begins, the patient has computed tomography

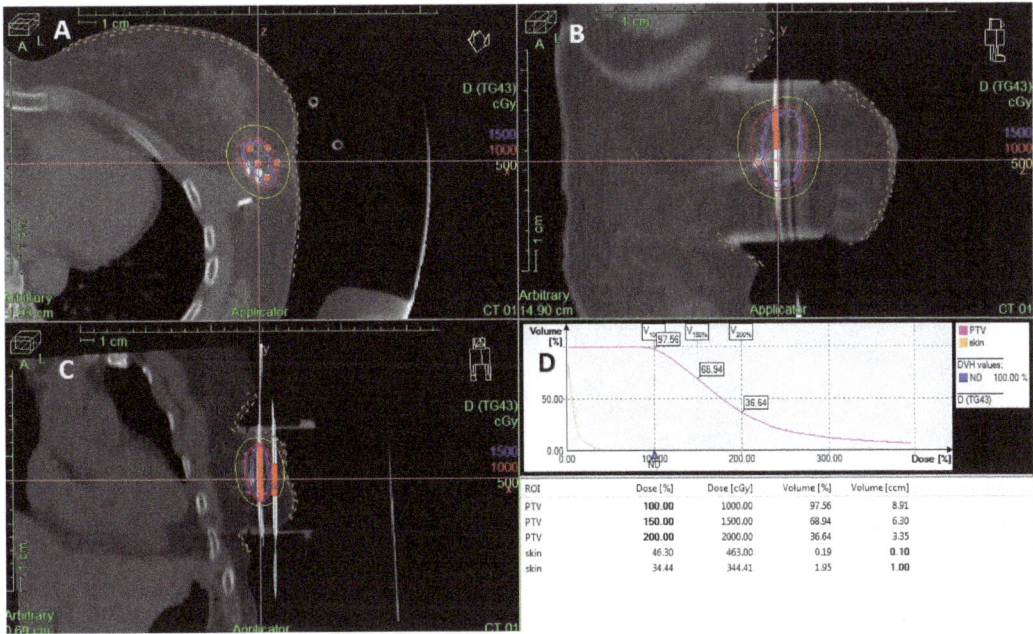

Figure 27. CT images and reconstruction on several planes (A, B, and C) and DVH (D).

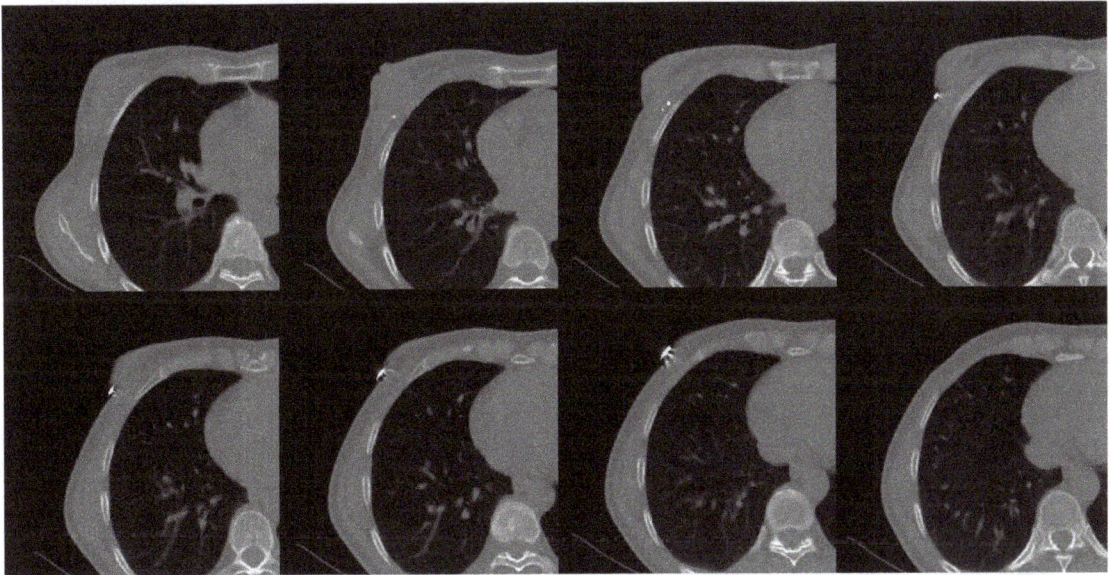

Figure 28. CT images before application with a marked scar.

(**Figure 37**). In the tumor bed was placed one applicator with seven channels. **Figure 38** shows scans with volume target contoured in TPS. Illustration from computerized planning system depicts three-dimensional reconstruction applicators, PTV, and dose distribution (**Figure 39**). Reconstruction on several planes and DVH is presented in **Figure 40**.

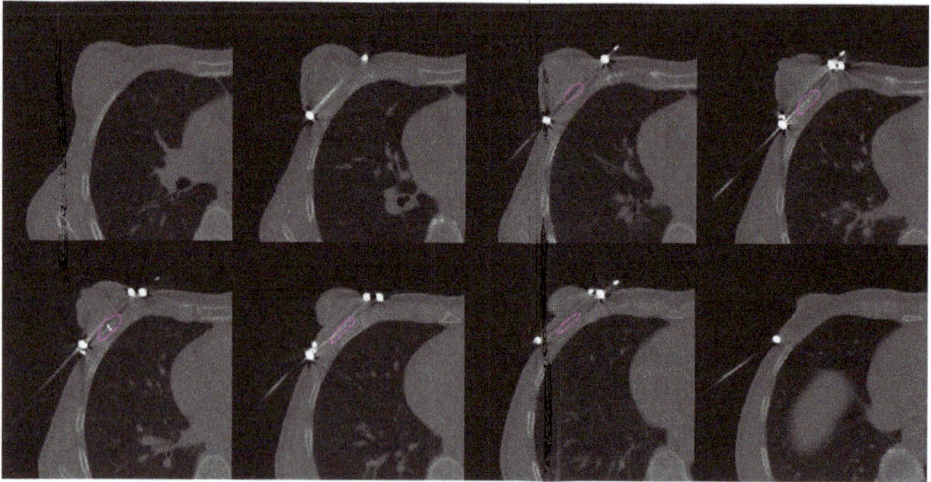

Figure 29. Images of the TPS with PTV.

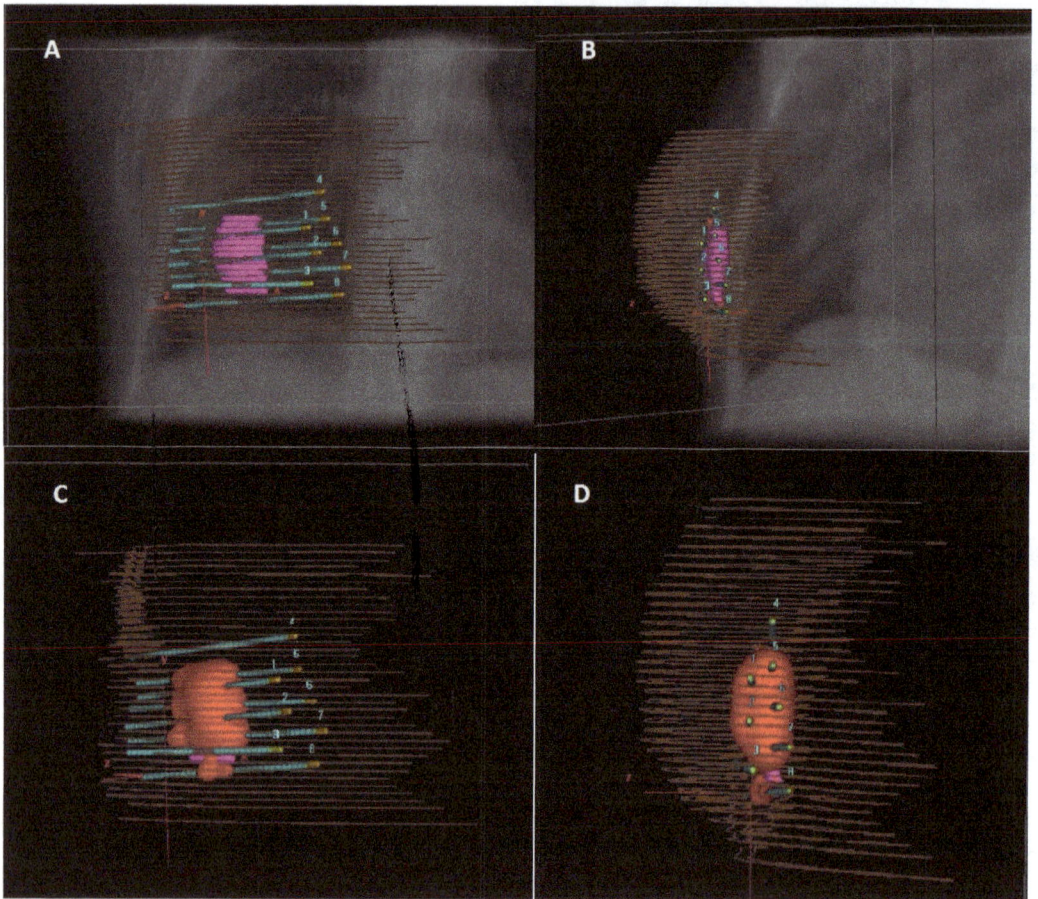

Figure 30. 3D reconstruction (A, C: front; B, D: side) of PTV applicators OARs and 3D dose reference distribution.

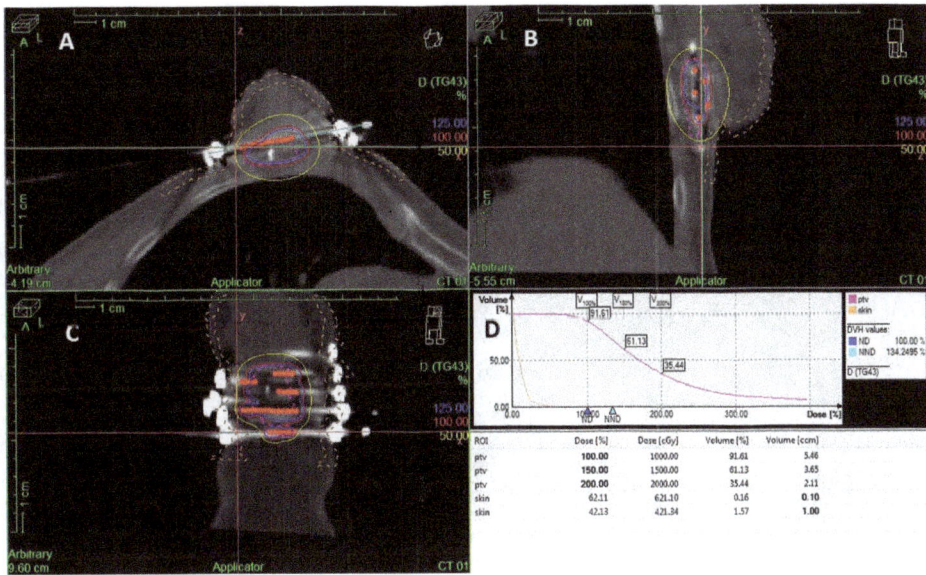

Figure 31. CT images and reconstruction on several planes (A, B, and C) and DVH (D).

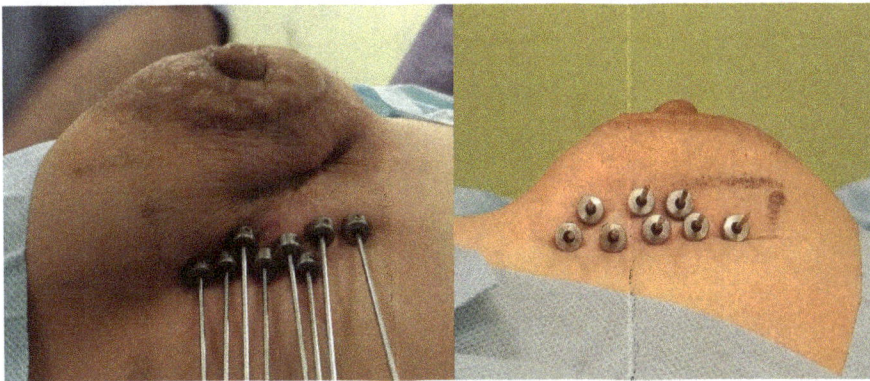

Figure 32. Patient with breast cancer treated using the free-hand technique.

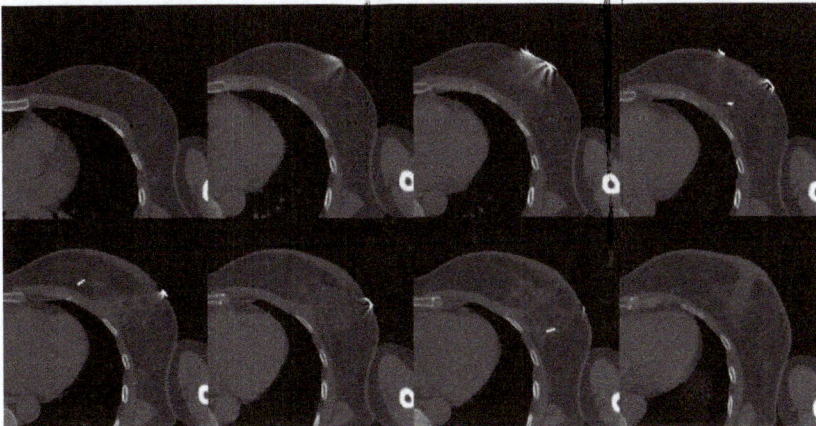

Figure 33. CT images before application with a marked scar.

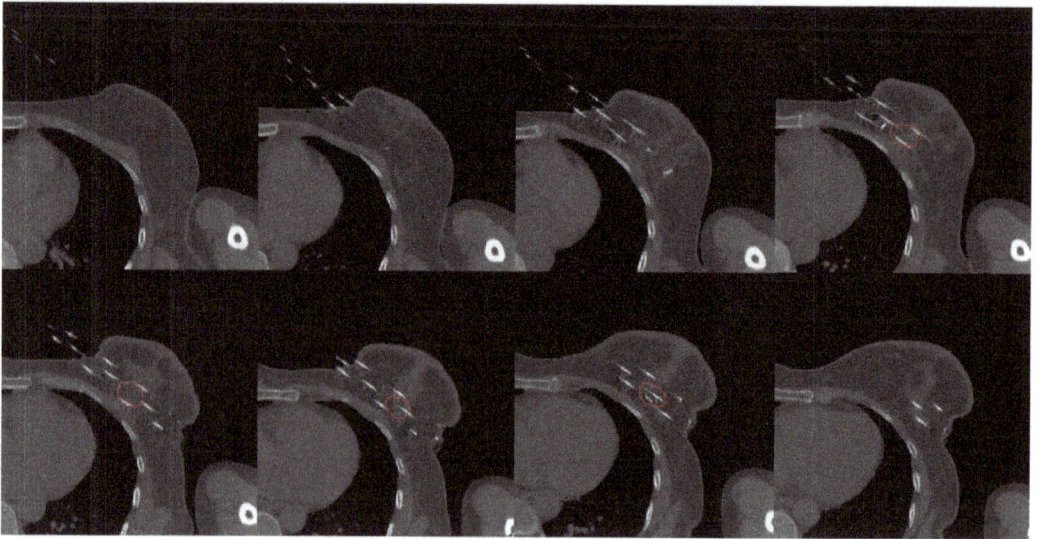

Figure 34. Images of the TPS with PTV.

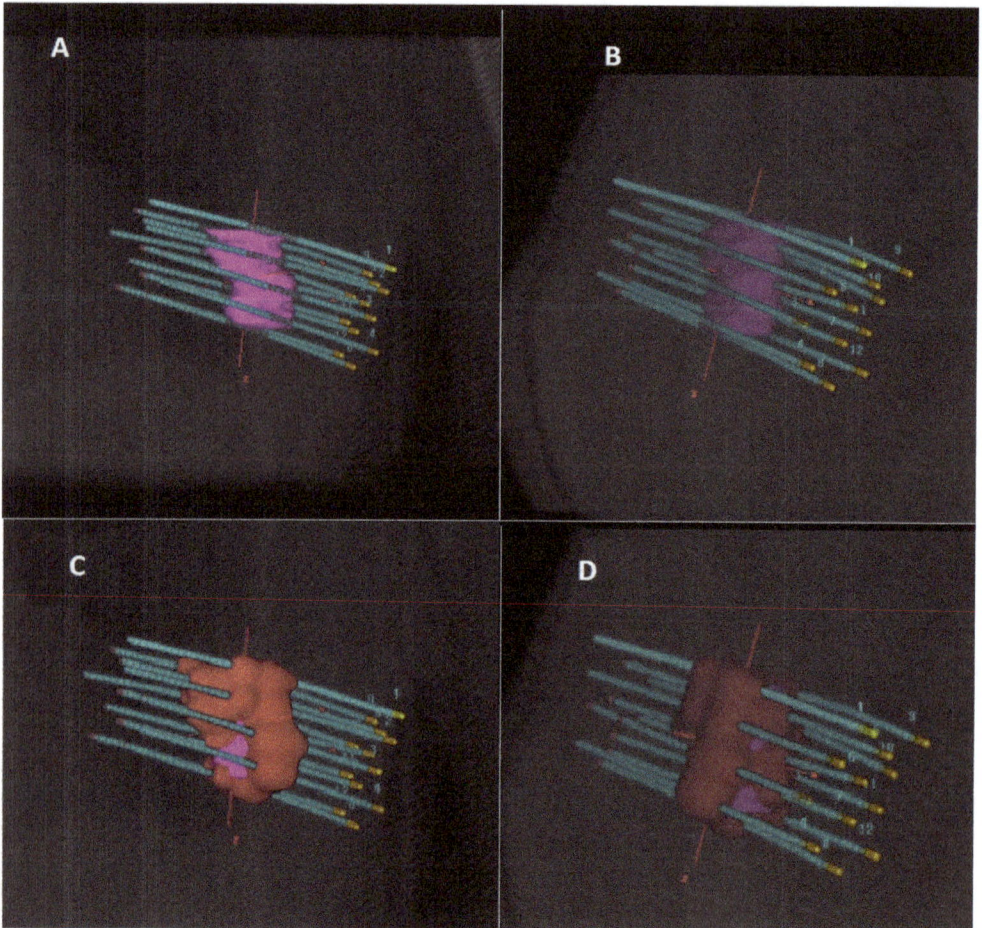

Figure 35. 3D reconstruction (A, C: front; B, D: side) of PTV applicators OARs and 3D dose reference distribution.

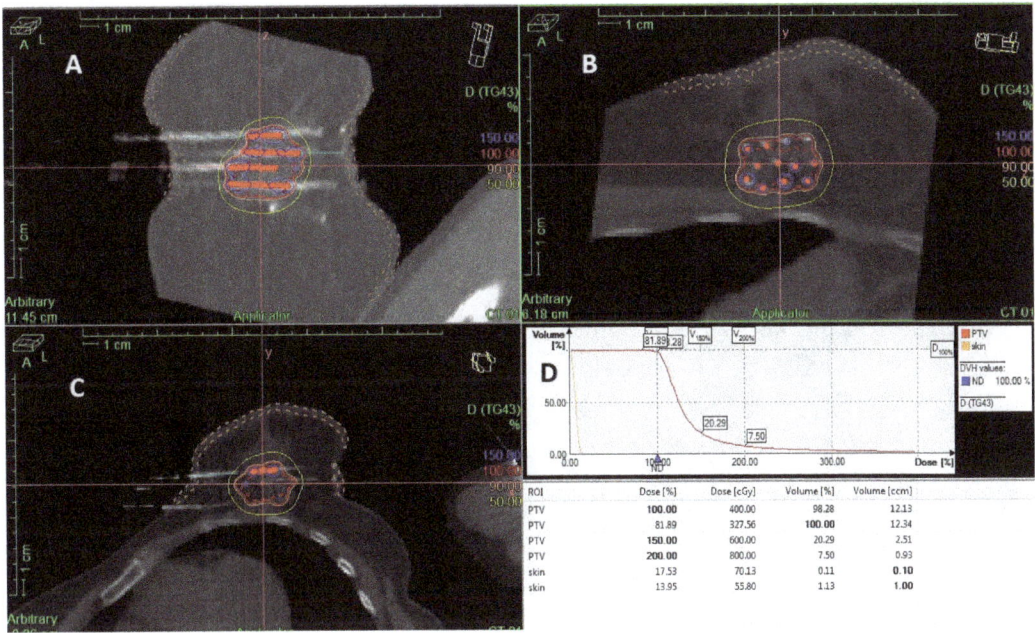

Figure 36. CT images and reconstruction on several planes (A, B, and C) and DVH (D).

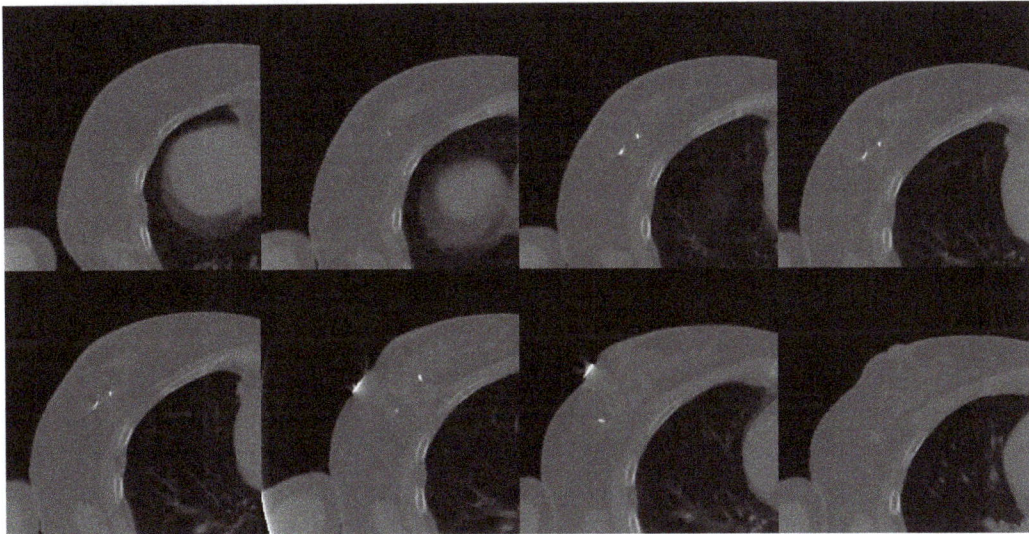

Figure 37. CT images before application with a marked scar.

2.4. Prostate cancer

Standard hospitalization procedure for patients suffering from prostate cancer in HDR brachytherapy is ultrasonographic imaging. Applicators used for the treatment are metal and plastic needles. Images are generated by Transrectal Ultrasound Scan (TRUS). Normally, the treatment kit consists of a transrectal probe that is mounted onto so-called stepper. A stepper is a set of mechanical lever system, a specialized stand with longitudinal boat for USG head at

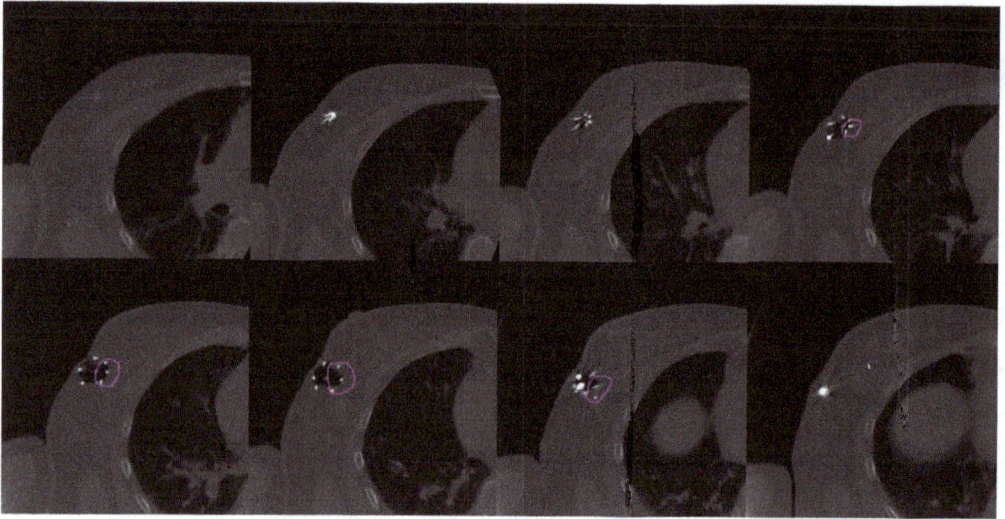

Figure 38. Images of the TPS with PTV.

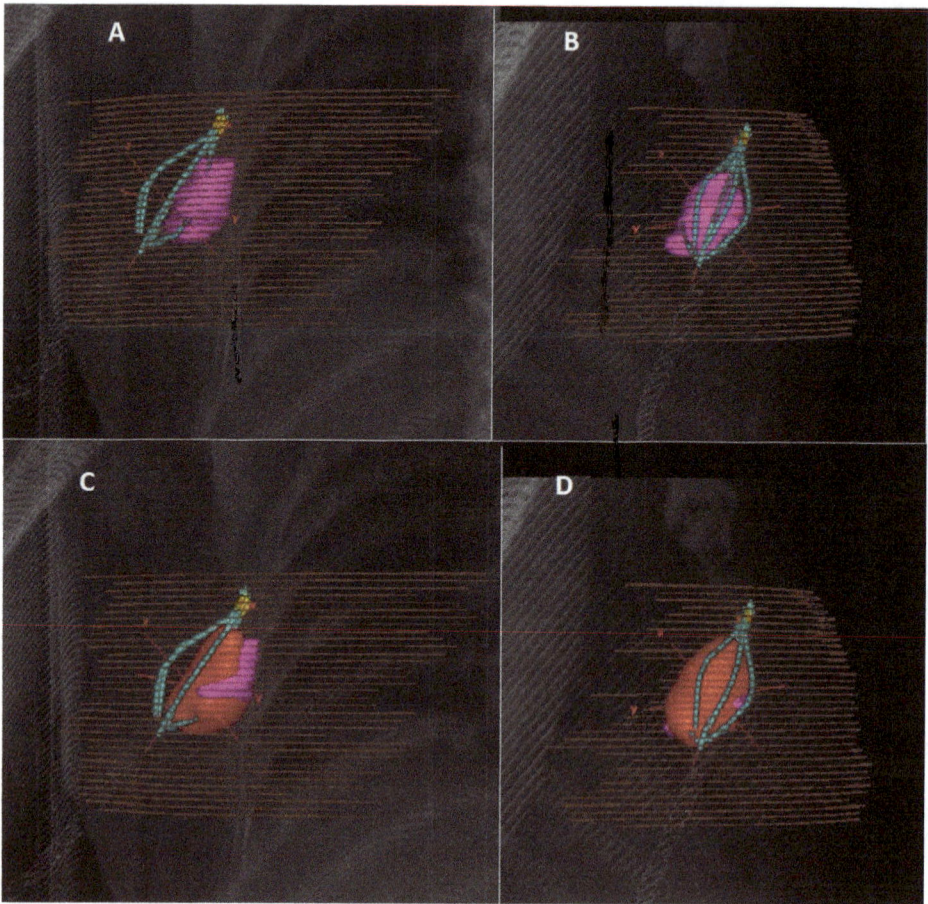

Figure 39. 3D reconstruction (A, C: front; B, D: side) of PTV applicators OARs and 3D dose reference distribution.

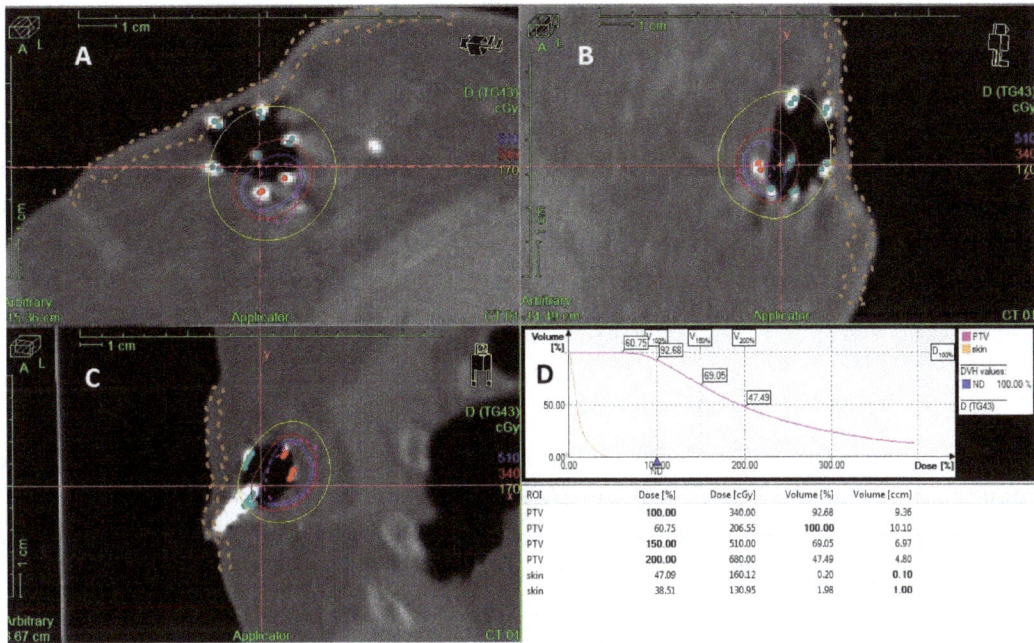

ROI	Dose [%]	Dose [cGy]	Volume [%]	Volume [ccm]
PTV	100.00	340.00	92.68	9.36
PTV	60.75	206.55	100.00	10.10
PTV	150.00	510.00	69.05	6.97
PTV	200.00	680.00	47.49	4.80
skin	47.09	160.12	0.20	0.10
skin	38.51	130.95	1.98	1.00

Figure 40. CT images and reconstruction on several planes (A, B, and C) and DVH (D).

its peak. During treatment, stepper was immobilized by being fixed to the floor. This prevents potential twists as well as target volume reading errors through planning system. Important function of the stepper was support of special ceramic targeting plate (template) and ultra-sonographic head. This plate has a grid of coordinate system correlating to this equivalently in the planning system. It is setting distance between the needles and the correct direction of the needle applicators is established. Gland images acquired from the ultrasonograph (1 mm intervals) were sent to the planning system simultaneously (on-line), enabling real-life change in volume target irradiation in reference to metal applicators and neighboring organs.

Prostate cancer can also be treated with means of HDR brachytherapy based on three-dimensional imaging from computer tomography. In this case, the procedure is more complicated compared to applying TRUS. This technique is usually applied with patients who already went through surgery where rectum was removed along the cancerous tumor. It is not possible to introduce transrectal probe after having undergone Miles surgery. Treatment is conducted with the help of computer tomography. We do not have an online preview while inserting catheters into the prostate area. The patient is laid in lateral position and not, as it is for standard treatment, in gynecological position. The reason for this comes from the fact that the treatment itself takes place on computer tomography. With patient laid like that, we can introduce applicators and perform CT imaging. They do not have to change the position between application and imaging processes. Hence, the danger of applicator relocation caused by patient's movement is eliminated. Furthermore, the position and inability to apply the stepper exclude the option of applying the ceramic plate. The needles are reviewed in the free-hand technique. Before the treatment begins, a three-dimensional imaging is performed to determine target's location as well as its volume. After the analysis of 3D images, the depth to which applicators will be introduced into patient's body can be determined. After first few needles have been applied, another computer tomography is performed to examine application geometry. The location as well as the depth, to which applicators have been introduced, is being inspected. Verification scheme is repeated after applying few applicators. After the application process is completed, a CT imaging is performed. Then, the images are sent to TPS with marked PTV and OAR areas. Prostate treatment planning based on CT imaging requires great experience from radiotherapist while introducing the needles into the prostate area. Medical physicists have to possess a wide experience in this type of procedures. In cases where needles are injected "free hand," it is common for catheters to intersect in patient's body, what in consequence can lead to difficulties when identifying individual applicators [12].

2.4.1. Case

The first case presents a patient with prostate cancer. Miles operation is a surgery for rectal cancer or anal cancer. The patient was treated with 30 Gy in two fractions twice a day. During application, the patient had twice CT examination for verification (**Figure 41**). In the tumor bed were placed 12 applicators. **Figure 42** shows scans with volume target contoured in TPS. Illustration from computerized planning system depicts three-dimensional reconstruction applicators, PTV, and dose distribution (**Figure 43**). Reconstruction on several planes and DVH is presented in **Figure 44**.

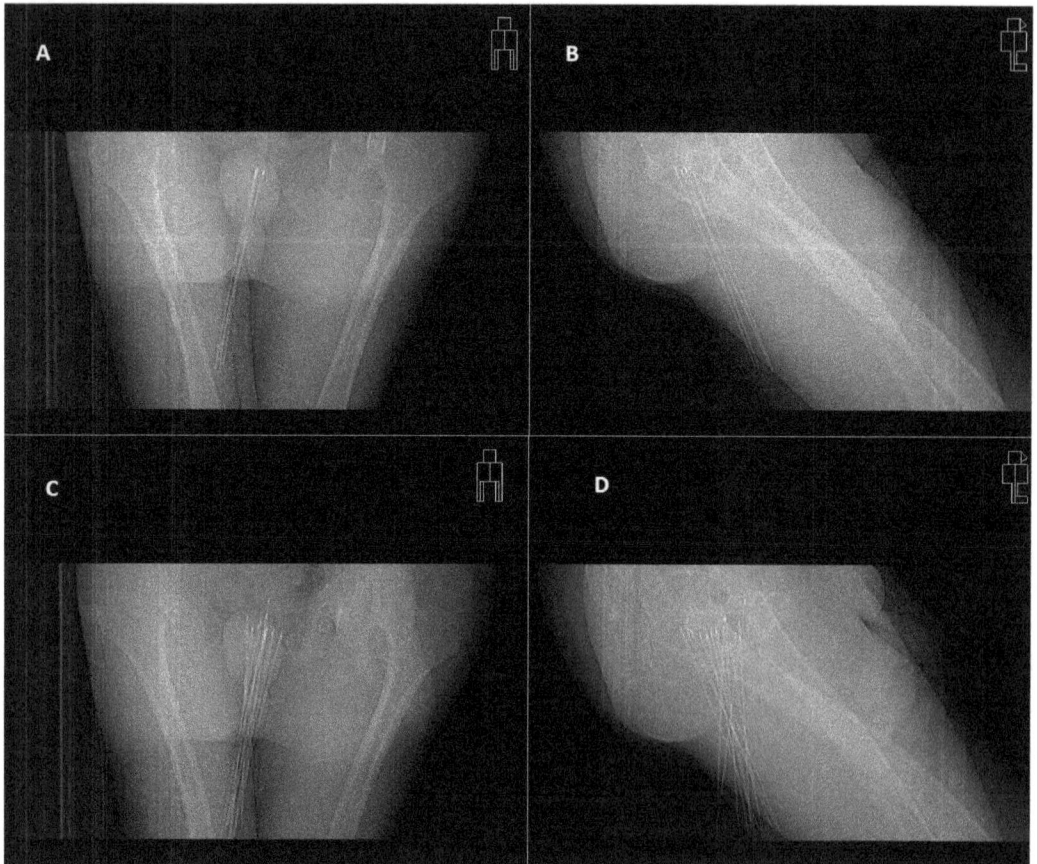

Figure 41. CT images: first imaging (A, B) and second imaging (C, D).

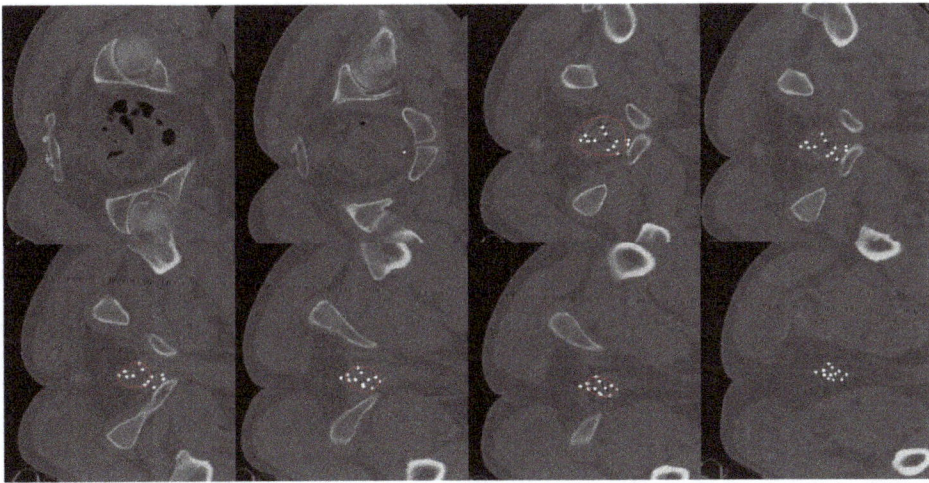

Figure 42. Images of the TPS with PTV.

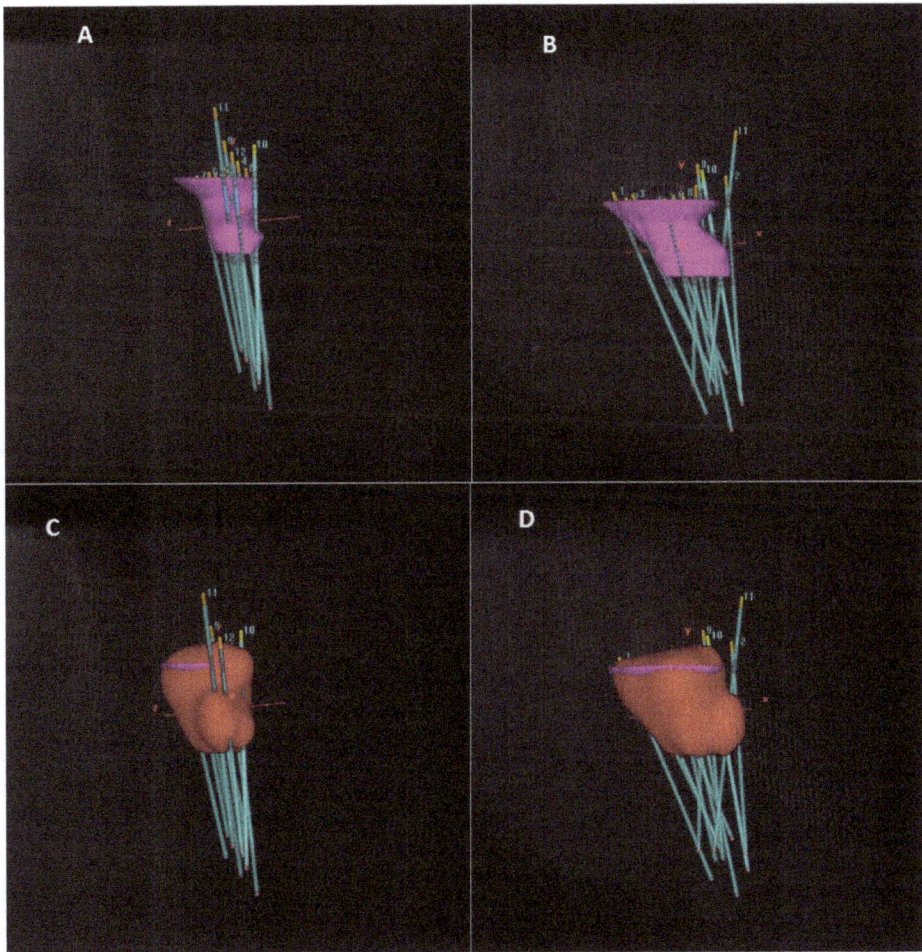

Figure 43. 3D reconstruction (A, C: front; B, D: side) of PTV applicators and 3D dose reference distribution.

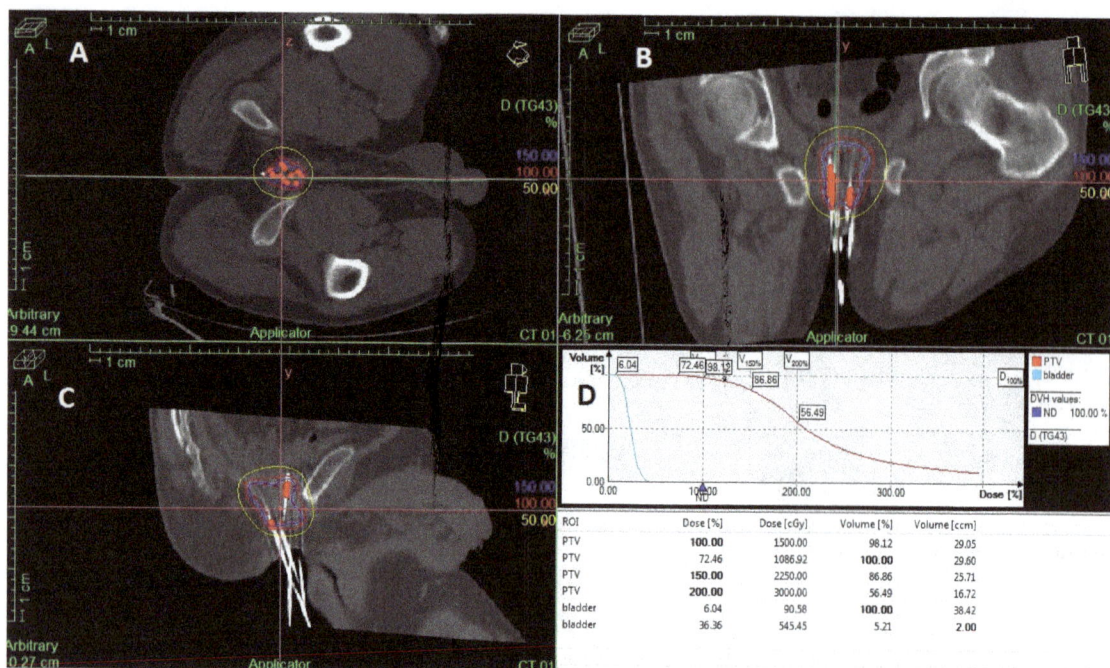

Figure 44. CT images and reconstruction on several planes (A, B, and C) and DVH (D).

3. Summary

Treatment planning in HDR brachytherapy based on three-dimensional imaging allows for prearranging and conducting optimal treatment in a given location. Routinely, in parts like the lung or esophagus, treatment plan is based on 2D imaging. Academic literature provides reports about incorporating 3D along with 2D imaging in lung cancer treatment. Significant differences are also pointed out when it comes to the coverage of the therapeutic area between these two methods. Thanks to the use of computer tomography, we have got the precise location of the irradiation area. We can adjust the most appropriate technique and applicators to conduct the most optimal treatment. What's more, the geometry of introduced implant allows for the ultimate target coverage with simultaneous protection of organs at risk

Utilizing three-dimensional imaging provides great possibility for treatment in location where previous access was hindered or impossible because of patient's anatomical structure or previously undergone procedures, i.e., Miles surgery.

Computer tomography allows for establishing individual treatment solutions that provide optimal approach to every patient as in skin cancer. With more and easier access to three-dimensional imaging, new ways of applying HDR brachytherapy open in new location as well as in form of radical treatment. With the use of imaging, we are now able to introduce catheters precisely into the tumor area with putting the patient at risk of posttreatment complications. It allows the treatment of people that no more qualify for other forms of treatment (radiotherapy). Because of the high gradient dose in HDR brachytherapy and patients with internal intracranial implants, i.e., pacemaker or cardioverter-defibrillator, we know exactly the dose the device will receive, so we can perform the procedures without exposing the patient to additional risk. Thanks to different optimization forms based on 3D images, HDR brachytherapy is applied not only in palliative treatment but also in new ways of radical treatment, i.e., in case of APBI.

Author details

Marcin Sawicki

Address all correspondence to: savi8307@poczta.fm

Brachytherapy Department, Subcarpathian Cancer Center, Brzozów, Poland

References

[1] Makarewicz R, editor. Brachyterapia HDR. Via Medica, Gdańsk; 2004

[2] Sawicki M. The evaluation of treatment plans in high-dose-rate endobronchial brachytherapy by utilizing 2D and 3D computed tomography imaging methods. Journal of Contemporary Brachytherapy. 2014;**6**(3):289-292

[3] Zvonarev PS. 2D/3D registration algorithm for lung brachytherapy. Medical Physics. 2013;**40**:021913

[4] Khan FM, Gibbons J, Mihailidis D, Alkhatib H, Khan's Lectures: Handbook of the Physics of Radiation Therapy. LWW, Gdańsk; 2009

[5] Melhus CS, Rivard MJ. Approaches to calculating AAPM TG-43 brachytherapy dosimetry parameters for Cs, I, Ir, Pd, and Yb sources. Medical Physics. 2006;**33**:1729

[6] Pérez-Calatayud J, Granero D, Casal E, Ballester F, Puchades V. Monte Carlo and experimental derivation of TG43 dosimetric parameters for CSM-type Cs-137 sources. Medical Physics. 2005;**32**(1):28-36

[7] Cavanaugh SX, Vidovic A, Law T, Bechara R, Parks C, Wei J, Swanson J. Multichannel endobronchial HDR catheter respiratory motion and resultant dosimetric variation. Brachytherapy. 2015;**14**:47

[8] Stewart A, et al. American Brachytherapy Society consensus guidelines for thoracic brachytherapy for lung cancer. Brachytherapy. 2016;**15**(1):1-11

[9] Łyczek J, et al. Comparison of the GTV coverage by PTV and isodose of 90% in 2D and 3D planning during endobronchial brachytherapy in the palliative treatment of patients with advanced lung cancer. Pilot study. Journal of Contemporary Brachytherapy. 2012;**4**:113-115

[10] Kowalik L, Lyczek J, Sawicki M, Kazalski D. Individual applicator for brachytherapy for various sites of superficial malignant lesions. Journal of Contemporary Brachytherapy. 2013;**5**(1):45-49

[11] Polgár C, Ott OJ, Hildebrandt G, Kauer-Dorner D, Knauerhase H, Major T, Slampa P. Late side-effects and cosmetic results of accelerated partial breast irradiation with interstitial brachytherapy versus whole-breast irradiation after breast-conserving surgery for low-risk invasive and in-situ carcinoma of the female breast: 5-year results of a randomised, controlled, phase 3 trial. The Lancet Oncology. 2017;**18**(2):259-268

[12] Łyczek J, Kazalski D, Sawicki M. Brachytherapy treatment planning for prostate cancer with the use of the computed tomography-based (CT-based) planning software in patients after total primary amputation of the rectum and EBRT (External Beam Radiation Therapy) due to rectal cancer. Physica Medica. 2016;**32**:227

Permissions

List of Contributors

Márcio Diniz-Freitas, Javier Fernández-Feijoo, Lucía García-Caballero, Maite Abeleira, Mercedes Outumuro, Jacobo Limeres-Pose and Pedro Diz-Dios
Special Needs Unit and OMEQUI Research Group, School of Medicine and Dentistry, Santiago de Compostela University, Santiago de Compostela, Galicia, Spain

Silvia Ruiz-España and David Moratal
Center for Biomaterials and Tissue Engineering, Universitat Politècnica de València, Valencia, Spain

Emine Kaygısız and Tuba Tortop
Faculty of Dentistry, Department of Orthodontics, Gazi University, Ankara, Turkey

Matthew Keane, Emily Paul, Cyril Rauch and Catrin Sian Rutland
School of Veterinary Medicine and Science, University of Nottingham, Nottingham, UK

Craig J Sturrock
The Hounsfield Facility, School of Biosciences, University of Nottingham, Nottingham, UK

Maximiliano Barahona, Jaime Hinzpeter and Cristian Barrientos
Orthopedic Surgery Department, Hospital Clinico Universidad de Chile, Chile

Mohammad Hammad Ather, Wasim Memon, Wajahat Aziz and Mohammad Nasir Sulaiman
Aga Khan University, Karachi, Pakistan

Karthik Ananthasubramaniam, Nishtha Sareen and Gjeka Rudin
Department of Medicine, Heart and Vascular Institute, Henry Ford Hospital, Detroit, Michigan, USA
Division of Cardiology, St. Joseph Mercy Hospital Oakland, Michigan, USA

Ufuk Tatli
Department of Oral and Maxillofacial Surgery, Faculty of Dentistry, Çukurova University, Adana, Turkey

Burcu Evlice
Department of Oral and Maxillofacial Radiology, Faculty of Dentistry, Çukurova University, Adana, Turkey

Miguel A. Vicente, Jesús Mínguez and Dorys C. González
Department of Civil Engineering, University of Burgos, Spain

Marcin Sawicki
Brachytherapy Department, Subcarpathian Cancer Center, Brzozów, Poland

Index

www.ingramcontent.com/pod-product-compliance
Lightning Source LLC
Chambersburg PA
CBHW061950190326
41458CB00009B/2838